AF614768

Nerve and Vascular Injuries in Sports Medicine

Venu Akuthota · Stanley A. Herring
Editors

Nerve and Vascular Injuries in Sports Medicine

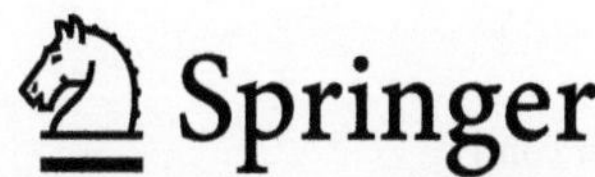

Editors
Venu Akuthota
University of Colorado
Denver School of Medicine
1635 N. Aurora Court
Aurora, CO 80045
The Spine Center
Denver, CO
USA

Stanley A. Herring
Department of Rehabilitation Medicine
University of Washington
401 Broadway
Seattle, WA 98122
USA

ISBN 978-0-387-76599-0 e-ISBN 978-0-387-76600-3
DOI 10.1007/978-0-387-76600-3
Springer Dordrecht Heidelberg London New York

Library of Congress Control Number: 2009921351

Printed on acid-free paper

Springer is part of Springer Science+Business Media (www.springer.com)

Foreword

The field of sports medicine covers a tremendous territory. Athletes present to their physician with everything from sprained ankles to bowel problems while running. Many of the classic textbooks in sports medicine cover many of these issues in a cursory way. Two major organ systems that account for many injuries in athletes are the nervous system and the vascular system. Because of their widespread, diffuse nature, athletes can present with myriad signs and symptoms related to these systems. Drs. Akuthota and Herring have done an outstanding job in their textbook *Nerve and Vascular Injuries in Sports Medicine* to produce a commonsense, yet thorough, approach to potential nerve and vascular injuries in athletes. The text provides any physician or clinician who evaluates and treats athletes with a clear path to an appropriate history, physical examination, imaging studies, and electrophysiologic and vascular examinations of any athlete with potential nerve or vascular injuries.

The first third of the book describes the appropriate evaluation of athletes with nerve and vascular symptoms and signs. Emphasis is placed on kinetic chain contributions to nerve and vascular injuries to address not only the cause of the injury but possible associated, contributing biomechanical deficiencies. The last two-thirds of the book cover regional specific nerve and vascular injuries with special attention to stingers, thoracic outlet syndrome, lumbar radiculopathy, and compartment syndromes.

In summary, *Nerve and Vascular Injuries in Sports Medicine* is the perfect complement to a sports medicine library and provides a thorough, practical text for any sports clinician who evaluates and treats athletes with potential nerve and vascular problems.

Joel Press, MD

Foreword

The field of sports medicine covers a tremendous breadth. Athletes present to their physician with everything from sprained ankles to bowel problems while running. Many of the classic textbooks in sports medicine cover many of these issues in a cursory way. Two major organ systems that account for many injuries in athletes are the nervous system and the vascular system. Because of their widespread influence, the athlete can present with myriad signs and symptoms related to these systems. Drs. Akuthota and Herring have done an outstanding job in their textbook *Nerve and Vascular Injuries in Sports Medicine* to produce a commonsense yet thorough approach to potential nerve or vascular injuries in athletes. The text provides any physician or clinician who evaluates and treats athletes with a clear path to an appropriate history, physical examination, imaging studies, and electrophysiologic and vascular examinations of the athlete with potential nerve or vascular injuries.

The first third of the book describes the appropriate evaluation of athletes with nerve and vascular symptoms and signs. Emphasis is placed on kinetic chain contributions to nerve and vascular injuries to address not only the cause of the injury but possible [illegible]. The last [illegible] special attention to [illegible]

[illegible]

Preface

At the 53rd Annual Meeting of the American College of Sports Medicine in Denver, Colorado in 2006, we hosted a symposium on neurovascular injuries in the athlete. The presentations and conversations that occurred as part of that symposium confirmed the challenges that sports medicine practitioners face when diagnosing and treating athletes with suspected vascular, peripheral nerve, or nerve root injuries ranging from the commonly occurring "stingers" and "handlebar palsies" to the rare but emergent effort vein thrombosis. These types of problems often do not receive much attention in the sports medicine literature.

After the symposium, we were presented with the opportunity to edit a textbook on nerve and vascular injuries in sports medicine. We gladly agreed and now have seen this project come to completion. This textbook is organized into three sections. The first section addresses anatomy, pathophysiology, and diagnosis, including physical examination and rehabilitation concepts for neurovascular injury as well as chapters devoted to electrodiagnostic evaluation, imaging, and vascular assessment. The second section of the book addresses upper limb neurovascular syndrome, including nerve entrapments, neurogenic and vascular thoracic outlet syndrome, and radicular and brachial plexus injury. The third section of the book approaches the lower extremity in the same comprehensive fashion, including peripheral nerve injury in the proximal and distal lower extremity, lumbar radiculopathy, compartment syndrome, and emergent vascular issues in the lower extremity.

We are grateful to our authors, who have busy professional and personal lives, for creating readable, practical, evidence-based work. Their contributions have produced a textbook that should serve as a helpful roadmap when treating problems that are often outside the mainstream of many sports medicine practices. Also, a thank you is certainly in order for Ms. Barbara Lopez-Lucio, developmental editor for Springer. Without her constant guidance (and gentle reminders), this publication would not exist.

It has been our pleasure and privilege to be involved in the creation of this textbook. We hope this reference serves as a useful guide to all of the sports medicine practitioners trying to help athletes with neurologic and vascular injuries.

Denver, Colorado
Seattle, Washington

Venu Akuthota
Stanley A. Herring

Contents

About the Editors

Venu Akuthota, MD
Associate Professor, Department of Physical Medicine and Rehabilitation; Director, The Spine Center of the University of Colorado Hospital; Pain Medicine Fellowship Director; University of Colorado School of Medicine, Aurora, CO; Team Physician, University of Colorado, Aurora, CO; Team Physician, University of Denver, Denver, CO, USA

Stanley A. Herring, MD
Medical Director of Spine Center and Clinical Professor, Departments of Rehabilitation Medicine, Orthopaedics and Sports Medicine, and Neurological Surgery, University of Washington, Seattle, WA; Team Physician, Seattle Seahawks, Seattle, WA; Team Physician, Seattle Mariners; Seattle, WA, USA

Contributors

Editors

Venu Akuthota Department of Physical Medicine and Rehabilitation, Aurora, CO, USA; The Spine Center of the University of Colorado Hospital, Aurora, CO, USA; University of Colorado School of Medicine, Aurora, CO, USA; University of Colorado, Aurora, CO, USA; University of Denver, Denver, CO, USA

Stanley A. Herring Departments of Rehabilitation Medicine, Orthopaedics and Sports Medicine, and Neurological Surgery, University of Washington, Seattle, WA, USA; Seattle Seahawks, Seattle, WA, USA; Seattle Mariners, Seattle, WA, USA

Authors

Andrea J. Boon Department of Physical Medicine and Rehabilitation, Mayo Clinic, Rochester, MN, USA

Jonathan T. Bravman Resident Physician in Orthopaedic Surgery, Department of Orthopaedics, University of Colorado, Aurora, CO, USA

Ellen Casey Resident Physician, Department of Physical Medicine and Rehabilitation, Rehabilitation Institute of Chicago/Northwestern Memorial Hospital, Chicago, IL, USA

Cynthia T. Chin Department of Radiology, University of California San Francisco, San Francisco, CA, USA

Mansour Y. Dib Department of Physical Medicine and Rehabilitation, AUBMC, Beirut, Lebanon

Mark E. Domroese Department of Physical Medicine and Rehabilitation, Gundersen Lutheran Medical Center, La Crosse, WI, USA

Peter Gonzalez Department of Physical Medicine and Rehabilitation, University of Colorado School of Medicine, Aurora, CO, USA

Mark A. Harrast Department of Rehabilitation Medicine, Department of Orthopaedics and Sports Medicine, University of Washington, Seattle, WA, USA

Anne Zeni Hoch Departments of Orthopaedic Surgery and Physical Medicine and Rehabilitation, Medical College of Wisconsin, Milwaukee, WI, USA

Joseph M. Ihm Rehabilitation Institute of Chicago, Chicago, IL, USA

Marla S. Kaufman Department of Rehabilitation Medicine and Department of Orthopaedics and Sports Medicine, University of Washington Medical Center, UW Medicine Sports and Spine Physicians, Seattle, WA, USA

Lisa S. Krivickas Department of Physical Medicine and Rehabilitation, Harvard Medical School, Boston, MA, USA

Scott Laker Department of Rehabilitation, University of Washington, Seattle, WA, USA

Paul H. Lento Rehabilitation Institute of Chicago, Chicago, IL, USA; Department of Physical Medicine and Rehabilitation, Northwestern University Medical School, Chicago, IL, USA

Gerard A. Malanga Pain Management, Overlook Hospital, Summit, NJ, USA; Atlantic Health, Summit, NJ, USA; New Jersey Medical School, Summit, NJ, USA

Erin Maslowski Resident, Department of Physical Medicine and Rehabilitation, University of Colorado Health Sciences Center, Aurora, CO, USA

Kelly C. McInnis Department of Physical Medicine and Rehabilitation, Harvard Medical School, Boston, MA, USA

Hector Mejia Department of Orthopaedics, University of Colorado, Aurora, CO, USA

Nayna Patel Physical Medicine and Rehabilitation, Core Orthopaedic Medical Center, Encinitas, CA, USA

Vikas V. Patel Department of Orthopaedic Surgery, University of Colorado, Denver, CO, USA

Heron Rodriguez Division of Vascular Surgery, Department of Surgery, Northwestern Memorial Hospital/Northwestern University, Chicago, IL, USA

William J. Sullivan Department of Physical Medicine and Rehabilitation, University of Colorado at Denver and Health Sciences Center, Aurora, CO, USA

Stuart M. Weinstein Department of Rehabilitation Medicine, University of Washington, Seattle, WA, USA

Jacqueline J. Wertsch Department of Physical Medicine and Rehabilitation, Medical College of Wisconsin, Milwaukee, WI, USA

Brian White Department of Orthopedics and Physical Rehabilitation, University of Massachusetts, Worcester, MA, USA

Thomas A. Whitehill Division of Vascular Surgery, University of Colorado Denver School of Medicine, Aurora, CO, USA

Part I
Anatomy, Pathophysiology, and Diagnosis

Chapter 1
Causes of Numbness and Tingling in Athletes

Venu Akuthota and Erin Maslowski

The Mystery Is in the History

The origins of numbness and tingling in athletes are not always as clear as they may seem. The terms *tingling* and *numbness* are often substitute descriptions for achiness and generalized discomfort. Particularly the sensation of tingling (this so-called positive sensory symptom is medically termed dysesthesias or paresthesias) is often vague and can be caused by a variety of pain generators. Although tingling can be due to nerve dysfunction, it can also be perceived when muscle or vascular structures are disturbed.

The sensation of numbness, on the other hand, is a negative sensory symptom precisely defined as a lack of sensation.[1] Numbness is thought to be more specific to nerve injury than is the sensation of tingling. Thus, when an athlete complains of numbness and especially tingling, the key to a diagnosis is to obtain a detailed history of the athlete's symptom perception. History taking becomes paramount because objective electrophysiologic or other testing is often lacking in many cases of athletes' tingling. This chapter examines the various causes and pathophysiology of numbness and tingling in athletes: nerve, vascular, or muscle disturbance.

Nerve Pain

Pain that originates in the nervous system itself is called neuropathic pain. A variety of uncomfortable sensations may occur because of nerve dysfunction. Positive sensory phenomena, such as *tingling* or *pins and needles* are thought to be caused by spontaneous ectopic discharges that originate in sensory nerves. In theory, latent depolarization-due to activation of sodium channels or dysfunction of rectifying potassium channels-produces ectopic discharges within sensory nerve pathways and the resultant symptoms.[2]

Athletics can cause a variety of nerve injuries depending on the sports played (Table 1.1). Traumatic peripheral nerve injury in particular has been shown to have histologic and electrophysiologic features leading to pain and paresthesias. Electron microscopy has shown that after nerve transection multiple unmyelinated sprouts grow out of each transected axon. Electrophysiologic recording reveals ongoing activity, abnormal excitability, and discharge characteristics arising from these neuron sprouts.[3] Cytokines secreted at the time of nerve injury-e.g., interleukin-1 (IL-1), tumor necrosis factor-α (TNFα)-may contribute to an inflammatory cascade.[3] Clinically, the Hoffman-Tinel sign (more commonly called the Tinel sign), in which paresthesias manifest when a peripheral nerve is percussed, is produced by the mechanical deformation of these excitable neuron sprouts. In fact, the Tinel sign was initially introduced to assess the progress of peripheral nerve regeneration after injury rather than as a diagnostic maneuver for peripheral nerve syndromes.

Deficits in central inhibitory mechanisms following nerve injury may also play a role in the production of nerve pain. One theory is that after nerve injury a few afferent intact sensory axons generate

V. Akuthota (✉)
Department of Physical Medicine and Rehabilitation, Aurora, CO, USA

V. Akuthota, S.A. Herring (eds.), *Nerve and Vascular Injuries in Sports Medicine*,
DOI 10.1007/978-0-387-76600-3_1, © Springer Science+Business Media, LLC 2009

Table 1.1 Nerve injuries in different sports

Sport	Upper extremity	Lower extremity
Archery	Digital nerve compression	–
	Median neuropathy at wrist	–
	Median neuropathy at pronator teres	–
	Long thoracic palsy	–
Arm wrestling	Radial nerve palsy	–
Auto racing	Brachial plexopathy	Sciatic neuropathy
	Median neuropathy (pronator syndrome)	Peroneal neuropathy
Backpacking/mountain climbing	Brachial plexus (backpack paralysis)	Tibial neuropathy (tarsal tunnel syndrome)
	Suprascapular neuropathy	
	Thoracic outlet syndrome	
Ballet dancing	Suprascapular neuropathy	Femoral neuropathy
		Peroneal neuropathy
		Sural neuropathy
		Dorsal cutaneous neuropathy
		Morton's neuroma
Baseball	Axillary neuropathy (quadrilateral space syndrome)	–
	Brachial plexopathy (pitcher's arm)	
	Digital neuropathy at the thumb	
	Median neuropathy (pronator syndrome and carpal tunnel syndrome)	
	Radial neuropathy	
	Suprascapular neuropathy	
	Thoracic outlet syndrome	
	Ulnar neuropathy (entrapment at medial epicondyle and cubital tunnel)	
Basketball	Suprascapular neuropathy	Peroneal neuropathy (traumatic)
	Median neuropathy at the wrist (wheelchair athletes)	Tibial neuropathy (tarsal tunnel syndrome)
	Stinger	
	Ulnar neuropathy (wheelchair athletes)	
Bicycling	Ulnar neuropathy (at Guyon's canal and elbow	Posterior cutaneous nerve of the thigh neuropathy
	Median neuropathy at the wrist (carpal tunnel syndrome)	Sciatic nerve palsy (unicyclist)
		Pudendal neuropathy
Bodybuilding and weightlifting	Ulnar neuropathy (multiple sites: deep motor branch, flexor carpi ulnaris, deep palmar branch, elbow)	Femoral neuropathy
	Stinger	
	Posterior interosseous neuropathy	
	Medial pectoral neuropathy	
	Suprascapular neuropathy	
	Median neuropathy (entrapment at the wrist, pronator syndrome)	
	Long thoracic neuropathy	
	Lateral antebrachial cutaneous neuropathy	
	Musculocutaneous neuropathy	
	Thoracodorsal neuropathy	
	Thoracic outlet syndrome	
	Dorsoscapular neuropathy	
Bowling	Digital neuropathy at the thumb	–
	Long thoracic nerve traction	
Boxing	Stinger	–
Cheerleading	Digital neuropathy	–
	Median neuropathy at the palmar branch	

Table 1.1 (continued)

Sport	Upper extremity	Lower extremity
Crew	Quadrilateral space syndrome, axillary nerve	–
Dancing	–	Morton's neuroma of a plantar nerve Tibial neuropathy (tarsal tunnel syndrome)
Football	Axillary neuropathy with or without dislocated shoulder Brachial plexopathy Cervical radiculopathy Long thoracic neuropathy Median neuropathy at the wrist Radial neuropathy Stinger Suprascapular neuropathy Thoracic outlet syndrome Ulnar neuropathy at the elbow Upper trunk brachial plexopathy	Iliohypogastric neuropathy Lumbosacral radiculopathy Peroneal neuropathy with knee dislocation Sciatic nerve (hamstring syndrome)
Frisbee	Posterior interosseous neuropathy	–
Golf	Median neuropathy distal to the wrist Carpal tunnel syndrome Long thoracic nerve traction Ulnar neuropathy at flexor carpi ulnaris	–
Gymnastics	Posterior interosseous neuropathy Long thoracic nerve traction	Lateral femoral cutaneous neuropathy Femoral neuropathy
Handball	Handball goalie's elbow	–
Hockey	Axillary neuropathy Stinger Long thoracic nerve traction	Tibial neuropathy (tarsal tunnel syndrome) Peroneal neuropathy
In-line skating, roller skating, skateboarding	–	Superficial peroneal neuropathy
Judo, karate, kickboxing	Ulnar neuropathy at trauma site Axillary neuropathy at trauma site Spinal accessory neuropathy at trauma site Long thoracic neuropathy at trauma site	Morton's neuroma of a plantar nerve Peroneal neuropathy at trauma site
Mountain climbing, hiking	Rucksack paralysis: brachial neuropathy involving upper and middle trunks Suprascapular neuropathy Axillary neuropathy Long thoracic neuropathy	Tibial neuropathy (tarsal tunnel syndrome)
Rifle shooting	Long thoracic nerve traction	–
Rowing	Musculocutaneous neuropathy (carpal tunnel syndrome)	–
Rugby, Australian rules football	Axillary neuropathy	Obturator neuropathy
Running	Thoracic outlet syndrome (long distance)	Peroneal neuropathy Lateral femoral cutaneous neuropathy Tibial neuropathy (tarsal tunnel syndrome) Posterior tibial neuropathy Morton's neuroma of a plantar nerve

Table 1.1 (continued)

Sport	Upper extremity	Lower extremity
		Interdigital neuropathies
		Plantar neuropathies
		Calcaneal neuropathy
		Sural neuropathy
		Superficial peroneal neuropathy
		Saphenous neuropathy
Scuba diving		Lateral femoral cutaneous neuropathy
Shooting	Long thoracic neuropathy	–
Skiing	Ulnar neuropathy (cross country)	Femoral neuropathy (cross country)
		Peroneal neuropathy (traumatic)
		Deep peroneal nerve (ski boots)
Snowmobiling, ATV riding	Brachial plexopathy	–
	Ulnar neuropathy at Guyon's canal	
Soccer	Long thoracic nerve traction	Peroneal neuropathy
Surfing	–	Common peroneal neuropathy
		Saphenous neuropathy
Swimming	Thoracic outlet syndrome	–
	Lateral antebrachial cutaneous neuropathy	
Tennis, raquetball	Digital neuropathy	–
	Distal ulnar neuropathy	
	Lateral antebrachial cutaneous neuropathy	
	Long thoracic neuropathy/traction	
	Median neuropathy (pronator syndrome, carpal tunnel syndrome)	
	Posterior interosseous neuropathy at the arcade of Frohse	
	Radial neuropathy secondary to fibrous arches at lateral head of triceps	
	Superficial radial neuropathy (sweatband)	
	Suprascapular neuropathy	
	Thoracic outlet syndrome	
Video gaming	Ulnar nerve at the wrist	–
Volleyball	Suprascapular neuropathy	–
	Axillary neuropathy	
	Long thoracic neuropathy/traction	
Wheelchair athletes	Median neuropathy (carpal tunnel syndrome)	–
	Ulnar neuropathy	
Windsurfing	Lateral antebrachial cutaneous neuropathy	–
Wrestling	Axillary neuropathy	–
	Brachial plexopathy	
	Cervical radiculopathy	
	Long thoracic neuropathy	
	Median neuropathy of the wrist	
	Stinger	
	Suprascapular neuropathy	
	Thoracic outlet syndrome	
	Ulnar neuropathy	

Data are from refs. 7, 8, 10, 21, 23, 33, 45–56

pain input to the spinal cord, whereas normal presynaptic inhibition of this input from the brain stem (in the periaqueductal gray and locus ceruleus) does not occur because most of the large fibers of the nerve have been destroyed.[3,4] *Central sensitization* is pain hypersensitivity due to post-nerve-injury changes in the central nervous system (CNS).[5] There appears to be decreased efficacy of the spinal opioid system after peripheral nerve transection.[3] There does not appear to be a direct correlation between the degree of nerve injury and the intensity of pain; that is, a minor lesion can cause severe pain.[3]

Vascular Pain

Vascular compromise, like neurologic injury, can cause pain, paresthesias, and paralysis. When these symptoms are accompanied by coolness, swelling, fatigue, pallor, pulselessness, and/or prolonged capillary refill, a vascular injury should be considered.[6] Because these injuries are not among the most common causes of pain in athletes, the clinician must have a high index of suspicion to recognize a vascular cause of dysfunction in an athlete.

The anatomic relation of certain vessels with their surrounding structures places them at risk of injury in the athlete.[6–9] The classic example is thoracic outlet syndrome (TOS). This syndrome may occur when an anatomic variant (e.g., a supernumerary rib) causes compression of the subclavian artery and vein when the arm is hyperabducted.[6,10] Symptoms of TOS include pain, paresthesias, numbness, and increased fatigability of the involved extremity.[7] Repetitive vascular injury in TOS can lead to arterial stenosis, arterial occlusion, poststenotic arterial dilatation, or aneurysm formation. Thrombus, capable of embolization, can form in the aneurysm or dilatation.[6]

Wilbourn and colleagues introduced the term *disputed TOS*. No anatomic variations or electrophysiologic dysfunction of nerves are found in this syndrome. The symptoms of paresthesias, coolness, and nerve pain are not thought to be due to vascular or nerve injury. Instead, symptoms are likely caused by soft tissue somatic referred pain.[11] Somatic referred pain often mimics neuropathic pain.

Muscle or Myofascial Pain

There are many causes of muscle pain as muscles are richly supplied with nociceptive fibers including thin, myelinated group III (Aδ) fibers and unmyelinated group IV fibers (C fibers). Muscle soreness can be caused by a well described syndrome called delayed-onset muscle soreness (DOMS). DOMS usually occurs after participation in a new activity. Symptoms appear 24–48 hours after the inciting event and resolve completely after several days. DOMS is thought to be due to excessive eccentric muscular contraction, which causes reversible ultrastructural changes in the muscle.[12,13] The most potent stimulator of muscle nociceptors is bradykinin, a nonapeptide released by damaged tissue in response to lowered pH, ischemia, and blood clots.[13] The release of nociceptor-sensitizing substances (e.g., bradykinin) during repair of this damage may lead to muscle soreness. Muscle pain and soreness are probably not related to mechanical muscle fiber damage as serum enzyme levels do not rise immediately.[13]

Muscle pain can also be associated with overuse injuries. In contrast to DOMS, this pain occurs in well trained muscles and is thought to be due to microtrauma that occurs at a faster rate than the muscle's repair mechanism. It is thought that excessive forces per muscle fiber leads to hypoxia, acidosis, and metabolic depletion, followed by calcium-mediated cellular damage.[13]

Finally, myofascial pain syndromes comprise a common muscle pain phenomenon believed to be caused by active trigger points or tender spots found in the belly of affected muscles. The etiology of trigger points is poorly understood. Proposed etiologies include localized truama, localized ischemia, and focal "energy crisis" resulting in release of nociceptor sensitizers.[13]

Basic Nerve and Muscle Anatomy

Peripheral nerves are composed of axons and structures that surround and support the axon. Peripheral nervous system cell bodies are located in either the anterior horn of the spinal cord (motor neurons) or dorsal root ganglion (sensory neurons).[14] Unmyelinated axons lie in an invagination of a

Schwann cell membrane. Myelinated axons are surrounded by a myelin sheath composed of many layers of a Schwann cell membrane. A single Schwann cell myelinates one segment of the axon. The small, unmyelinated segments between Schwann cells are called nodes.[15] Myelinated fibers propagate nerve signals faster than unmyelinated fibers because the action potential jumps from node to node by saltatory conduction.[15] The internodal region houses a concentration of sodium and potassium channels.

Multiple axons run together in a unit called a fascicle. Endoneurium is the connective tissue that surrounds the axons within the fascicle. Fibrous perineurium surrounds each fascicle. Epineurium binds the fascicles into a bundle, called a nerve trunk.[14,15] These connective tissues play an important role in protecting the nerve and supporting appropriate regeneration if the nerve is damaged. In fact, when nerve trunks are elongated, the initial stretch occurs through the "unwrinkling" of the connective tissue undulations rather than through nerve axons.[15] Clinically, this connective tissue becomes important in the susceptibility of the nerve roots (often lacking connective tissue) to avulsion when compared to more peripheral nerves, which have robust connective tissue.[16]

Nerves may be classified by fiber types: types A, B, and C. Sensory neurons may also be classified by another scheme, with types I–IV. These classifications schemes are summarized in Tables 1.2 and 1.3.

A motor unit consists of an alpha motor neuron, its axon, the neuromuscular junction, and the muscle fibers innervated by the alpha motor neuron. A single axon may give rise to multiple terminal axons, each of which innervates a single muscle fiber. Within the motor unit, all muscle fibers are histologically identical.[16] When a nerve fires, all of the muscle fibers in that motor unit depolarize.

Table 1.2 Classic nerve fiber classifications

Fiber type	Supplies
Aα	Sensory: proprioception and motor
Aβ	Sensory: pressure and touch
Aγ	Motor: muscle spindles
Aδ	Sensory: pain, temperature, touch
B	Preganglionic autonomic
C	Dorsal root fibers: pain and reflex responses
C	Postganglionic sympathetic fibers

From ref. 16

Table 1.3 Modern nerve fiber classifications

Fiber type	Supplies	Corresponds to
Ia	Muscle spindles, annulospiral endings	Aα
Ib	Golgi tendon organ	Aα
II	Muscle spindles, touch, pressure	Aβ
III	Supply pain, temperature, and touch receptors	Aδ
IV	Pain and other receptors	C

From ref. 16

Skeletal muscle fibers, or myocytes, are multinucleated cells. The nuclei are found close to the cell's plasma membrane, or sarcolemma. The cytoplasm of muscle fibers is filled with myofilaments, which together comprise the contractile apparatus of myofibrils. Myofibrils are composed of identical, repeating units called sarcomeres.[17] Each sarcomere is comprised of actin (thin filaments) and myosin (thick filaments) oriented in a longitudinal direction. In addition, there are perpendicularly oriented Z bands.[17] The T-tubule system runs parallel to the Z bands with sarcoplasmic reticulum on each side. It is this system that facilitates calcium release during excitation.[17]

Individual muscle fibers are surrounded by connective tissue called endomysium. Perimysium groups muscle fibers into primary and secondary bundles called fasciculi. Finally, epimysium refers to connective tissues that surround single muscles or large groups of fibers.[17] Muscle spindles are structures comprised of specialized muscle and nerve fibers that respond to stretch in muscles and maintain tone.[17]

Muscle fibers are divided into three types: type I (red), type IIa (intermediate), and type IIb (white). Type I fibers are slow twitch and slow to fatigue; type IIa fibers are fast twitch with intermediate fatigability; and type IIb fibers are fast twitch and fatigue rapidly. Fiber types are present in varying amounts in various muscles, giving each muscle unique contractile properties.[16]

Pathophysiology of Athletic Peripheral Nerve Injury

Athletic nerve injury is a unique beast, and its pathophysiology should not be merely extrapolated from literature on traumatic peripheral nerve injury

Table 1.4 Classification of nerve injury

Seddon	Sunderland	Affected structure (s)	Intact structure(s)
Neurapraxia	Class 1	Myelin	Axon, endoneurium, perineurium, epineurium
Axonotmesis	Class 2	Axon	Endoneurium, perineurium, epineurium
Neurotmesis	Class 3	Axon, endoneurium	Perineurium, epineurium
Neurotmesis	Class 4	Axon, endoneurium, perineurium	Epineurium
Neurotmesis	Class 5	Axon, endoneurium, perineurium, epineurium	None

Data are from refs. 14, 19, 22, 24, 35

Table 1.5 Mechanisms of nerve injury and associated pathology

Compression (chronic)	Traction	Hypoxia/ischemia	Laceration
Neurapraxia Axonotmesis	Neurapraxia Axonotmesis	Neurapraxia	Neurontmesis

Table 1.6 Entrapment neuropathies

Quadrilateral space syndrome	Axillary nerve at the quadrilateral space
Suprascapular nerve syndrome	Suprascapular nerve compression at the suprascapular notch (supraspinatus and infraspinatus weakness); suprascapular nerve compression at the spinoglenoid ligament (isolated infraspinatus weakness)
Carpal tunnel syndrome	Median nerve compression at the wrist
Pronator syndrome	Anterior interosseous nerve/median nerve compression at the bicipital aponeurosis, pronator teres, or flexor digitorum superficialis
Cubital tunnel syndrome	Ulnar nerve compression at the elbow
Ulnar tunnel syndrome	Ulnar nerve compression at the wrist (Guyon's canal)
Tardy ulnar palsy	Ulnar nerve stretched at elbow
Arcade of Struthers	Ulnar nerve compression in the distal arm
Supinator syndrome	Radial nerve compression at the supinator muscle
Radial tunnel syndrome	Posterior interosseous nerve at the radial tunnel (sensory deficit)
Posterior interosseous nerve syndrome	Posterior interosseous nerve at the radial tunnel (motor deficit)
Meralgia paresthetica	Lateral femoral cutaneous nerve compression
Tarsal tunnel syndrome	Medial and lateral plantar nerve compression
Thoracic outlet syndrome	Angulation of lower trunk/medial cord of brachial plexus over cervical rib or band
Pudendal nerve entrapment	Pudendal nerve entrapment either between the sacrospinous and sacrotuberous ligaments vs. the pudendal canal (unknown)
Piriformis syndrome	Compression of the sciatic nerve in the piriformis muscle
Common peroneal nerve syndrome	Compression of the common peroneal nerve at the fibular neck (peroneal tunnel)
Wartenberg's syndrome	Compression of radial nerve between brachioradialis and extensor carpi radialis longus and by external forces

Data are from refs. 22, 25, 49–54, 56–58

in which high kinetic energy forces typically occur (e.g., motor vehicle accidents). In athletics, a few cases of nerve injury are due to acute presentations, such as with joint dislocations. Yet even in these cases the kinetic energy forces are much lower than with motor vehicle accidents. Instead, most cases of athletic nerve injury are due to chronic compression or traction.

The classic descriptions of nerve injury (Table 1.2), described by Seddon in 1943,[18] serve as a good conceptual model but become inadequate for understanding and prognosticating athletic nerve injury presentation and recovery. Seddon described three major classes of nerve injury.

- *Neurapraxia* (nonaction) describes an injury that is incomplete, with the axon intact. Neurapraxia may involve *conduction block* or *conduction slowing*. The observed conduction failure across the lesion is due to segmental demyelination[18,19] or ischemia.[20] Recovery occurs when the nerve is remyelinated.[21] Recovery from neurapraxia is spontaneous and relatively rapid.[18,19,21,22]
- *Axonotmesis* describes an injury in which there is an interruption of the axons and myelin sheaths, but the nerve stroma is intact.[19] Wallerian degeneration occurs, and as a result there is an absence of nerve conduction in the distal, degenerating segment.[22,23] In the case of axonotmesis, regeneration occurs spontaneously and is functional because the endoneurium guides the regenerating axon to the correct destination.[19]
- *Neurotmesis* describes a nerve that either has been completely severed or is so affected by scar tissue that regeneration without surgical intervention is not possible.[18,19] The axon, endoneurium, perineurium, and epineurium are no longer in continuity.[22]

Because most athletic nerve injuries produce a neuropraxic lesion and also often display axonal involvement, the Seddon classification appears to be inadequate. Moreover, athletic nerve injury is usually due to a chronic model of nerve pathophysiology. The Seddon classification system is more appropriate for an acute nerve injury. A second classification scheme, developed by Sir Sydney Sunderland and published in 1951,[24] describes five types of nerve injury with distinctions between the classes of injury based on the connective tissues involved. The Sunderland system is even less relevant to athletic nerve injury except in those rare cases where there has been acute neurotmetic injury that requires surgical planning and intervention.

Myelin Injury (Conduction Block and Conduction Slowing)

Athletic myelin injury (neuropraxia) primarily causes symptoms when there is *segmental demyelination* of the internodal membrane. The demyelinated membrane leaks current, leaving insufficient current across the internodal membrane.[15] When the myelin is only slightly damaged, there is widening of the nodal areas and *conduction slowing* of nerve action potential. Conduction slowing may or may not cause symptoms. When myelin is severely damaged, there is destruction of the internodal segment and a *conduction block* results. Conduction block, unlike conduction slowing, inevitably causes symptoms such as weakness and sensory loss. Electrodiagnostic studies reveal conduction slowing or conduction block at the site of the lesion, whereas proximal and distal segment nerve conduction remains normal.[21] Because there is no Wallerian degeneration and the axon is intact, muscle atrophy is not seen except that due to disuse.[22] Complicating matters, if conduction block is severe, axonal loss may be seen.[25] The deficits associated with conduction block are somewhat predictable. Large, myelinated fibers are more susceptible to compression than fibers with little or no myelination because there are is a relative paucity of sodium channels in the internodal segments of myelinated nerves.[20] In general, motor fibers are affected more severely than sensory and sympathetic fibers with conduction block. If sensory fibers are affected, touch sensation is often more affected than pain fibers.[22]

Axonal Injury and Wallerian Degeneration

If the axon or cell body is involved, Wallerian degeneration occurs 3–5 days after the initial insult. Wallerian degeneration describes dissolution of the axon into ovoids and secondary degeneration of myelin along the entire length of the nerve distal to the site of injury. It occurs when the axon distal to a lesion loses its connection with its cell body.[21] The effects of Wallerian degeneration are not seen on nerve conduction studies (NCSs) until 7–10 days after injury because the axon distal to the site of injury is capable of normal conduction initially.[23] Degeneration of the axon and associated myelin is accompanied by proliferation of Schwann cells on the proximal end and phagocytic removal of axonal and myelin debris.[15,26] After Wallerian degeneration is complete, the only occupant of the endoneurial sheath distal to the lesion is a row of Schwann cells.[24] Athletes can be advised that if their nerve injury includes an axonal process with Wallerian degeneration nerve regrowth occurs at a rate of 1 mm/day, 1 cm/week, or 1 inch/month.[15]

Mechanisms of Athletic Nerve Injury

Athletic nerve injury can occur acutely or chronically owing to the following.

- Compression (pressure)
- Ischemia (hypoxia)
- Traction (stretch, angulation)
- Friction

Compression (pressure) and ischemia appear to be the primary mechanisms involved in athletics. Pressure seems to be the responsible agent of injury with chronic entrapment of nerves, although ischemia may also play a small role. *Acute* athletic nerve injury may cause damage with high pressure for a short period of time (e.g., acute radial nerve injury from a humeral shaft fracture). In addition, a rapidly reversible physiologic block of conduction can occur in athletics when a brief period of suprasystolic pressure is applied to a nerve (e.g., peroneal nerve compression from cross-legged sitting, causing a reversible sensation of the foot "falling asleep"). This rapidly reversible physiologic block of conduction is due to ischemia. *Chronic* athletic nerve injury may cause damage with moderate or low pressure for long or intermittent periods of time (e.g., ulnar nerve injury from long distance bicycling riding). This chronic compression appears to be the most common mechanism of injury in athletics.

Compression

Animal models have been developed to understand the effects on nerves with acute and chronic compression. Compression, rather than ischemia, appears to be the primary mechanism of nerve injury in these models. Animal models of acute neural compression by pneumatic tourniquet have suggested that the pressure gradient itself creates the injury.[2,14,27] In these studies, the site of injury was found at the edges of the site of compression rather than areas of the lowest perfusion. Paranodal ortions of the injured myelin infold and cause paranodal demyelination.[15,22,27] More severe injury causes segmental demyelination (loss of myelin within the entire segment between two nodes).[15] The resultant shortening of the internodal distances causes conduction velocity slowing.[15,28]

In other animal models created for chronic compression of nerves, the histopathologic appearance of myelin is different from that found with acute compression. The myelin for each internode region tapers toward the lesion, whereas the opposite end of the internode accumulates into a bulbous collection of myelin.[29] This bulbous paranodal swelling end is always directed away from the site of entrapment, creating a tadpole appearance. Under the compression zone, demyelination and occasionally Wallerian degeneration are seen.[22] Unlike the acute model, myelin abnormalities are found in the entire region of the entrapment,[15] not just the edges. In chronic compression models, axonal degeneration is a secondary phenomenon occurring late in the course of nerve injury.[30]

Human nerve pathophysiology may be different from that of animal models. Surgical observations have demonstrated swelling proximal to and thinning within the zone of entrapment. Chronic secondary effects such as edema, hemorrhage, and neural fibrosis can follow the initial insult and cause proximal swelling.[24] Extensive demyelination and remyelination are present in the zone of entrapment.[31] Human nerves are susceptible to acute compression when they lie in a superficial, unprotected location or when they are subjected to increased pressure because of anatomic constraints.[10] Human peripheral nerves may also be more susceptible to injury with older age, the presence of systemic illness, connective tissue disorders, and vascular disorders.[32]

Ischemia

Ischemic injury is rarely the sole cause of peripheral nerve injury in the athlete but likely plays an important secondary role, particularly with acute injury. This is because the vascular anastomoses on the nerve surface and in the perineurium provide ample blood flow.[10] Lundborg and Rydevik showed that after 6 hours of ischemia there is rapid restoration of action potential amplitude and conduction velocity with reperfusion.[14] As mentioned earlier, this is termed *rapidly reversible physiologic block of conduction*. In contrast, after 8 hours of ischemia, there is irreversible damage[10] due to nerve axonal infarction. Prolonged ischemia of this nature has occurred in athletes owing to fracture/dislocations or compartment syndromes.[10] Notably, compartment syndromes should cause more injury to muscle than to nerves as muscle tissue is more vulnerable to limb ischemia than is peripheral nerve tissue.[32]

Ischemia and endoneurial edema may contribute to injury of nerves that are chronically and moderately compressed.[2,14] The transperineurial vessels (vaso nervorum) are subject to compression as they traverse the perineurium at oblique angles. Compression is caused by endoneurial edema and elevated endoneurial fluid pressure, both of which are consequences of external nerve compression.[2,14] Constriction of these vessels results in venous congestion, leakage of endoneurial capillaries, and elevated endoneurial fluid pressures. In turn, resultant local metabolic disturbances interfere with nerve function.[14] The obstruction of venous return and accumulation of blood, such as that described with lumbar spinal stenosis, can lead to further ischemia owing to blockage of the vaso nervorum.[32] Local ischemia of a susceptible nerve is thought to cause acute exacerbation of pain and paresthesias,[2,15] whereas chronic pressure is thought to cause motor presentations (e.g., weakness, atrophy, fasciculations, myokymia) and numbness. This goes to the point that numbness and tingling are distinct symptomatic entities.

Traction

Stretch-related (traction) injuries to peripheral nerves are common in athletics. To wit, it has been reported that 15% of all grade II and III lateral ankle sprains have damage to the peroneal nerve on electrodiagnostic studies.[33] Peripheral nerves are elastic owing to their collagenous endoneurium, as demonstrated when a nerve is transected and the two ends separate.[14] When a nerve is stretched beyond its capacity, injury occurs. Although most nerves can stretch 10%–20% without significant damage, there is an elongation at which mechanical failure occurs (approximately 30%–70%).[10,34] A nerve's tensile strength is determined by the strength of the tough perineural layer that surrounds its fascicle.[14,35,36] The rate of force in application also affects the degree of injury to the nerve. Experimentally, slow stretch over a number of years can increase the length of a nerve significantly without any loss of function.[34] On the other hand, if significant force is applied acutely, complete transection may occur (although more often the nerve remains intact).[37]

Nerve fibers have a redundant course when viewed in longitudinal section. This property allows the nerve to accommodate increased tension with changes in body position, especially when the nerve traverses a joint. When placed under tension, the nerve first slides within its tissue bed before it takes up its intrinsic slack.[14,36] A force that pulls the nerve beyond its limit of elasticity and slack can disrupt the axon, myelin, and microcirculation of the nerve and damage the nerve irreversibly.[36] Severe stretch injuries can result in intraneural and extraneural scar formation, which can compress and tether a peripheral nerve along its course, further complicating the injury.[14,36]

In sports, an example of acute traction causing nerve injury is seen in the *burner* or *stinger*, the most common sports-related peripheral nerve injury.[10,23] Several mechanisms for this injury have been proposed. One theory is that the brachial plexus is stretched when there is lateral deviation of the neck away from the involved side with accompanied ipsilateral shoulder depression. Shoulder and neck separation with the athlete's arm at his or her side increases tension on the superior trunk (C5 and C6) of the brachial plexus.[7] If traction is severe, it may be accompanied by cervical root avulsion.[23] An example of athletic injury due to repetitive nerve traction is found in the long thoracic nerve injury when an athlete repeatedly assumes a position with his or her head tilted or rotated laterally away from the affected nerve and the arm raised overhead. This position may double the length of the nerve between points of relative fixation, and over time repetitive microtrauma results in long thoracic neuropathy.[8]

Laceration

Laceration of the nerve is a rare traumatic event in sports. This type of nerve injury can be a complete transection or, as is seen more often, have some remaining continuity.[36] After nerve transection, apoptosis occurs followed by cell death. As many as 20%–50% of neurons in the dorsal root ganglia are lost. Motor neurons also die but probably to a lesser extent.[38] Factors that influence neuronal loss in the dorsal root ganglia after transection include age, time from injury to surgical repair, and proximity of the injury to the spinal cord. Immediate repair of a nerve may reduce neuronal loss.[38]

Double Crush Syndrome

In 1973, Upton and McComas presented their theory of the *double crush syndrome*. They proposed that when a single axon is compromised in one region it becomes more vulnerable to damage at another site.[14,25,39,40] The theory was based on the idea that many of their patients with carpal tunnel syndrome or ulnar neuropathy at the elbow also had evidence of compression of the corresponding nerve root. Critics of the theory argue that a cervical radiculopathy should not have an effect on distal conduction or myelination and that the presence of a cervical radiculopathy should have minimal effect on distal motor axon function of the median nerve because the median nerve is comprised of multiple cervical nerve roots.[41] Several studies using electrophysiologic data have suggested that the relation between cervical radiculopathy and carpal tunnel syndrome is associational rather than causative.[41,42] As such, the supposition of a double crush syndrome for compressive neuropathies appears dubious and is rare if it occurs at all.

For generalized peripheral neuropathies, there does exist inconclusive support for "double crush susceptibility." For example, patients with diabetes clearly have an increased incidence of carpal tunnel syndrome. However, it has been demonstrated that the severity of peripheral neuropathy did not predict the prevalence of carpal tunnel syndrome, nor did diabetic patients with carpal tunnel syndrome have more severe peripheral neuropathy.[43]

Nerve Recovery

Unlike most CNS processes, the peripheral nervous system has a unique ability to regenerate after injury. Overall, the peripheral nerve's capacity to initiate regeneration persists for at least 1 year after injury.[37] Survival of a peripheral neuron is not ensured after severe injury. Current research suggests that trophic molecules in the peripheral nerve microenvironment-e.g., nerve growth factor (NGF), brain-derived neurotrophic factor (BDNF), cytokines-play a role in cell survival[37] and axonal regeneration.[26] Interestingly, functional changes in the CNS after peripheral nerve injury repair are also key factors in functional recovery.[38,44] Much more has been described about the recovery from traumatic axonal injury than from a chronic compression injury causing segmental demyelination. Many nerve lesions are mixed processes in that there is both demyelinative and axonal involvement. Mixed lesions are thought to recover in approximately the following order.

1. Resolution of conduction block
2. Distal axon sprouting of spared axons
3. Muscle fiber hypertrophy
4. Redistribution of sensory function
5. Axonal regeneration of injured axons

The resolution of any conduction block is the initial process to achieve nerve recovery. Being that athletic nerve injuries are either acute ischemia or chronic phenomena involving segmental demyelination, knowledge of the time frame of this part of nerve recovery is important for prognosticating return to play. Ischemia-producing conduction block reverses rapidly, usually within a few minutes or hours.[20] Compression that produces conduction block can also be reversed provided the offending etiology is mitigated. Typically, it takes up to 3 months to reverse this type of conduction block.[20] If the length of segmental demyelination is significant, it may take longer to alleviate the block.

Shortly after axonal injury (approximately 3–5 days), the distal stump of the nerve undergoes Wallerian degeneration. Schwann cells and macrophages are recruited to the site of the injury to remove the axonal and myelin fragments.[26] Schwann cells produce numerous growth factors; and macrophages release interleukin-1 (IL-1), which up-regulates other growth factors.[38] Axonal regeneration starts proximal to the site of the injury, with the axon in its intact endoneurial tube. One dominant axon emerges as other axonal sprouts are reabsorbed. The expansion of the distal axon tip, or growth cone, is directed by the cell body and increases the length of the axoplasm.[37] Extensions of the growth cone, called filopodia or neurites, form and elongate the regenerating axon by ameba-like advancement of the filopodia.[22] In a simple injury without disruption of the endoneurial tube, axon tips arrive at the injury site within 4–10 days after injury.[22]

If there is scar formation and a space between the nerve ends, the potential for functional regeneration depends on the length of time since the injury, the age of the subject, and the content of the scar.[22] The growth cone may secrete a protease to dissolve debris in its path.[37] After nerve transection, approximately one of every six or seven nerve fibers arrive at the appropriate destination. If the gap is narrow, neurites follow fibroblastic bridges to unite the nerve ends. If the gap is wide, a neuroma forms and only a few axons actually bridge the gap.[22] The rate of growth of the regenerating axon has been reported to be 0.5–9.0 mm/day.[37] Growth can reach 2.5–4.0 mm/day once the distal portions are in the endoneurial tube.[22] The rate varies by nerve: The median nerve grows 2–4 mm/day, the ulnar nerve 1.5 mm/day, and the radial nerve 4–5 mm/day.[22] Another convenient estimate, as mentioned earlier, is 1 mm/day, 1 cm/week, and 1 inch per month.[15,25] The rate of growth is inversely proportional to the distance from the cell body; that is, growth is slower for more distal injuries, and the growth rate slows as the growth cone advances distally.[22,37] The axonal regeneration process may be faster for a crush injury than for a laceration injury. Clinically, the distal progress of a regenerating nerve may be followed by an advancing Tinel sign.[37]

Remyelination begins when the axon tip reaches the distal portion of the endoneurial tube that contains Schwann cells. Schwann cells align around the regenerating axon. Each Schwann cell rotates around the axon to form the myelin sheath. This process lags 9–20 days behind the advancing front of the axon.[22] Myelination advances at 4 mm/day. It may take 1 year for the myelin to mature fully.[22,26] Remyelination by Schwann cells during nerve regeneration appears to be under the control of three major players: extracellular matrix proteins, neurotrophic factors, and hormones such as progesterone, thyroid hormone, and erythropoietin.[26]

The end organs for peripheral nerves are muscles or skin. Denervated muscle fibers are viable and available for only 18–24 months after an injury.[20] Thus, with complete injuries to the lower brachial plexus, hand function is not expected to recover despite surgical drafting, as the length segment is too long.[20] For sensory nerves, the end organ (skin) is always viable and has a longer window of opportunity to reinnervate the cutaneous supply of the injured nerve.

References

1. Misulis K. In: Bradley WG, ed. Neurology in Clinical Practice. 4th ed. Philadelphia: Butterworth Heineman; 2004:409.
2. Dyck PJ, Thomas P, eds. Peripheral Neuropathy. 4th ed. Philadelphia: Elsevier Saunders; 2005.
3. Zimmermann M. Pathobiology of neuropathic pain. Eur J Pharmacol 2001;429(1–3):23–37.
4. Melzack R, Wall PD. Pain mechanisms: a new theory. Science 1965;150(699):971–9.
5. Stanos S, Tyburski M, Harden R. Management of chronic pain. In: Braddom RL, ed. Physical Medicine and Rehabilitation. 3rd ed. Philadelphia: Elsevier; 2007: 951–88.
6. Arko FR, Harris EJ, Zarins CK, Olcott CT. Vascular complications in high-performance athletes. J Vasc Surg 2001;33(5):935–42.
7. Koffler KM, Kelly JDT. Neurovascular trauma in athletes. Orthop Clin North Am 2002;33(3):523–34, vi.
8. Safran MR. Nerve injury about the shoulder in athletes. Part 2: Long thoracic nerve, spinal accessory nerve, burners/stingers, thoracic outlet syndrome. Am J Sports Med 2004;32(4):1063–76.
9. Edwards PH Jr, Wright ML, Hartman JF. A practical approach for the differential diagnosis of chronic leg pain in the athlete. Am J Sports Med 2005;33(8):1241–9.
10. Feinberg JH, Nadler SF, Krivickas LS. Peripheral nerve injuries in the athlete. Sports Med 1997;24(6):385–408.
11. Wilbourn AJ. Thoracic outlet syndromes. Neurol Clin 1999;17(3):477–97, vi.
12. Meleger AL, Krivickas LS. Neck and back pain: musculoskeletal disorders. Neurol Clin 2007;25(2):419–38.
13. Thompson JM. Diagnosis and treatment of muscle pain syndromes. In: Braddom RL, ed. Physical Medicine and Rehabilitation. 2nd ed. Philadelphia: Saunders; 2000: 934–56.
14. Lundborg G, Rydevik B. Effects of stretching the tibial nerve of the rabbit: a preliminary study of the intraneural

circulation and the barrier function of the perineurium. J Bone Joint Surg Br 1973;55(2):390–401.
15. Dawson DM, Hallett M, Wilbourn AJ, eds. Entrapment Neuropathies. 3rd ed. Philadelphia: Lippincott Raven; 1999.
16. Buschbacher L. Rehabilitation of patients with peripheral neuropathies. In: Braddom RL, ed. Physical Medicine and Rehabilitation. 2nd ed. Philadelphia: Saunders; 2000: 1024–44.
17. Cotran RS, Kumar V, Collins T. Robbins Pathologic Basis of Disease. 6th ed. Philadelphia: Saunders; 1999.
18. Seddon H. Three types of nerve injury. Brain 1943; 66:238–87.
19. Seddon H. Surgical Disorders of the Peripheral Nerves. Edinburgh: Churchill Livingstone; 1972.
20. Robinson LR. Traumatic injury to peripheral nerves. Muscle Nerve 2000;23(6):863–73.
21. Wilbourn AJ. Plexopathies. Neurol Clin 2007;25(1): 139–71.
22. Dumitru D, Amato AA, Zwarts M, eds. Electrodiagnostic Medicine. Philadelphia: Hanley & Belfus; 2001.
23. Elman L, McCluskey L. Occupational and sport related traumatic neuropathy. Neurologist 2004;10(2):82–96.
24. Sunderland S. Nerve Injuries and their Repair. Edinburgh: Churchill Livingstone; 1991.
25. Campbell WW. AAEE case report #18: ulnar neuropathy in the distal forearm. Muscle Nerve 1989;12(5): 347–52.
26. Chen ZL, Yu WM, Strickland S. Peripheral regeneration. Annu Rev Neurosci 2007; 30:209–233.
27. Ochoa J, Danta G, Fowler TJ, Gilliatt RW. Nature of the nerve lesion caused by a pneumatic tourniquet. Nature 1971;233(5317):265–6.
28. Ochoa J, Fowler TJ, Gilliatt RW. Anatomical changes in peripheral nerves compressed by a pneumatic tourniquet. J Anat 1972;113(Pt 3):433–55.
29. Neary D, Ochoa J, Gilliatt RW. Sub-clinical entrapment neuropathy in man. J Neurol Sci 1975;24(3):283–98.
30. Aguayo A, Nair CP, Midgley R. Experimental progressive compression neuropathy in the rabbit: histologic and electrophysiologic studies. Arch Neurol 1971;24(4): 358–64.
31. Thomas PK, Fullerton PM. Nerve fibre size in the carpal tunnel syndrome. J Neurol Neurosurg Psychiatry 1963; 26:520–7.
32. Werner RA, Andary M. Carpal tunnel syndrome: pathophysiology and clinical neurophysiology. Clin Neurophysiol 2002;113(9):1373–81.
33. Lorei MP, Hershman EB. Peripheral nerve injuries in athletes: treatment and prevention. Sports Med 1993; 16(2):130–47.
34. Sunderland S. Stress-strain phenomena in human peripheral nerve trunks. Brain 1961;84:102–19.
35. Sunderland S. The anatomy and physiology of nerve injury. Muscle Nerve 1990;13(9):771–84.
36. Grant GA, Goodkin R, Kliot M. Evaluation and surgical management of peripheral nerve problems. Neurosurgery 1999;44(4):825–39; discussion 39–40.
37. Burnett MG, Zager EL. Pathophysiology of peripheral nerve injury: a brief review. Neurosurg Focus 2004; 16(5):E1.
38. Lundborg G, Rosen B. Hand function after nerve repair. Acta Physiol (Oxf) 2007;189(2):207–17.
39. Upton AR, McComas AJ. The double crush in nerve entrapment syndromes. Lancet 1973;2(7825):359–62.
40. Hochman MG, Zilberfarb JL. Nerves in a pinch: imaging of nerve compression syndromes. Radiol Clin North Am 2004;42(1):221–45.
41. Richardson JK, Forman GM, Riley B. An electrophysiological exploration of the double crush hypothesis. Muscle Nerve 1999;22(1):71–7.
42. Kwon HK, Hwang M, Yoon DW. Frequency and severity of carpal tunnel syndrome according to level of cervical radiculopathy: double crush syndrome? Clin Neurophysiol 2006;117(6):1256–9.
43. Richardson JK. Session C169: double crush syndromes: do they exist? In: American Academy of Physical Medicine and Rehabilitation Annual Meeting Notes; 2000.
44. Lundborg G. Richard P. Bunge memorial lecture: nerve injury and repair—a challenge to the plastic brain. J Peripher Nerv Syst 2003;8(4):209–26.
45. Toth C, McNeil S, Feasby T. Peripheral nervous system injuries in sport and recreation: a systematic review. Sports Med 2005;35(8):717–38.
46. Safran MR. Nerve injury about the shoulder in athletes. Part 1: Suprascapular nerve and axillary nerve. Am J Sports Med 2004;32(3):803–19.
47. Krivickas LS, Wilbourn AJ. Sports and peripheral nerve injuries: report of 190 injuries evaluated in a single electromyography laboratory. Muscle Nerve 1998;21(8): 1092–4.
48. Krivickas LS, Wilbourn AJ. Peripheral nerve injuries in athletes: a case series of over 200 injuries. Semin Neurol 2000;20(2):225–32.
49. Bencardino JT, Rosenberg ZS. Entrapment neuropathies of the shoulder and elbow in the athlete. Clin Sports Med 2006;25(3):465–87, vi–vii.
50. Aldridge JW, Bruno RJ, Strauch RJ, Rosenwasser MP. Nerve entrapment in athletes. Clin Sports Med 2001; 20(1):95–122.
51. Goslin KL, Krivickas LS. Proximal neuropathies of the upper extremity. Neurol Clin 1999;17(3):525–48, vii.
52. McCrory P, Bell S, Bradshaw C. Nerve entrapments of the lower leg, ankle and foot in sport. Sports Med 2002;32(6):371–91.
53. Aoki M, Takasaki H, Muraki T, et al. Strain on the ulnar nerve at the elbow and wrist during throwing motion. J Bone Joint Surg Am 2005;87(11):2508–14.
54. Cutts S. Cubital tunnel syndrome. Postgrad Med J 2007; 83(975):28–31.
55. Dickerman RD, Stevens QE, Cohen AJ, Jaikumar S. Radial tunnel syndrome in an elite power athlete: a case of direct compressive neuropathy. J Peripher Nerv Syst 2002;7(4):229–32.
56. Izzi J, Dennison D, Noerdlinger M, et al. Nerve injuries of the elbow, wrist, and hand in athletes. Clin Sports Med 2001;20(1):203–17.
57. Levine BP, Jones JA, Burton RI. Nerve entrapments of the upper extremity: a surgical perspective. Neurol Clin 1999;17(3):549–65, vii.
58. Spinner RJ. Outcomes for peripheral nerve entrapment syndromes. Clin Neurosurg 2006;53:285–94.

Chapter 2
Diagnostic Tests for Nerve and Vascular Injuries

Venu Akuthota and Ellen Casey

Clinical Pearls

- Nerve conduction studies study the faster myelinated nerve fibers. Thus, if small fiber or autonomic neuropathies are suspected, electrodiagnostic studies may not be sensitive.
- Fasciculations are often seen in athletes after exercise owing to release of free radicals and muscle fatigue. Coffee consumption and dehydration are thought to exacerbate these benign fasciculations. They can be seen with needle electromyography.
- For sports-related cases, ankle brachial pressure index measurements at rest are rarely useful. What is usually needed are measurements before and after exercise or postexercise measurements compared to the asymptomatic contralateral side.
- Just as with vascular physical examination maneuvers, the clinician must keep in mind the high rate of false-positive results, particularly when using provocation tests or "functional" tests.

Introduction

Sports medicine practitioners often need to supplement the history and physical examination with other diagnostic tests as examination maneuvers often have low sensitivity and specificity. For nerve and vascular injuries, the most important tests are electrodiagnostics (also referred to as *electromyography*, or EMG) and vascular diagnostics.

Electrodiagnostic Testing

Electrodiagnostic (EDX) testing can be an important tool when evaluating athletes with nerve issues. Whereas imaging studies identify structural integrity, EDX studies evaluate the physiology and function of the peripheral nervous system. The EDX examination, however, evaluates the physiology of nerves and muscles only at a particular time. Furthermore, a negative EDX examination does not rule out the possibility of pathology because electrophysiologic studies are time- and severity-dependent. In this light, the EDX impression must be based on the entire clinical picture. Clinical judgment is needed in EDX consultations, and therefore EDXs are highly dependent on the quality of the electromyographer.[1]

Typically, EDX testing is divided into nerve conduction studies (NCSs) and the needle examination (NE). The NE is also referred to as electromyography (EMG). Many clinicians use the term electromyography for all components of the EDX examination.

Anatomy

Electrodiagnostic studies evaluate the integrity of the peripheral nervous system or lower motor neuron pathway. The peripheral nervous system

V. Akuthota (✉)
Department of Physical Medicine and Rehabilitation,
Aurora, CO, USA

V. Akuthota, S.A. Herring (eds.), *Nerve and Vascular Injuries in Sports Medicine*,
DOI 10.1007/978-0-387-76600-3_2, © Springer Science+Business Media, LLC 2009

includes both afferent sensory pathways and efferent motor pathways. The sensory pathway begins with cutaneous receptors forming sensory axons. These sensory axons coalesce in either pure sensory or mixed nerves. The sensory fibers travel through specific portions of nerve plexi (e.g., brachial plexus, lumbosacral plexus) and house their cell bodies in the dorsal root ganglion, usually located within the intervertebral foramina. The sensory fibers then form dorsal roots as they synapse into the dorsolateral spinal cord. NCSs of pure sensory and mixed nerves are used to evaluate this aspect of the peripheral nervous system.

The efferent motor pathway starts at the level of the spinal cord with anterior horn cells. The motor axons, originating from the cell bodies of anterior horn cells, exit the spinal canal as spinal nerves and divide into ventral and dorsal rami. The motor fibers in the ventral rami traverse their respective plexi ending as peripheral motor nerves.[1] Peripheral motor nerves synapse at specific muscles through individual neuromuscular junctions, where acetylcholine is transported to the muscle membrane to induce an all-or-none action potential. NCSs of pure motor or mixed nerves are used to evaluate this aspect of the peripheral nervous system from the point of stimulation to the recording site. Motor units can be evaluated during needle EMG with voluntary muscle activation. A motor unit represents the lower motor neuron pathway, including a single anterior horn cell, motor axons traversing through a plexus and peripheral nerves, and muscle fibers.

Specific Electrodiagnostic Studies

Nerve Conduction Studies

Nerve conduction studies may be performed on motor, sensory, or mixed nerves. There are numerous pitfalls with NCSs (Table 2.1); therefore, it is imperative that well trained consultants perform the EDX studies.[1] Both motor and sensory nerve conduction studies test only the fastest myelinated axons of a nerve; thus, the lightly myelinated or unmyelinated C fibers are not examined with EDX.[2] Motor nerves are stimulated at accessible sites, and the compound muscle action potential (CMAP) is recorded over the motor points of innervated muscles. Deep motor nerves and deep proximal muscles are more difficult to study and interpret.[3] Sensory nerves can be studied along the physiologic direction of the nerve impulse (orthodromic) or opposite the physiologic direction of the afferent input (antidromic). Stimulated and recorded sensory nerves produce a sensory nerve action potential (SNAP). Frequently, sensory axons are tested in mixed nerves, such as plantar nerves, and produce a mixed nerve action potential (MNAP).

Table 2.1 Sources of error in nerve conduction studies

- Temperature
- Inadequate or excessive stimulation
- Improper placement of electrodes
- Tape measurement error
- Not adjusting values for age
- Anomalous innervation
- Volume conduction of impulse to nearby nerve
- Improper filter settings
- Improper electrode montage setup
- Involuntary muscle contractions

CMAP, SNAP, and MNAP waveforms are analyzed and interpreted by the clinician. Waveform parameters include amplitude, latency, and conduction velocity. In general, amplitude measurement evaluates the number of functioning axons in a given nerve and, for motor studies, the number of muscle fibers activated. Latency refers to the time from the stimulus to the recorded action potential. With motor NCSs, latency takes into account peripheral nerve conduction (distal to the site of stimulation), neuromuscular junction transmission time, and muscle fiber activation. With sensory nerves, latency measures only the conduction of the segment of nerve being stimulated. Conduction velocity across a segment of nerve can also be calculated when nerves are stimulated at a distal site and a proximal site.

Proximal Nerve Conduction Studies

Sports-related nerve injuries often involve proximal nerves such as the suprascapular, long thoracic, axillary, and femoral nerves. The proximal nerves are not always accessible to stimulation and recording as they lie deeply. In the upper limb, many of the proximal nerves can be stimulated at Erb's point, located just superior to the clavicle and lateral to the sternocleidomastoid. Stimulation at this location is often painful, and supramaximum stimulation is often in the range of 60 mA. Erb's point stimulation volume conductance produces depolarization of the upper brachial plexus. Surface or needle recording can be utilized. If needle recording is used, the amplitude measurement to assess for an axonal injury becomes less reliable. Also, short segment evaluation is unavailable with proximal nerve conduction studies. Therefore, proximal nerve conduction studies may not be able to distinguish a demyelinating injury (e.g., conduction block) from an axonal injury. Latency measurements can also be difficult to interpret because the exact course of the proximal nerve cannot be measured as it is in the distal extremity. To help mitigate measurement error, authors have suggested obstetric calipers and comparisons to the unaffected contralateral side.[4]

Late Responses

The H reflex is the electrophysiologic analog to the ankle stretch reflex. Its measurement looks at afferent and efferent conduction mainly along the S1 nerve root pathway.[5] Thus, the H reflex test looks at the afferent and efferent pathways and provides information about the sensory pathway that is not tested by standard needle EMG. An S1 nerve injury can be due to S1 radiculopathy from a herniated lumbar disc or lumbar stenosis, peripheral neuropathy (usually with bilateral abnormal H reflexes), or sciatic/tibial nerve injuries.[6] Therefore, evaluation of other peripheral nerves through standard NCSs may be helpful to sort out the differential diagnosis.

The F wave is a late muscle potential that results from a motor nerve volley created by supramaximally stimulated anterior horn cells.[7] Unlike the H reflex, the F wave can be elicited at many spinal levels and from any muscle. F-wave studies, like H reflexes, look at a long pathway. Consequently, small focal abnormalities tend to be obscured by the longer segments. Abnormal F-wave values may be due to nerve injury anywhere along the long pathway evaluated.

Needle Examination

The NE evaluates the entire motor unit (lower motor neuron pathway) but not the sensory pathway. This component of the EDX evaluation includes needle EMG of muscles at rest (to detect axonal injury) and during volitional activity (to evaluate voluntary motor unit morphology and recruitment). The NE must be timed such that abnormalities are optimally detected. If the NE is performed too early (i.e., less than 2–3 weeks after the initial injury), spontaneous muscle fiber discharges (denervation potentials) may not have had time to develop. If the NE is performed too late (i.e., more than 6 months after the initial injury), reinnervation via collateral sprouting may have halted spontaneous muscle fiber discharges.[6]

When muscles are studied at rest, the electromyographer studies the electrical activity of selected muscles for abnormal waveforms. Among these abnormal waveforms, the most common abnormal finding is the presence of fibrillations and positive waves. They are typically found when the muscle tested has been denervated or the muscle is inflamed.[8] Fibrillations and positive sharp waves are graded on a scale from 0 to 4+. Complex repetitive discharges (CRDs) are also common. They represent a group of single muscle fibers that are time-linked because of crosstalk between neighboring muscle fibers. Fasciculation potentials can be found in a variety of benign and malignant conditions. They represent spontaneous discharges of an entire motor unit; thus, they are much larger than fibrillations and positive waves. Sometimes fasciculations are grossly observed as muscle twitches. Benign fasciculations may be found in athletes following heavy exercise, dehydration, anxiety, fatigue, coffee consumption, or smoking. When muscles are studied while contracting, motor units may be analyzed. Motor unit analysis offers an opportunity to distinguish between neuropathic and myopathic conditions.[1]

Needle examination also may help differentiate acute from chronic neuropathic conditions. The amplitude of fibrillations can grade a nerve injury as being present for less than or more than 1 year.[9] This can be particularly useful for distinguishing an athlete's acute-on-chronic nerve injury. Chronic nerve injuries, without significant ongoing denervation, additionally show large-amplitude, long-duration, polyphasic motor unit potentials.[6]

Provocation Electrodiagnostics

Some authors advocate performing EDX after exercise or with the limbs in provocative positions. These techniques have not been validated with sound research and are subject to measurement error. Anecdotally, however, they appear to have a limited use. Leach and colleagues described peroneal nerve entrapment in runners that was detected only with EDX testing following exercise.[10] Athletes diagnosed with compartment syndrome and potential nerve entrapment (e.g., superficial peroneal nerve entrapment as it exits the fascia of the lateral compartment) have also been postulated as requiring EDX following exercise.[11] Fishman et al. have suggested that electrophysiologic evidence of piriformis syndrome is more apparent when an H reflex is tested with the sciatic nerve on stretch (hip flexed to 90°, maximally adducted, and knee flexed to 90°).[12] Other studies have not supported the notion that EDX sensitivity is improved with dynamic positions, such as after pronator syndrome provocation maneuvers.[13] Spuriously slow and fast nerve conduction velocities can be recorded with the limb in various positions, most famously ulnar nerve studies around the elbow.[14] Therefore, these techniques need to be interpreted with caution as many "abnormal" readings occur based on measurement error alone.

Dynamic or Quantitative Electromyography

Numerous studies have employed electrophysiologic techniques to demonstrate the sequence of muscle recruitment and muscle force. Dynamic and quantitative EMG does not constitute a diagnostic test and is available only in specialized laboratories. Quantitative EMG employs surface or needle (fine wire) electrodes placed in muscles to record EMG signals through multiple channels. Often fine wire electrodes are used to record signals in deeper muscles. Caution should be used when correlating the EMG signal amplitude with muscle force because the relation is not consistently linear. Quantitative EMG has also been used to assess the degree of muscle fatigue and biomechanics of sports activities. The kinesiology of athletic maneuvers, such as running and throwing, has been elucidated with dynamic EMG. Surface EMG can be used as a biofeedback device in athletes.[15]

Indications for Electrodiagnostic Testing

The utility of EDX testing in a given athlete may be estimated (following a thorough history and physical examination) by a review of supplemental information (e.g., imaging studies) and a thorough appreciation for the chronology of electrophysiologic changes that occur following nerve injury. Some useful generalizations about the indications for EDX[6] are worthy of review and are discussed below.

- Establish and/or confirm a diagnosis. A thorough EDX examination can rule out a competing diagnosis. Nerve injury localization often needs to be confirmed objectively prior to contemplating invasive or surgical treatment. Additionally, EDX studies may alert the examiner to the possibility of an unsuspected concomitant pathologic process-for example, a runner with tarsal tunnel syndrome with superimposed lumbosacral radiculopathy.
- Localize nerve lesions. For nerve injuries to be precisely treated, the exact location of nerve injury must be elucidated. For example, an athlete presenting with plantar foot numbness and tingling may have a sciatic nerve lesion anywhere along the course of the nerve or its branches. EDX studies can then be used to determine if the sciatic nerve injury is occurring at the piriformis or its terminal branches.
- Determine the extent and chronicity of nerve injury. Properly timed EDX studies can differentiate a neuropraxic injury from axonal degeneration. This information may have a significant impact on the aggressiveness of the treatment for

a nerve injury. The acuteness and chronicity of a nerve lesion may also be assessed using fibrillation amplitude measurement and motor unit analysis as well as the patient's clinical history.[1,9]

- Correlate the findings of anatomic studies. When so-called abnormal findings are found on imaging tests, EDX studies are useful for correlating nerve function with the anatomic abnormalities. This may be particularly useful in the spine because disc herniations effacing nerve roots can be seen in asymptomatic individuals.[16]
- Assist in prognosis and return to play.

Nerve Recovery and Return to Play

By determining the degree of nerve injury, the clinician can predict nerve function recovery. In general, neuropraxic (conduction slowing and conduction block) injuries recover sooner than axonal (axontmesis and neurotmesis) injuries. When ordering EDX studies, the timing of the findings should be kept in mind (Table 2.2). Nerve conduction studies can determine if neuropraxic injury is present, and needle examination can analyze motor units. Most athletic nerve lesions are neuropraxic or a mix of neuropraxic and axonal injuries.

If an axonal injury is present, EDX performed around the 1-month mark can help quantify the number of surviving axons. EDX performed before postinjury day 9 may show normal distal segment motor nerve conduction parameters (or before postinjury day 11 in the case of sensory nerve conduction). Motor (CMAP) and sensory (SNAP) axon amplitudes can be compared to those on the other side to estimate the number of surviving axons. However, there may be 30%–50% side-to-side variability. The greater the percentage of axons lost, the poorer the prognosis. It has been estimated that if 30%–50% of axons are preserved, recovery is excellent. If 10%–30% of axons survive, recovery is good but not complete. If less than 10% of axons are preserved, recovery is poor.[17]

Needle EMG examination of volitional motor units can also help predict prognosis. Of course, if no motor units are detected during the early stages and nerve conduction studies do not reveal conduction block, a severe axonal injury is present and recovery can be predicted to be poor. After a couple

Table 2.2 Axonal injury: timing of Wallerian degeneration and nerve recovery

Time	Nerve degeneration	Nerve recovery	NCS correlate	NE correlate
Day 0	None	None	Proximal-recorded segment ABI Distal segment normal	Decreased recruitment
Day 3	NMJ impaired	Nodal and terminal sprouts		
Day 9	Motor axons lost		Distal segment CMAP decrease	Increased insertional activity
Day 11	Sensory axons lost		Distal segment SNAP decrease	
Day 14				Large denervation potentials
Day 21		Increased fiber density		Denervation in distal muscles
Weeks 6–8		Axonal sprouting	CMAP/SNAP increasing	Nascent reinnervation potentials
Week 16		Axonal regrowth		Maturing reinnervation proximal
Week 20		Axonal 1 mm/day		Maturing reinnervation distal
Year 1				Smaller denervation potentials
Year 2		Muscle no longer viable		

NCS, nerve conduction study; NE, needle examination; ABI, ankle brachial pressure index; NMJ, neuromuscular junction; CMAP, compound muscle action potential; SNAP, sensory nerve action potential of months, motor unit morphology analysis can indicate acute and chronic reinnervation.[18] If spontaneous reinnervation is occurring, surgery is rarely needed.[17] However, EDX studies should not be the sine qua non for return to play because they may lag behind clinical recovery. The best determination of return to play remains the athlete's functional performance in simulated sports activities.[3]

Limitations of Electrodiagnostic Testing

Electrodiagnostic testing is not perfect and should not be performed in every athlete with neurologic signs or symptoms. Some diagnoses are unequivocal, and treatment should be initiated without delay. If the athlete has progressive neurologic deficits, such as after a traumatic posterior knee dislocation, the results of EDX studies would be unimportant, as the patient requires emergent care. Relative contraindications to EDX include a pacemaker (no Erb's point stimulation), arteriovenous fistula, open wound, coagulopathy, lymphedema, anasarca, and/or pending muscle biopsy.

Electromyography Report

The electrophysiologic report should include a number of important pieces of data for the referring physician. The electrophysiologic findings should correlate with physical findings, and any discrepancies should be identified. Inconsistencies may have as much importance in the clinical treatment of the patient as consistent results. Also, the degree of definitiveness of findings needs to be conveyed to the referring physician. A diagnosis of S1 radiculopathy by H reflex changes carries different weight than abundant spontaneous activity in the S1 myotomal distribution. EDX examiners and referring physicians need to remember that one abnormal finding does not make the diagnosis if all other evidence is pointing to a different diagnosis. There should also be sufficient evidence to rule out alternative possibilities and to identify superimposed conditions. The EMG interpretation should mention the degree of injury and chronicity if possible. Prognosis is critical for referring physicians to know-if a prognosis is obtainable. Finally, results should be compared with previous EDX data whenever possible.[15]

Vascular Diagnostic Tests

The diagnosis of sports-related vascular injuries is often challenging owing to the lack of obvious physical examination signs and the lack of an appropriate index of suspicion. This is partly due to the relatively low incidence of vascular injuries in the realm of sports medicine as well as the paucity of sports medicine literature dedicated to vascular injuries in sports. Both arterial and venous injuries can occur in sports. Subclavian vein thrombosis (Paget–von Schroetter syndrome) appears to be the most common venous injury in athletes, and axillary artery and popliteal artery entrapments appear to be the most common arterial injuries in sports.[19] With athletes, arterial vascular injury typically results from nonocclusive injury in which some arterial flow continues distal to the injury rather than traumatic occlusive injury in which all distal perfusion is lost. With these rare traumatic occlusive injuries, delaying definitive treatment of an obvious arterial injury that is approaching the 6-hour limit of warm ischemia time to obtain vascular tests is ill-advised. However, when nonocclusive injury (Table 2.3) is suspected, a variety of vascular diagnostic tests can be utilized.

Table 2.3 Types of nonocclusive vascular injury in sports

- Dissection
- Aneurysm
- Injury
- Intermittent compression/entrapment
- Stenosis
- Thrombosis

Anatomy

Upper Limb

Of course, the emanation of the entire arterial supply is from the heart and aorta. The arch of the aorta gives off the left subclavian artery, whereas the right subclavian artery arises from the brachiocephalic artery. The subclavian arteries, as suggested by their name, course inferior to the clavicles to the outer margins of the first ribs, where they become the axillary arteries.[20] In the shoulder region, the axillary artery, relatively fixed to the lateral edge of the pectoralis minor, gives off the anterior and posterior circumflex humeral arteries and forms the brachial artery in the upper arm. The axillary artery can become injured with shoulder dislocations or reductions; yet the distal pulses may be intact owing to the extensive anastomotic arterial connections around the shoulder, permitting good collateral flow.[20] The mechanism of injury is that the axillary artery becomes taut with an abducted and externally rotated shoulder. When the humeral head dislocates in this position, the axillary artery is forced anteriorly, and the pectoralis minor acts as a fulcrum over which the artery is deformed and injured.[21]

The cords of the brachial plexus lie juxtaposed to the axillary vessels. The arterial branching then becomes more complex, giving off various branches, which eventually form the radial and ulnar arteries. These arteries form the arterial arches of the hand, which then sprout the digital arteries. The venous structures lie close to the arterial structures. In particular, the subclavian vein can develop thromboses from repetitive shoulder activity (e.g., throwing sports) because of external compression due to thoracic outlet anomalies and stress from exercise temporarily causing hypercoagulability and microscopic intimal tears in the vessel wall (Fig. 2.1).[22]

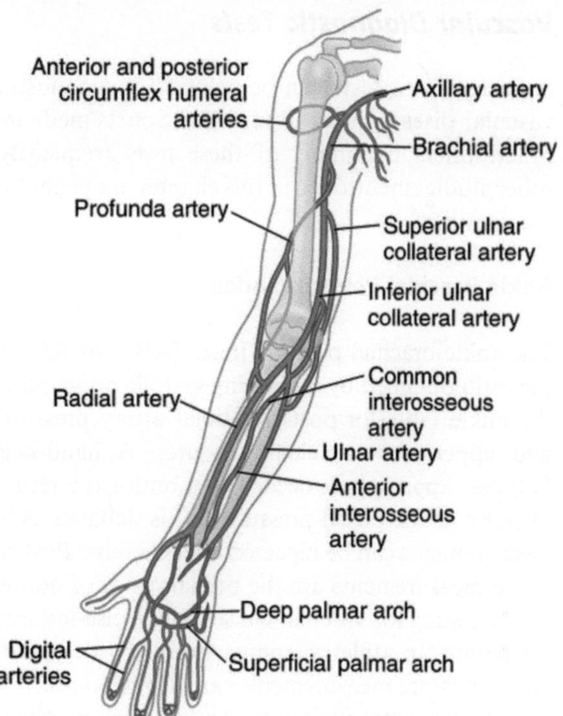

Fig. 2.1 Upper limb vasculature supply

Lower Limb

The arterial supply of the leg begins with the iliac arteries. Specifically, the external iliac artery, prone to impingement with hip flexion in bicyclists, traverses underneath the inguinal ligament and then becomes the common femoral artery. The femoral artery is the major artery of the thigh. The common femoral artery splits into the superficial and deep (profunda) femoral arteries, which give off the circumflex arteries supplying the femoral head and neck. Interruption of the circumflex arteries at the femoral neck, as with hip dislocations or fractures, can jeopardize the arterial supply to the femoral head. The superficial femoral artery becomes the popliteal artery after it exits the adductor (Hunter's) canal at the superior edge of popliteal fossa. The popliteal artery is particularly vulnerable owing to tethering at the adductor hiatus and soleus arch. After the popliteal artery gives off the geniculate arteries, it trifurcates into the anterior tibial (then forming the doralis pedis artery), posterior tibial, and peroneal arteries.[20] The posterior tibial artery passes behind the medial malleolus and divides into the medial and lateral plantar arteries that anastomose with the dorsalis pedis artery.

The venous anatomy of the lower extremity is divided into the deep and superficial systems. The deep venous system follows the arterial system, with the external iliac vein descending into the thigh becoming the femoral vein until it exits the adductor canal where it turns into the popliteal vein. The popliteal vein branches into the anterior tibial, posterior tibial, and peroneal veins, collectively referred to as the calf veins. The superficial venous system consists of the great and small saphenous veins as well as smaller perforating veins. The lower limb veins are particularly vulnerable to deep vein thromboses.

Vascular Diagnostic Tests

An assortment tests can be helpful for diagnosing vascular disease in the lower limb. Sports medicine practitioners use many of these tests frequently; other studies mentioned in this chapter are probably less familiar.

Ankle Brachial Pressure Index

The ankle brachial pressure index (ABPI or ABI) is the ratio obtained by measuring systolic pressures at the ankle (anterior/posterior tibial artery pressure) and upper arm (brachial pressure). A hand-held Doppler apparatus is needed to monitor the return of pulse as the blood pressure cuff is deflated. ABI measurements can be repeated after exercise. Postexercise measurements are the primary tool of noninvasive testing for vascular causes of exercise-induced leg pain.[23] In athletes, comparisons of side-to-side ankle pressure measurements can also be useful.

Athletes with moderate arterial lesions likely have a normal resting ABI. However, increasing the blood flow through an area of stenosis via high-intensity exercise augments the pressure gradient through the lesion and facilitates the diagnosis of moderate to severe arterial lesions.[24] Patients with nontraumatic, exercise-induced leg pain with an ABI 1 minute after maximum exercise of < 0.5 or a side-to-side difference of > 0.18 should be referred for further arterial investigation.[25] There are some caveats to using the ABI when evaluating vascular disease in the lower limb.

- Lack of consensus on the ABI cutoff point to indicate vascular disease
- Ambiguity regarding the normal values of the ABI in elite athletes
- Logistical difficulty of obtaining simultaneous serial ABIs rather than consecutive measurements that may not occur quickly enough to detect the rapidly resolving postexercise differences

Even so, the ABI, particularly with postexercise testing, can be a valuable screening test for vascular problems in athletes. Limiting angiography to patients with either an abnormal physical examination (e.g., a pulse deficit) or ABI abnormalities appears to be an effective strategy for detecting arterial injury.[20]

Duplex Ultrasonography

Another commonly used noninvasive test is duplex ultrasonography, which uses sound waves to produce images of arteries and veins. It is used to identify a variety of vascular pathologies including thrombi, stenosis, inflammation, and vessel wall thickening. Some of the advantages of duplex ultrasonography are the ease of use, lack of side effects, and minimal expense. Ultrasonography has been shown to have a sensitivity of 82%–95% and a specificity of 96% in the diagnosis of stenosis $> 50\%$ of the luminal diameter and a sensitivity of 90%–95% and specificity of 96%–97% in the diagnosis of complete occlusions.[26] It is important to note that vascular ultrasonography is highly operator-dependent; and virtually all the available information is based on studies of patients with atherosclerotic disease rather than exercise-related vascular disease.

Duplex ultrasonography is the modality of choice for evaluating patients suspected of having deep venous thrombosis. A positive test demonstrates thrombus-filled veins that lose the compressibility observed in normal veins. On rare occasions, venography is needed for cases when ultrasonography fails to define the presence of thrombus.[27] Currently, venography has been effectively supplanted by duplex ultrasonography. Venography has some utility in sports cases, as with subclavian vein thrombosis, because images can be obtained in various "kinking" positions.

Angiography

Angiography (or arteriography) is the gold standard for diagnosing arterial disease. Conventional angiography involves use of a guidewire and catheter, which are inserted percutaneously into an artery (most commonly the femoral artery). Radiopaque contrast material is injected to highlight vessel abnormalities with x-ray imaging. Digital subtraction angiography (DSA) is another adaptation that allows better visualization of blood vessels in a bony or dense soft tissue environment. Precontrast images are subtracted from postcontrast images, and the final product is a clear picture of the vessels without the overlying background. The advantages of this technique are that it provides better overall visualization of the arterial tree and allows simultaneous therapeutic interventions that may be required.[28] The downsides to angiography are that it is rather invasive and potentially morbid, as well as expensive (Table 2.4). Angiography, particularly intraarterial DSA with vasodilatation-induced pressure measurements, is the most useful confirmatory test for athletic vascular conditions, such as external iliac artery endofibrosis.[29]

Table 2.4 Complications of angiography

- Cost
- Bleeding
- Thrombosis
- Arteriovenous (AV) fistula
- Pseudoaneurysms
- Allergic reaction to contrast
- Nephrotoxicity due to contrast
- False-positive results (~5%)

The most familiar vascular injury in sports is popliteal artery injury after knee dislocation. The proper algorithm of vascular tests for suspected popliteal artery injury is controversial. In the past, routine arteriography of every knee dislocation was suggested. Now, however, a selected approach in which only individuals meeting screening criteria undergo angiography is recommended. If physical examination detects asymmetry of pulse, color, and temperature, further testing is likely needed. If the ABI or screening ultrasonography is judged abnormal, arteriography can be used in these equivocal cases. Knee dislocations from high-energy trauma (e.g., motor vehicle crashes) are more likely to produce popliteal artery injury than low-energy sports mechanisms; hence, angiography is rarely needed for a sports-related popliteal artery injury.[20]

Advanced Imaging Angiography

In most of today's vascular centers, traditional angiography used solely for diagnostic purposes has been virtually replaced by computed tomography angiography (CTA) and magnetic resonance angiography (MRA). These techniques allow simultaneous visualization of the vasculature and any surrounding anatomic abnormalities; moreover, the side effect profile is more favorable because the contrast medium is injected intravenously rather than intraarterially. CT scanning is reportedly the most sensitive test for congenital popliteal artery entrapment syndrome (PAES); and a novel vascular diagnostic test, photoplethysmography, is most sensitive for functional PAES. Photoplethysmography, an optically obtained measurement of the volume and vascular perfusion of various organs, can be performed with dynamic ankle plantar flexion and dorsiflexion to show functional arterial occlusion. However, the high false-positive rate for this test must be considered, as 50%–60% of the normal population have transient popliteal artery occlusion with knee extension and plantar flexion.[30]

Magnetic Resonance Imaging

Magnetic resonance imaging (MRI) can also be used as a vascular diagnostic test, particularly for such conditions as compartment syndromes. Some authors have suggested that MRI be used in preference to traditional measurement of compartment pressures because of the wide range of compartment pressure normal values and the invasiveness of the test. MRI in the setting of compartment syndrome can show edema, hemorrhage, hematoma, and vessel injury and inflammation.

Magnetic resonance angiography is being increasingly used in the diagnosis of thoracic outlet syndrome. It appears to be more sensitive with the arms abducted. MRI of the brachial plexus is increasingly being used to assess for a mass effect or soft tissue abnormalities within or around the neurologic structures.[31]

References

1. Robinson LR, Stolp-Smith KA. Parasthesias and focal weakness: the diagnosis of nerve entrapment. In: AAEM Annual Assembly Handouts. Vancouver: Johnson Printing; 1999.
2. Gooch CL, Weimer LH. The electrodiagnosis of neuropathy: basic principles and common pitfalls. Neurol Clin 2007;25:1–28.
3. Feinberg JH. The role of electrodiagnostics in the study of muscle kinesiology, muscle fatigue and peripheral nerve injuries in sports medicine. J Back Musculoskel Med 1999;12:73.

4. Casazza BA, Young JL, Press JP, Heinemann AW. Suprascapular nerve conduction: a comparative analysis in normal subjects. Electromyogr Clin Neurophysiol 1998;38(3):153–60.
5. Fisher MA. H reflexes and F waves: fundamentals, normal and abnormal patterns. Neurol Clin 2002;20(2): 339–60.
6. Press JM, Young JL. Electrodiagnostic evaluation of spine problems. In: Gonzalez G, Materson RS, eds. The Nonsurgical Management of Acute Low Back Pain. New York: Demos Vermande; 1997:191.
7. Fisher MA. The contemporary role of F wave studies. Muscle Nerve 1998;21:1098.
8. Dumitru D, Amato AA, Zwarts MJ, eds. Electrodiagnostic Medicine. Philadelphia: Hanley & Gelfus; 2002.
9. Kraft GH. Fibrillation potential amplitude and muscle atrophy following peripheral nerve injury. Muscle Nerve 1990;13:814.
10. Leach RE, Purnell MB, Saito A. Peroneal nerve entrapment in runners. Am J Sports Med 1989;17:287.
11. Bachner EJ, Friedman MJ. Injuries to the leg. In: Nicholas JA, Hershman EB, eds. The Lower Extremity and Spine in Sports Medicine. St. Louis: Mosby; 1995.
12. Fishman LM, Dombi GW, Michaelsen C, et al. Piriformis syndrome: diagnosis, treatment, and outcome-a 10-year study. Arch Phys Med Rehabil 2002;83:295–301.
13. Mysiew WJ, Colachis SC. The pronator syndrome: an evaluation of dynamic maneuvers for improving electrodiagnostic sensitivity. Arch Phys Med Rehabil 1991; 70:274–7.
14. Checkles NS, Russakov AD, Piero DL. Ulnar nerve conduction velocity-effect of elbow position on measurement. Arch Phys Med Rehabil 1971;53:362.
15. Akuthota V, Chou L, Press J. Electrodiagnostic testing in runners. In: O'Connor F, Wilder R, eds. Textbook of Running Medicine. New York: McGraw-Hill; 2001.
16. Jensen MC, Brant-Zawadzki MN, Obuchowski N, et al. Magnetic resonance imaging of lumbar spine in people without back pain. N Engl J Med 1994;331:69.
17. Robinson LR. Traumatic injury to peripheral nerves. AAEM Minimonograph #28. AAEM: Rochester, MN; 2000.
18. Rogers CJ. Electrodiagnostic Medicine Handbook. San Antonio, TX: University of Texas Health Sciences Center; 1996.
19. Arko FR, Harris EJ, Zarins CK, Olcott C 4th. Vascular complications in high-performance athletes. J Vasc Surg 2001;33(5):935–42.
20. Newton EJ. Peripheral vascular injury. In: Rosen's Emergency Medicine: Concepts and Clinical Practice. 6th ed. St. Louis: Mosby; 2006.
21. Brown FW, Navigato WJ. Rupture of the axillary artery and brachial plexus palsy associated with anterior dislocation of the shoulder: report of a case with successful vascular repair. Clin Orthop 1968;60:195–9.
22. Bhimji S, Ugbarugba S, Nzerue CM. Subcalvian vein thrombosis. E-Medicine. http://www.emedicine.com/med/topic2772.htm/. Accessed April 2, 2008.
23. Abraham P, Chevalier JM, Leftherios G, et al. Lower extremity arterial disease in sports. Am J Sports Med 1997; 25:581–4.
24. Le Faucheur A, Noury-Desvaux B, Jaquinandi V, et al. Simultaneous arterial pressure recordings improve the detection of endofibrosis. Sci Sports Exerc 2006;38: 1889–94.
25. Taylor AJ, George KP. Ankle to brachial pressure index in normal subjects and trained cyclists with exercise-induced leg pain. Med Sci Sports Exerc 2001;33:1862–7.
26. Favaretto E, Pili C, Amato A, et al. Analysis of agreement between duplex ultrasound scanning and arteriography in patients with lower limb artery disease. J Cardiovasc Med 2007;8:337–41.
27. Hyers TM. Management of venous thrombembolism: past, present, and future. Arch Intern Med 2003;163: 759–68.
28. Cossman DV, Ellison JE, Wagner WH, et al. Comparison of contrast arteriography to arterial mapping with colorflow duplex imaging in the lower extremities. J Vasc Surg 1989;10:522–8.
29. Bender MHM, Schep G, de Vries WR, et al. Sports-related flow limitations in the iliac arteries in endurance athletes: aetiology, diagnosis, treatment and future developments. Sports Med 2004;34(7):427–42.
30. Schep G, Schmikli SL, Bender MHM, et al. Recognising vascular causes of leg complaints in endurance athletes. Part I: Validation of a decision algorithm. Int J Sports Med 2002;23:313–21.
31. Demondion X, Bacqueville E, Paul C, et al. Thoracic outlet: assessment with MR imaging in asymptomatic and symptomatic populations. Radiology 2003;227(2): 461–8.

Chapter 3
Magnetic Resonance Neurography

Cynthia T. Chin

Introduction

Evaluation of peripheral nerve disorders has relied primarily on an accurate clinical history, thorough physical examination, and electrodiagnostic (EDX) testing. This information often allows determination of the location and severity of the underlying peripheral nerve problem. However, while EDX studies are sensitive, they do not display the anatomic detail needed for precise localization and treatment planning. Additional limitations of these EDX studies include difficulty performing these studies in young children and infants, difficulty accessing deep muscles, and having to wait several weeks after nerve injury before changes can be detected.

The radiologic study of peripheral nerve disorders was initially limited to secondary skeletal changes on plain radiographs and computed tomography (CT) myelography for demonstrating nerve root avulsion in patients with severe proximal brachial plexus injuries.

Routine CT and magnetic resonance imaging (MRI) have been useful to exclude the possibility of mass lesions in the vicinity of a peripheral nerve. Recent technical improvements in MRI have resulted in improved visualization of both normal and abnormal peripheral nerves.

The ability to image peripheral nerves can significantly change the diagnosis and treatment of peripheral nerve disease and can lead to improved understanding of the pathophysiology of peripheral nerve disease.

Technique of Magentic Resonance Neurography

Magnetic resonance neurography (MRN) is tissue-selective imaging directed at identifying and evaluating characteristics of nerve morphology. Visualization of the fascicular structure of the nerves is made possible by exploiting differences in the water content and connective tissue structure of the fascicles and perineurium compared with the surrounding epineurium.[1]

Standard MRI techniques allow the detection of nerves. However, there is low conspicuity of these structures from the surrounding tissues. The inherent problems of low signal intensity and low conspicuity are addressed by suppressing signal from the adjacent nonneural structures such as blood vessels and fat in muscle and marrow. The use of T2-weighted fat-saturated and inversion recovery sequences allows optimal conspicuity of peripheral nerves. Standard T1- and T2-weighted sequences can display the anatomy of the adjacent muscle, bone, vessels, and nerves as they are outlined by fat planes.

Because of its small size, an abnormal signal on T2-weighted sequences within a nerve is often obscured by signal in adjacent fat. Fat suppression techniques are crucial for identifying normal and abnormal nerve tissue. Frequency-selective fat resonance saturation and short-inversion-time inversion

C.T. Chin (✉)
Department of Radiology, University of California San Francisco, San Francisco, CA, USA

V. Akuthota, S.A. Herring (eds.), *Nerve and Vascular Injuries in Sports Medicine*,
DOI 10.1007/978-0-387-76600-3_3, © Springer Science+Business Media, LLC 2009

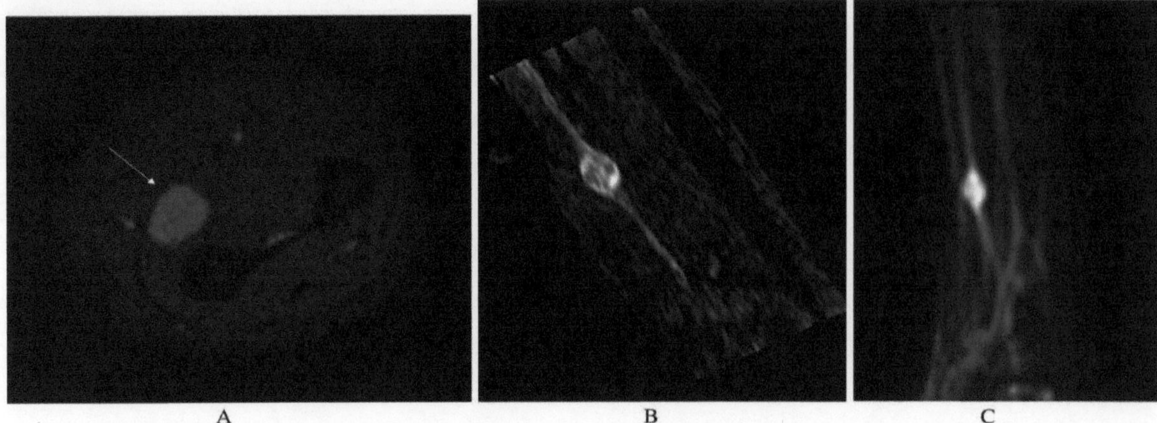

Fig. 3.1 Median nerve schwannoma. (**A**) Axial postgadolinium T1-weighted image demonstrates an enhancing schwannoma (*arrow*) in the mid-forearm. (**B**) Three-dimensional water-selective sequences (3D WATS) reformatted image demonstrates the origin of the tumor arising from the median nerve along its longitudinal plane with maintenance of adjacent muscle and bone detail. (**C**) Diffusion-weighted imaging (DWI) demonstrates the median nerve and tumor and additional nerves in the forearm in isolation of the adjacent structures

recovery (STIR) are common techniques used for fat saturation. The STIR method, which provides uniform, consistent fat saturation and maintains high T2 contrast, is therefore more reliable compared to the frequency-selective fat-saturation method. The disadvantages of the STIR sequences include a relatively lower signal-to-noise ratio (SNR) and sensitivity to blood flow artifacts. Flow saturation bands may be utilized to attenuate the accompanying blood flow phase shift artifacts.[1] Iterative decomposition of water and fat with echo asymmetry and least squares estimation (IDEAL) is an MRI sequence combining the advantages of both the STIR and frequency-selective fat saturation techniques, offering both reliable uniform fat saturation and an optimal SNR. It has been used for musculoskeletal imaging and at our institution is being applied to image peripheral nerves as well.[2,3]

Multiplanar reformations allow mapping of the extent of nerve involvement and can be performed with various sequences. Three-dimensional (3D) volumetric gradient sequences with T2 weighting-e.g., 3D double-echo steady-state sequences (3D DESS) or 3D water-selective sequences (3D WATS)-have been used for ligamentous evaluation in musculoskeletal imaging. When applied to the peripheral nervous system, these sequences allow image acquisition in the axial plane with multiplanar reformations, which allow anatomic detail of adjacent structures such as muscle and bone to be demonstrated while maintaining sensitivity in detecting an abnormal nerve signal (Fig. 3.1).[4] Reformations with the nerves in isolation can also be displayed similar to magnetic resonance angiography (MRA) utilizing maximum intensity projection sequences and postprocessing.

Diffusion Weighted Imaging

Magnetic resonance diffusion-weighted imaging (DWI) has been extremely helpful for evaluating lesions in the brain such as acute infarction, abscess, and neoplasm. The image contrast it provides is dependent on detecting random microscopic molecular water motion, which can be significantly altered in various disease states.[5] Its use in spine imaging is being developed for evaluating the spinal cord and potential etiologies of myelopathy.[6] DWI is being applied to the peripheral nervous system and can detect and demonstrate normal and abnormal ganglia and proximal roots.[7–9] Its potential utility is being demonstrated for evaluating normal and abnormal nerve anatomy related to trauma, neoplasm, and radiation injury (Fig. 3.1).

Coils

Phased-array coils have produced images with an improved SNR and improved resolution, thereby enhancing the ability to visualize both normal and abnormal peripheral nerves. Compared with MRI with standard coils, phased-array coils allow higher resolution, thinner sections, and faster acquisition of images. Phased-array coils integrate data from multiple small coils to produce a single image, which has a high SNR and a composite field of view (FOV) similar to that of a larger surface coil. The images produced from phased-array coils compare favorably with those from larger surface or whole-body coils.[10] However, it is necessary to target the area of clinical interest accurately because only a relatively small FOV can be imaged with high spatial resolution.[1]

Magnetic resonance neurography has diagnostic utility because it is effective for demonstrating continuity, morphology, and response to injury (edema) associated with many kinds of pathology. It is useful for evaluating segments of peripheral nerve that are routinely difficult to evaluate electrophysiologically. First, nerve segments involving the brachial or lumbosacral plexuses can be difficult to evaluate with conventional nerve conduction studies (NCSs). Second, concomitant peripheral polyneuropathy can make interpretation of the NCSs difficult. Third, abnormalities detectable on clinical motor and sensory examinations following acute nerve injury may not be detectable on needle electromyography (EMG) and NCSs for 2–5 weeks, but anatomic changes in the nerve may be seen much earlier.

Anatomy and Imaging Appearance of The Peripheral Nerve

Peripheral nerves can be subdivided into three components: (1) conducting axons; (2) insulating Schwann cells; (3) a surrounding connective tissue matrix that can support axonal regeneration.

Nerve fibers are sheathed by Schwann cells individually or in groups. A basal lamina layer envelops Schwann cells and is important in supporting axonal regeneration.

The nerve fibers are embedded within a connective tissue compartment called the endoneurium. Nerve fibers and surrounding endoneurium are grouped together into fascicles and encircled by compact, concentrically arranged, elongated perineural cells (the perineurium). These fascicles are grouped together to form the peripheral nerve and are embedded within a connective tissue compartment called the epineurium, which contains fibroblasts, macrophages, mast cells, blood vessels, and fat (Fig. 3.2).

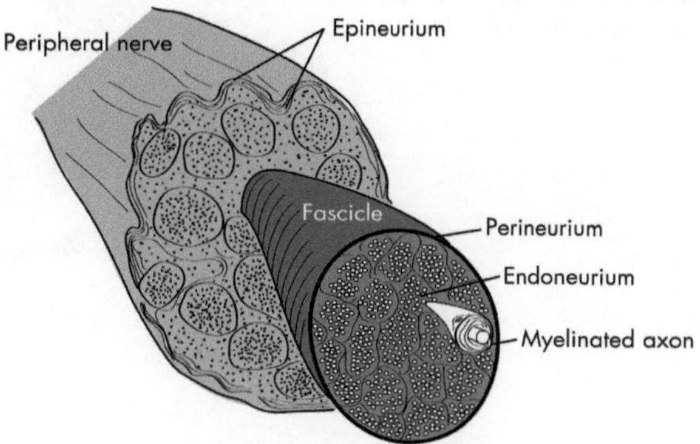

Fig. 3.2 Normal peripheral nerve anatomy

Imaging Appearance of Normal Nerves

T1-weighted images show the size and location of the nerve. A normal nerve on cross-sectional imaging is oval or round. The size of a particular nerve varies along its course and from person to person. The fascicles within the nerve are visible on high-resolution, cross-sectional images. On T2-weighted sequences, the nerves appear uniform in size, intermediate in signal, and in general slightly hyperintense compared to adjacent muscle.

Depiction of the nerve fascicular pattern is based on differences in the MR signal of the fascicles within the perineurium compared to that of the interfascicular epineurium. The fascicular signal is dominated by endoneurial fluid and axoplasmic water. The interfascicular image signal is dominated by fibrofatty connective tissue, which is susceptible to fat suppression (Figs. 3.3, 3.4).[1]

Imaging Appearance of Abnormal Nerves

Compressive or infiltrative lesions of the peripheral nerve may produce three abnormalities.

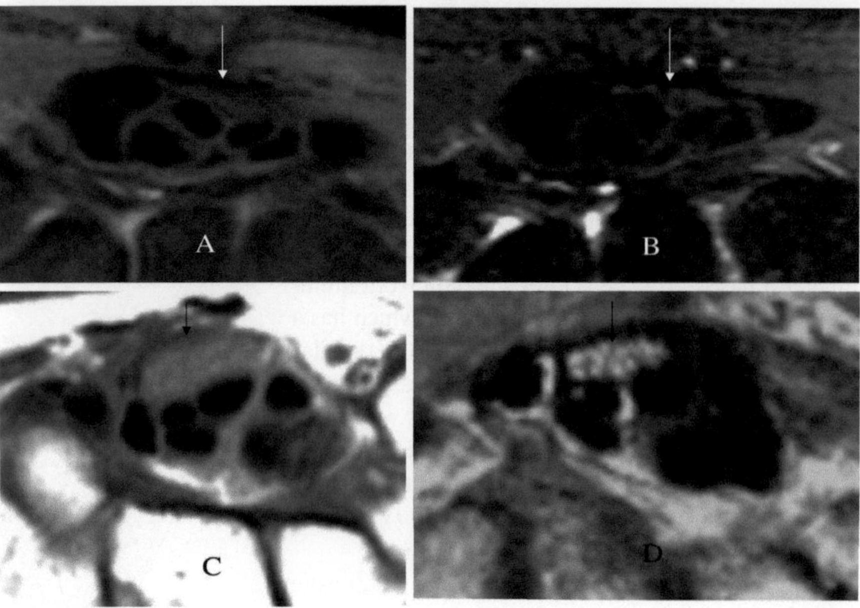

Fig. 3.3 Median nerve. Normal axial T1-weighted (**A**) and short-inversion-time inversion recovery (STIR) (**B**) sequences of the median nerve in an asymptomatic patient (*arrows*). Abnormal increased fascicular size and signal of the median nerve in a patient with carpal tunnel syndrome on axial T1-weighted (**C**) and STIR (**D**) sequences (*arrows*)

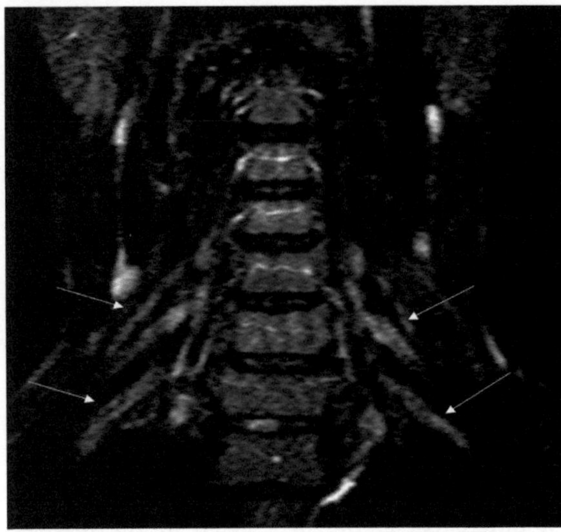

Fig. 3.4 Normal cervical plexus. Coronal STIR sequence through the cervical plexus demonstrates a normal intermediate signal and normal oblique linear orientation of the roots of the bilateral brachial plexus (*arrows*)

- Distort the normal nerve course and configuration
- Disrupt the fascicular pattern described above
- Produce homogenous prolongation of the T2 relaxation time (increased T2 signal intensity) in the nerve

In the latter circumstance, increased signal is probably related to increased water content or breakdown of myelin.[11]

Diffuse or focal enlargement of a nerve and a diffuse or focal hyperintense T2 signal in the nerve are abnormal findings. At present, no reliable quantitative method for evaluating signal intensity of normal and abnormal nerves has been developed. An altered fascicular pattern is another abnormal finding that may manifest as marked enlargement or abnormal increased signal of individual fascicles in the nerve in a nonuniform pattern (Figs. 3.3, 3.5).

The pathogenesis of a focal signal abnormality is not known but may represent localized edema or increased fluid accumulation in the endoneurial spaces. Possible mechanisms for an abnormal, increased T2 signal in the nerve include interruption of normal axoplasmic flow resulting in increased axoplasm proximal and distal to the site of injury, increased endoneurial fluid as a result of venous obstruction allowing accumulation within the fascicles, and demyelination.[12–14]

The characteristic temporal nature of MR signal abnormalities may be used to evaluate the extent of nerve injury and provide valuable information that correlates with improved clinical function. In animal studies involving laboratory-induced crush injuries to the sciatic nerve, increased T2 signal

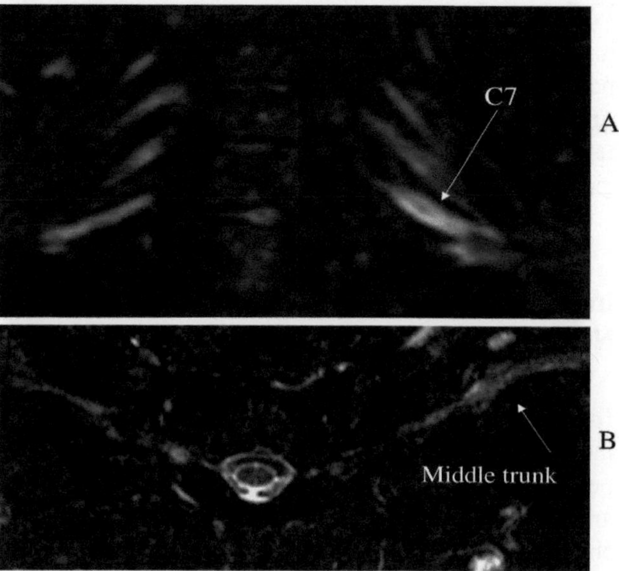

Fig. 3.5 Brachial neuritis. Coronal (**A**) and axial (**B**) STIR sequences through the cervical plexus demonstrate an abnormally increased size and signal of the left C7 root and middle trunk in a patient with brachial neuritis

changes were seen as early as 7 days before normalizing by 10 days. In severed sciatic nerves that were prevented from regenerating, there were prolonged T2 signal abnormalities that persisted for up to 42 days. These abnormalities normalized by 60 days despite an absence of axonal regeneration.[15] There are numerous case reports where axonal loss distal to the site of injury following traumatic nerve injury correlates with high signal MRI abnormalities that slowly normalize over many months. The evolution of the MR signal correlates with regeneration of axons and functional recovery.[13,16] It can be useful to follow nerve injury and recovery with MRN, given that MR signal changes in nerves normalize rapidly with regeneration.

Mechanisms of Injury

Both direct mechanical distortion and microvascular compromise contribute to the pathophysiology underlying peripheral nerve dysfunction. Usual mechanisms consist of compression, ischemia, and traction. Nerves often course in neurovascular bundles; and vascular trauma can occur concomitantly with neural injury and cause further damage through ischemia.[17] Compared to the central nervous system (CNS), the peripheral nervous system is relatively resistant to ischemia. An important feature of the peripheral nervous system is its ability to recover via both remyelination and axonal regeneration.

Entrapment syndromes represent the most common type of chronic nerve injury. Mass lesions can cause nerve injury through direct compression or actual infiltration. Nerves may also be affected by such systemic diseases as diabetes mellitus, gout, systemic amyloidosis, hypothyroidism, and renal failure. Genetic or environmental factors include alcoholism, malnutrition, and toxin exposure.

Susceptibility of peripheral nerves to acute or chronic compressive and tensile forces is a function of internal anatomy and location. The tough perineural layer surrounding each fascicle is composed of elastin and collagen. This layer is normally under a certain amount of resting tension longitudinally, as demonstrated by the nerve shortening that occurs after transection. Nerves can stretch 10%–20% before structural damage occurs.[18] Certain nerves are vulnerable at specific anatomic locations—i.e., where they are superficial, fixed in position, or coursing across a joint. The nerve fibers within fascicles have an undulating course, allowing accommodation of levels of tension produced by normal changes in body position. With increasing tension, the nerve slides and then takes up internal slack provided by its undulating course; any further tension can disrupt axons and myelin sheaths.

Connective tissue damage may occur with stretch injuries, which can lead to intraneural and extraneural scar formation. Extraneural scar may distort or compress peripheral nerves along their course or tether a nerve, interfering with its normal physiologic gliding.[19]

Indications for Imaging of Peripheral Nerves

Indications are evolving in response to improvements in MRI techniques and methods for treating peripheral nerve disease. The localization, extent, and severity of nerve injury are some important characteristics that can be demonstrated by MRN.[12–14]

Trauma

Traumatic peripheral nerve injury ranges from disruption of axonal conduction with preservation of anatomic continuity of the nerve connective tissue sheaths (neurapraxic injury) to transection with complete loss of nerve continuity (neurotmetic injury). Most serious peripheral nerve injuries do not lead to actual transection of the nerve but, rather, leave the nerve in continuity. Clinically, it may be difficult to distinguish closed nerve injuries that ultimately recover on their own from those that do not and therefore require surgical repair. Serial clinical and EDX evaluations over a period of months have traditionally been the mainstay of decision making in the management of closed traumatic peripheral nerve injuries. MRN may be used noninvasively to localize traumatic peripheral nerve injury and perhaps help determine whether surgery would be of benefit in a more expeditious manner (Fig. 3.6). MRN complements electrophysiologic data when determining the exact site and type of nerve injury and can show the relation of the intact nerve to posttraumatic lesions such as neuromas as well as focal or diffuse perineural fibrosis.

Brachial Plexus Injuries

Posttraumatic plexopathy may be the sequela of laceration, compression, stretching, perineural fibrosis, or nerve root avulsion. A useful classification for surgical management divides the injured region into the more common supraclavicular and infraclavicular (including retroclavicular) levels. Traumatic meningocele, or pseudomeningocele, may occur with or without avulsion. Pseudomeningoceles and fusiform retraction of the distal plexus may suggest avulsion injury, although simple dural

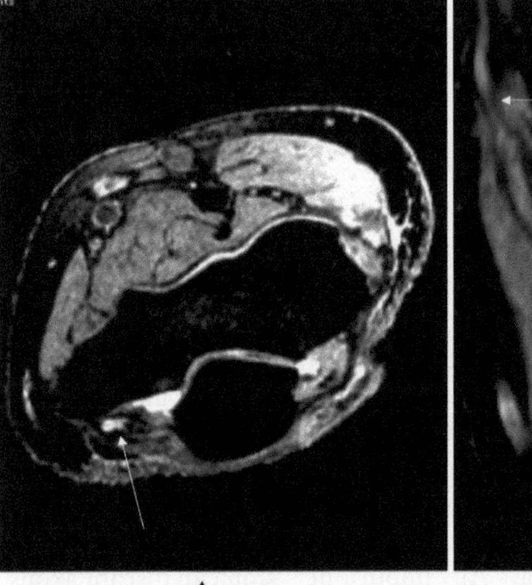
A

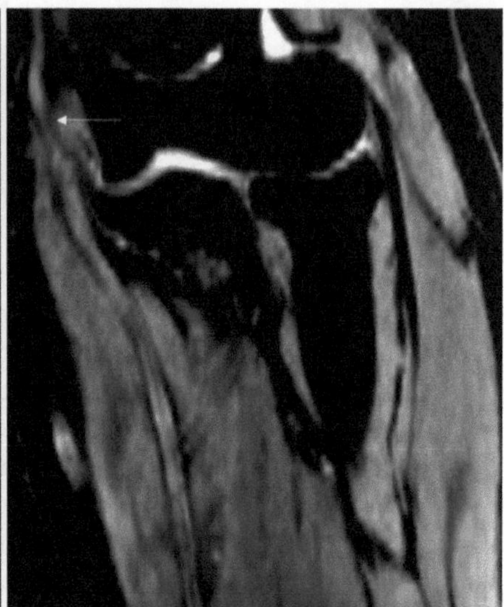
B

Fig. 3.6 Nerve transection. Three-dimensional double-echo steady-state sequences (3D DESS). Axial (**A**) and coronal (**B**) reformatted sequences through the elbow demonstrates abnormal increased signal, size, and discontinuity of the ulnar nerve, compatible with a transection injury in a patient whose arm was caught in an elevator door (*arrows*)

tears or partial avulsion injuries can also result in a pseudomeningocele.[20]

Adult Brachial Plexus Trauma

In adults, brachial plexus injuries can be caused by various mechanisms including penetrating injuries, falls, and most commonly motor vehicle trauma (up to 70% involving motorcycles or bicycles). Often the diagnosis is delayed or ignored as the clinician waits for signs of clinical recovery (Fig. 3.7).

Three-dimensional volumetric acquired sequences allow reformations that can demonstrate peripheral nerve continuity or disruption, which is important in determining whether surgical treatment is required. 3D volumetric acquired sequences and diffusion sequences can also aid in identifying pre- and postganglionic injury, which is also important for prognosis and appropriateness of surgical repair. Postganglionic injuries are located distal to the dorsal root ganglion (DRG), whereas preganglionic lesions are located proximal to the DRG. With preganglionic injuries the nerve is avulsed from the spinal cord, and repair requires a neurotization procedure; in contrast, postganglionic injuries may be surgically repaired or grafted. MR DWI, a method for detecting random microscopic motion (diffusion) of water protons, has recently been applied to the evaluation of peripheral nerves. The spinal cord, ganglia, and proximal peripheral nerves can be demonstrated with this technique, which may prove useful for distinguishing preganglionic from postganglionic avulsion[7,8] (Fig. 3.8).

Birth-Related Trauma

An infrequent injury to the brachial plexus can occur in newborn infants manifested by an inability to move one upper limb. When the C5 and C6 cervical roots are involved it is called Erb's palsy, and there is an associated flaccid upper arm with a lower arm that is extended and internally rotated.

An important concept of MR neurography is the ability to detect not only an abnormal increased signal on T2 sequences in the nerve but also to look for an abnormal course of the nerves, which may be present as a sequela of traction injury. The loss of the normal oblique orientation of the cervical plexus in the absence of a pseudomeningocele is an important indicator of severe traction injury

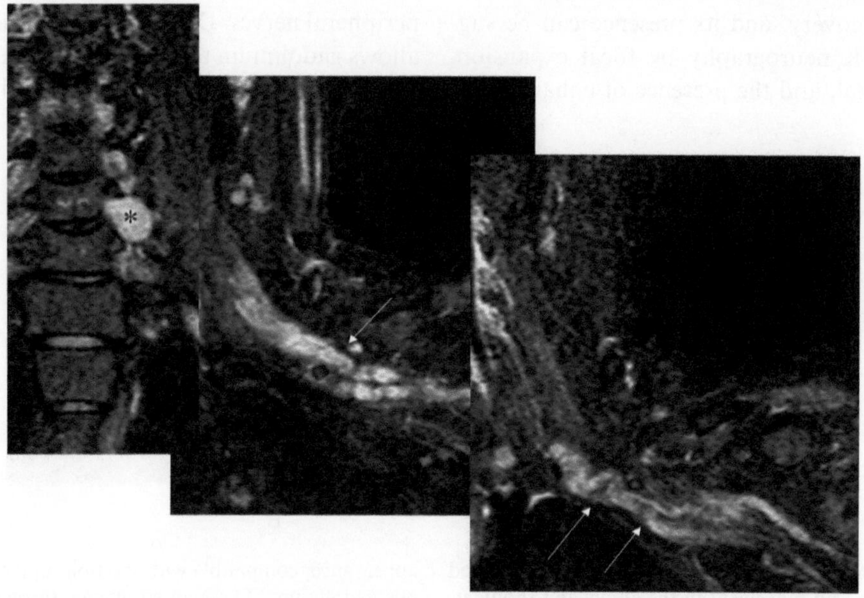

Fig. 3.7 Avulsion injury. Coronal STIR sequence through the left brachial plexus in a 19-year-old man following a motorcycle accident demonstrates a C7 pseudomeningocele (*asterisk*) and fusiform retraction of the distal C7 root and middle trunk (*double arrows*) and C6 root (*arrow*) compatible with avulsion and a traction injury

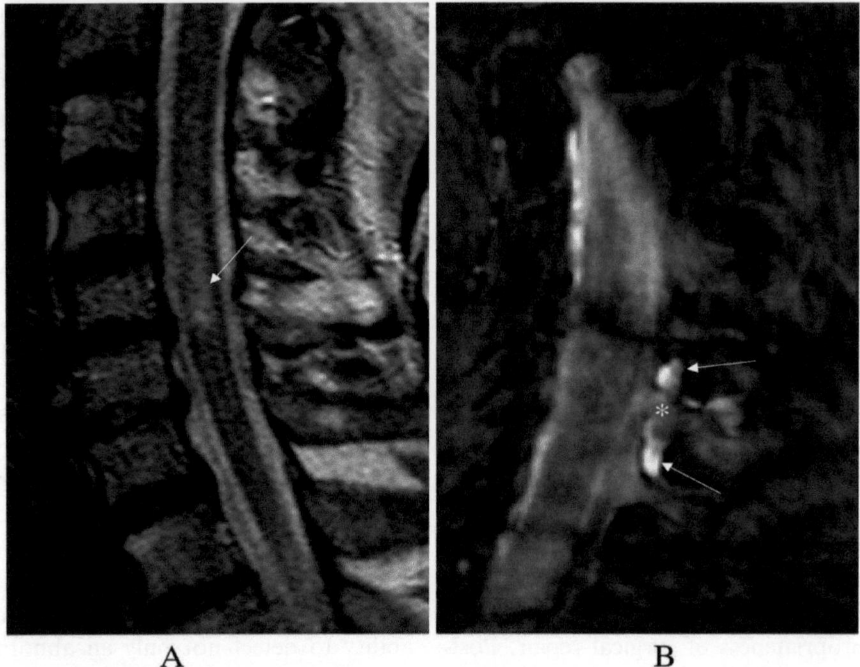

Fig. 3.8 Preganglionic avulsionin a 55-year-old man after a motor vehicle accident with cervical spinal cord contusion (*arrow*) on the sagittal T2-weighted sequence (**A**). The sagittal oblique 3D WATS sequence (**B**) demonstrates the C7 pseudomeningocele (*arrows*) and preganglionic C7 avulsion (*asterisk*)

without avulsion and can result in a relatively lax appearance of the cervical roots (Fig. 3.9).[21]

Posttraumatic neuroma formation may interfere with nerve recovery, and its presence can be suggested on MR neurography by focal expansion, increased signal, and the presence of enhancement with gadolinium. A normal ganglion enhances with gadolinium; and a normal nerve–blood barrier results in no appreciable enhancement of the peripheral nerves. Disruption of this normal barrier allows gadolinium to leak into the epineural tissues, with resultant enhancement that can be homogeneous;

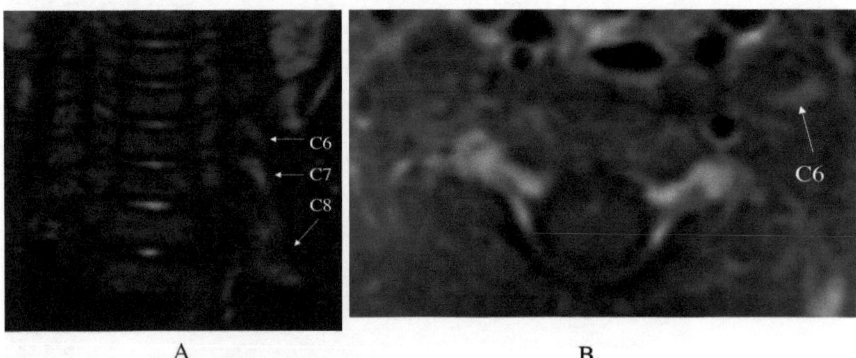

Fig. 3.9 An 11-month-old male infant had a birth-related plexus injury and no movement in the elbow and shoulder. Coronal STIR sequence (**A**) demonstrates increased size and signal of the C6, C7, and C8 roots of the left brachial plexus. The orientation of the roots is abnormal with a lax appearance, compatible with traction injury (*arrows*). Axial postgadolinium T1-weighted image through the cervical plexus demonstrates abnormal enhancement of the left C6 root in the interscalene space (**B**), compatible with a neuroma, which was confirmed at surgery (*arrow*)

in the correct clinical setting, it suggests the presence of neuroma formation, which is important for surgical planning in patients who no longer demonstrate clinical recovery (Fig. 3.9).

Radiculopathy

Radiculopathy is usually caused by compression of the proximal portion of a spinal nerve or roots by a disc or osteophyte. MRI has been used extensively to evaluate cervical and lumbar radiculopathy because of its sensitivity in visualizing degenerative changes. However, its specificity is limited as changes may be found in a large percentage of asymptomatic patients. On MRN, abnormal increased signal on T2 and STIR sequences are observed in symptomatic spinal nerves. This increased signal in symptomatic patients may be seen associated with or without EDX abnormalities and may therefore be a highly sensitive technique for increasing the specificity of selecting patients who might benefit most from surgical decompression.

Magnetic resonance neurography is a more sensitive technique than standard spine MRI for detecting signal changes in proximal lumbar and cervical nerve roots. Among patients with clinical evidence of cervical radiculopathy,[22] significant signal change was observed 2–3 cm distal to the site of nerve root compression on STIR sequences in the affected nerve roots. MRN may be particularly helpful for assessing the structural integrity of specific nerve roots in patients with diffuse anatomic changes in the spine (i.e., multilevel degenerative disc or spondylotic changes). Abnormal nerve root signal in this setting draws further diagnostic attention to a specific segment of the spine (i.e., lateral recess syndrome detected by CT myelography) (Fig. 3.10).

Entrapment Syndromes

Magnetic resonance neurography can localize the site of nerve entrapment by demonstrating an abnormal signal at the site of entrapment. Common locations include the median nerve in the carpal tunnel, the ulnar nerve in the cubital tunnel, the lower trunk of the brachial plexus in the thoracic outlet, and the sciatic nerve at the greater sciatic foramen. Abnormal nerve morphology and signal abnormalities may be detected and identified along with denervation and atrophy.[23]

Extraspinal Sciatica

Conventional MRI techniques may provide excellent visualization of the spinal cord, the central

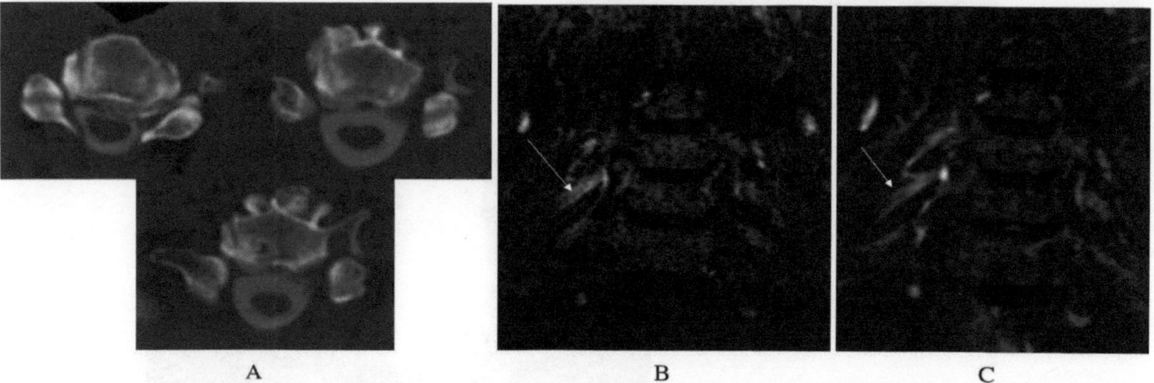

Fig. 3.10 Radiculopathy. Axial images through the cervical spine from a myelogram (**A**) demonstrate multilevel, severe neuroforaminal narrowing in a patient with right upper extremity pain. (**B**) Preoperative coronal STIR sequence demonstrates increased size and signal of the right C6 cervical root (*arrow*). (**C**) Postoperative coronal STIR sequence after a right C6 foraminotomy demonstrates an interval decrease in size and signal of the right C6 root (*arrow*)

canal, and the neuroforamina in patients with back and leg pain. However these techniques do not evaluate the extraforaminal lumbosacral plexus and sciatic nerves. In some patients with leg pain resembling lumbosacral radicular sciatica and normal routine lumbar MRI, symptoms may be attributable to extraforaminal sciatic nerve injury or compression. MRN may identify causative anatomic abnormalities and direct clinical treatment.[24–26]

The lumbar plexus is anatomically located behind the psoas muscle and composed of the L1-4 ventral rami. The lumbosacral trunk, formed by the ventral ramus of L5 combined with a minor branch of L4, descends over the sacral ala and joins with the S1, S2, and S3 ventral rami and a branch of S4 to form the sacral plexus. The sciatic nerve originates from the upper division of the sacral plexus and exits the pelvis through the greater sciatic foramen. The sciatic nerve continues into the thigh and is composed of the common peroneal and tibial nerves, which remain distinct yet travel together until the sciatic nerve bifurcates proximal to the knee into the separate common peroneal and tibial nerves.[25]

Some patients with leg pain resembling lumbosacral radicular sciatica have normal lumbar MRI results. In such patients, the symptoms have often been attributed to entrapment of the sciatic nerve in the buttock by the overlying piriformis muscle or by an adjacent band of fascia. However, the diagnosis of piriformis syndrome is controversial; and it has been difficult to obtain objective evidence for the existence of such an entity. MRN may reveal signal abnormalities within the sciatic nerve in some patients with extraspinal sciatica (Fig. 3.11).[26]

For patients with extraforaminal sciatica, the spectrum of abnormal plexus and sciatic nerve findings is diverse. They may include fibrous and muscular entrapment, vascular compression, trauma, neoplasm, ischemia, postradiation changes, and hypertrophic neuropathy.[25]

Brachial Plexus Entrapment

There are three potential sites of compression along the course of the brachial plexus or the subclavian/axillary artery or vein: the interscalene triangle; the costoclavicular space between the first thoracic rib and the clavicle; and the retropectoralis minor space posterior to the pectoralis minor muscle. Clinical

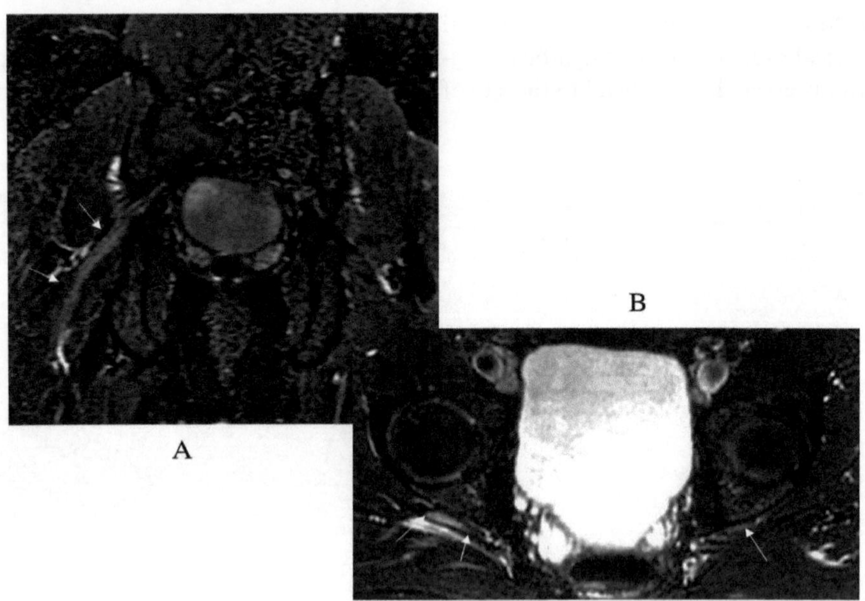

Fig. 3.11 Extraspinal sciatica. Coronal (**A**) and axial (**B**) STIR sequences through the pelvis of a patient with right sciatica and normal routine MRI of the lumbar spine demonstrates abnormal increased size and signal in the right sciatic nerve (*double arrows*) as it exits the sciatic notch. The left sciatic nerve is normal (**B**) (*single arrow*)

symptoms of entrapment or compression (thoracic outlet syndromes) may be due to venous or arterial compression, brachial plexus compression, or combined neurovascular compression.

Classic neurologic thoracic outlet syndrome (TOS) usually manifests as a chronic lower trunk plexopathy with paresthesias and atrophy affecting the arm, forearm, and hand. Compression or entrapment is usually the result of a congenital fibrous band extending from an elongated transverse process or rudimentary cervical rib to the first thoracic rib with resultant stretching, angulation, and distortion of the usual course and orientation of the brachial plexus. Routine MR coronal T1 sequences may demonstrate the osseous and fibrous anomalies.[27] MRN is useful for demonstrating distortion of the course of the brachial plexus and, in cases of significant compression, the associated intraneural edema (Fig. 3.12).

Traumatic TOS results from clavicular injury, usually a midshaft fracture with resultant injury to the subjacent blood vessels and brachial plexus. There may be compression by displaced fracture fragments, hematoma, or pseudoaneurysm formation. Symptoms frequently present in a relatively delayed fashion, days to even years after the initial

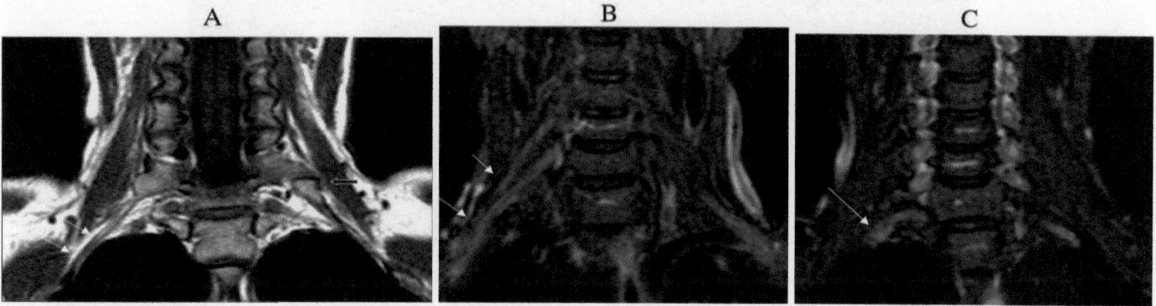

Fig. 3.12 Thoracic outlet syndrome in a 57-year-old woman with right upper extremity pain and paresthesias. (**A**) Coronal T1 sequence through the cervical plexus demonstrates a left cervical rib (*arrow*) and right C7 fibrous band (*double arrows*). The coronal STIR sequences (**B**, **C**) demonstrates the right C6 and C7 roots splayed laterally by the fibrous band (*double arrows*) and an expanded edematous right C8 root compressed by the fibrous band (*single arrow*)

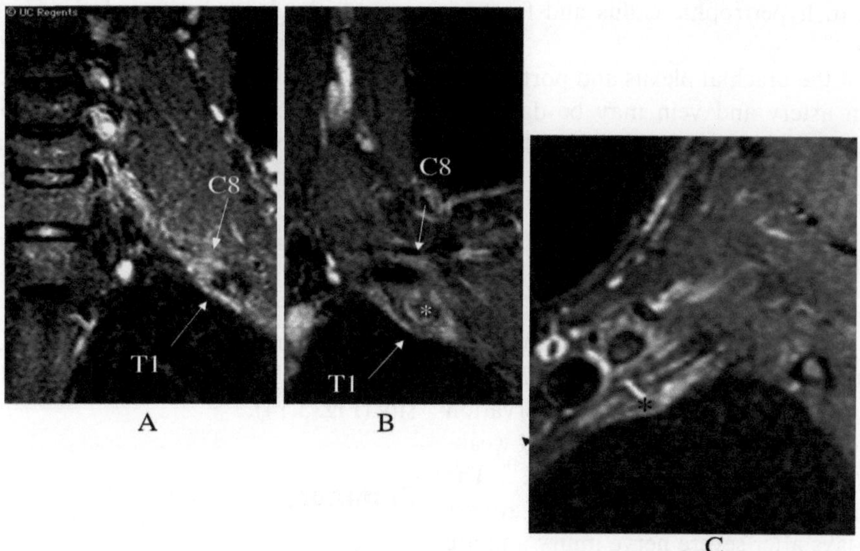

Fig. 3.13 Nonunion rib fracture in a 22-year-old man with delayed diagnosis of a C8 neuropathy months following a snowboarding accident. Coronal (**A**, **B**) and sagittal (**C**) STIR sequences of the cervical–thoracic junction demonstrates callus formation around a nonunionized left T1 rib fracture (*asterisks*) that splays the adjacent left C8 and T1 nerve roots (*arrows*)

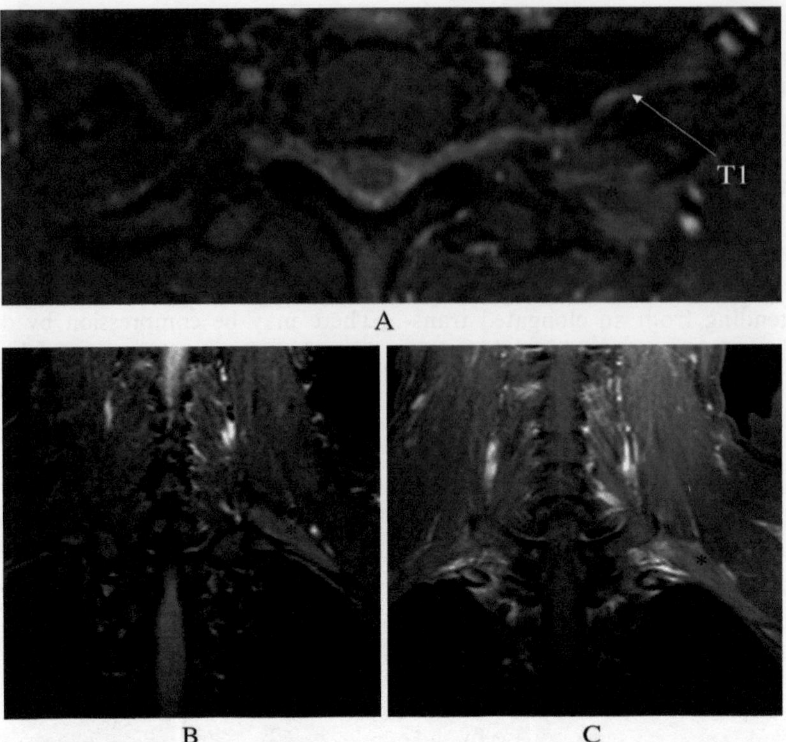

Fig. 3.14 Muscle denervation in a 71-year-old man with brachial neuritis of the left T1 root. Axial (**A**) and coronal (**B**) STIR sequences and coronal postgadolinium T1-weighted sequence(**C**) of the upper thoracic spine demonstrates increased signal of the left T1 nerve root (*arrow*). There is associated increased signal and enhancement of the left T1 intercostal muscle compatible with denervation (*asterisks*)

injury, owing to hypertrophic callus and fracture nonunion.

The cords of the brachial plexus and portions of the subclavian artery and vein may be damaged alone or in various combinations (Fig. 3.13).[28]

Muscle Denervation

Increased T2 signal change on STIR sequences has been demonstrated in denervated muscles. The signal change correlates with the degree of denervation found on needle EMG and with the clinical weakness observed on neurologic examination.[18] The signal changes in the denervated muscle can appear as early as 4 days after severe nerve injury and are accompanied by gadolinium contrast enhancement.[29] Signal change is found in muscles supplied by nerves sustaining axonal injury only; it is not seen with demyelinative lesions. Although the pathophysiology of increased muscle signal is not completely understood, it is thought to be related to an acute increase in blood flow associated with a loss of sympathetic vasoconstriction and a shift in protons (water) from the intracellular to the extracellular space. It appears that MRI of muscle can provide valuable information regarding the type of nerve injury (i.e., axonal versus demyelinative) that, in turn, can help predict the clinical prognosis. Chronic denervation shows decreased volume and fatty atrophy, manifesting as high T1 signal intensity (Fig. 3.14).

Summary

Treatment of spinal and peripheral nerve lesions relies on localizing the pathology. Current evaluation of such pathology mainly involves the use of conventional MRI and EMG. MRN is a novel technique used for directly imaging spinal and peripheral nerves. Features of intraneural topography can be displayed, and the morphology and signal intensity characteristics that distinguish a normal from an abnormal nerve can be demonstrated. MRN is a valuable complementary adjuct for the evaluation of spinal and peripheral nerve pathologies.

References

1. Maravilla KR, Bowen BC. Imaging of the peripheral nervous system: evaluation of peripheral neuropathy and plexopathy. AJNR Am J Neuroradiol 1998;19(6): 1011–23.
2. Fuller S, Reeder S, Shimakawa A, et al. Iterative decomposition of water and fat with echo asymmetry and least-squares estimation (IDEAL) fast spin-echo imaging of the ankle: initial clinical experience. AJR Am J Roentgenol 2006;187(6):1442–7.
3. Siepmann DB, McGovern J, Brittain JH, Reeder SB. High-resolution 3D cartilage imaging with IDEAL SPGR at 3 T. AJR Am J Roentgenol 2007;189(6):1510–5.
4. Rajeswaran G, Lee JC, Healy JC. MRI of the popliteofibular ligament: isotropic 3D WE-DESS versus coronal oblique fat-suppressed T2W MRI. Skeletal Radiol 2007;36(12):1141–6.
5. Schaefer PW, Grant PE, Gonzalez RG. Diffusion-weighted MR imaging of the brain. Radiology 2000; 217(2):331–45.
6. Demir A, Ries M, Moonen CT, et al. Diffusion-weighted MR imaging with apparent diffusion coefficient and apparent diffusion tensor maps in cervical spondylotic myelopathy. Radiology 2003;229(1):37–43.
7. Skorpil M, Karlsson M, Nordell A. Peripheral nerve diffusion tensor imaging. Magn Reson Imaging 2004; 22(5):743–5.
8. Tsuchiya K, Imai M, Tateishi H, et al. Neurography of the spinal nerve roots by diffusion tensor scanning applying motion-probing gradients in six directions. Magn Reson Med Sci 2007;6(1):1–5.
9. Takahara T, Imai Y, Yamashita T, et al. Diffusion weighted whole body imaging with background body signal suppression (DWIBS): technical improvement using free breathing, STIR and high resolution 3D display. Radiat Med 2004;22(4):275–82.
10. Roemer PB, Edelstein WA, Hayes CE, et al. The NMR phased array. Magn Reson Med 1990;16(2):192–225.
11. Does MD, Snyder RE. Multiexponential T2 relaxation in degenerating peripheral nerve. Magn Reson Med 1996;35(2):207–13.
12. Britz GW, Haynor DR, Kuntz C, et al. Carpal tunnel syndrome: correlation of magnetic resonance imaging, clinical, electrodiagnostic, and intraoperative findings. Neurosurgery 1995;37(6):1097–103.
13. Filler AG, Kliot M, Howe FA, et al. Application of magnetic resonance neurography in the evaluation of patients with peripheral nerve pathology. J Neurosurg 1996; 85(2):299–309.
14. Aagaard BD, Maravilla KR, Kliot M. MR neurography: MR imaging of peripheral nerves. Magn Reson Imaging Clin N Am 1998;6(1):179–94.
15. Cudlip SA, Howe FA, Griffiths JR, Bell BA. Magnetic resonance neurography of peripheral nerve following experimental crush injury, and correlation with functional deficit. J Neurosurg 2002;96(4):755–9.
16. Dailey AT, Tsuruda JS, Filler AG, et al. Magnetic resonance neurography of peripheral nerve degeneration and regeneration. Lancet 1997;350(9086):1221–2.
17. Gilliatt RW. Physical injury to peripheral nerves: physiologic and electrodiagnostic aspects. Mayo Clin Proc 1981;56(6):361–70.
18. Grant GA, Goodkin R, Kliot M. Evaluation and surgical management of peripheral nerve problems. Neurosurgery 1999;44(4):825–39; discussion 839–40.
19. McLellan DL, Swash M. Longitudinal sliding of the median nerve during movements of the upper limb. J Neurol Neurosurg Psychiatry 1976;39(6):566–70.
20. Sunderland S. Mechanisms of cervical nerve root avulsion in injuries of the neck and shoulder. J Neurosurg 1974;41(6):705–14.
21. Smith AB, Gupta N, Strober J, Chin C. Magnetic resonance neurography in children with birth-related brachial plexus injury. Pediatr Radiol 2008;38(2):159–63.
22. Dailey AT, Tsuruda JS, Goodkin R, et al. Magnetic resonance neurography for cervical radiculopathy: a preliminary report. Neurosurgery 1996;38(3):488–92, discussion 492.
23. Bordalo-Rodrigues M, Rosenberg ZS. MR imaging of entrapment neuropathies at the elbow. Magn Reson Imaging Clin N Am 2004;12(2):247–63, vi.
24. Filler AG, Haynes J, Jordan SE, et al. Sciatica of nondisc origin and piriformis syndrome: diagnosis by magnetic resonance neurography and interventional magnetic resonance imaging with outcome study of resulting treatment. J Neurosurg Spine 2005;2(2):99–115.
25. Moore KR, Tsuruda JS, Dailey AT. The value of MR neurography for evaluating extraspinal neuropathic leg pain: a pictorial essay. AJNR Am J Neuroradiol 2001; 22(4):786–94.
26. Lewis AM, Layzer R, Engstrom JW, et al. Magnetic resonance neurography in extraspinal sciatica. Arch Neurol 2006;63(10):1469–72.
27. Wilbourn AJ. Thoracic outlet syndromes. Neurol Clin 1999;17(3):477–97, vi.
28. Bowen BC, Pattany PM, Saraf-Lavi E, Maravilla KR. The brachial plexus: normal anatomy, pathology, and MR imaging. Neuroimaging Clin N Am 2004;14(1): 59–85, vii–viii.
29. Bendszus M, Koltzenburg M, Wessig C, et al. Sequential MR imaging of denervated muscle: experimental study. AJNR Am J Neuroradiol 2002;23(8):1427–31.

Chapter 4
Physical Examination of the Peripheral Nerves and Vasculature

Brian White, Peter Gonzalez, Gerard A. Malanga, and Venu Akuthota

Systematic Examination

A thorough physical examination begins with a detailed history followed by inspection, palpation, and testing of muscle strength, tone, reflexes, and sensation. This systematic approach to the physical examination is useful for the peripheral nervous system and vascular system so pertinent details are not missed. When inspecting neurovascular structures, the physical examination is the primary initial clinical assessment. In addition to these fundamental aspects of the physical examination, many "special" provocation or relief tests and signs have been developed. The clinician then forms an impression from the information gathered during the history and physical examination and may use more advanced diagnostic tests to rule in or rule out a diagnosis.

Inspection

The physical examination begins with an inspection of the athlete that is both global and specific in nature. The specific component is targeted by the history and assists in identifying injury or pathology affecting the neurovascular structures in question. The global examination acts as an adjunct to the specific examination by looking at other areas of potential injury not identified in the history. The global examination covers the kinetic chain and may highlight areas that can biomechanically affect the primary pain generator. Specific items to note during the inspection include signs of trauma, lacerations, ecchymosis, muscle atrophy, fasciculations, gross deformity of normal anatomy, areas on the body compressed by clothing or equipment, and signs of prior injury and scars. Fasciculations may be present in athletes when muscles are weak and fatigued. Rarely, they represent a neurologic disorder of the motor unit.

Palpation

Once this thorough inspection is completed, the examiner should proceed to palpation. The areas targeted have been identified through both the history and inspection. Again, as with inspection, there should be both a targeted and a more global palpatory examination. The targeted examination attempts to identify tender structures or masses associated either regionally or functionally. When evaluating vascular injuries, the pulses should be palpated for strength and quality and compared to those on the contralateral side.

Neurologic Examination

The physical examination then proceeds to components often collectively identified as being part of the neurologic examination, including manual muscle testing (MMT), muscle stretch reflexes (MSRs),

B. White (✉)
Department of Orthopedics and Physical Rehabilitation, University of Massachusetts, Worcester, MA, USA

V. Akuthota, S.A. Herring (eds.), *Nerve and Vascular Injuries in Sports Medicine*,
DOI 10.1007/978-0-387-76600-3_4, © Springer Science+Business Media, LLC 2009

muscle tone, and the sensory examination. This constellation of examination elements may allow the examiner to localize the site and extent of injury or lesion.

Strength Testing

Testing this element of the neurologic examination is generally done by MMT with the examiner placing a force along the length of a muscle and the patient being instructed to resist. This is, by its very nature, a subjective maneuver as it relies on both patient effort and estimation of force applied on the part of the examiner. Early descriptions of MMT were made in polio patients by Robert Lovett in 1912.[1] Proper performance of MMT requires that a force be applied to the muscle tested in direct opposition to its primary action just proximal to the next distal joint beyond the muscle's insertion. Care is taken to prevent motor substitution by the patient, which may be subtle, especially in the case of injured athletes. For example, triceps weakness can be disguised by using shoulder external rotator substitution. The astute clinician, therefore, isolates muscle action as specifically as possible. In the above example, triceps can be tested in a supine position rather than a seated position to avoid this substitution pattern.

Many systems have been described in an attempt to quantify measurement of muscle strength. However, that of the Medical Research Council is the mostly commonly employed grading scale (Table 4.1).[1] There are many variations on this basic scale, and many have used modified scales that include (−) and (+) designations to record subtle variances in muscle power. Particular subjectivity is noted with the 4/5 MMT designation. Also, in the setting of injury, pain may cause involuntary motor inhibition that may mimic true neurogenic weakness. It is important to remember that MMT is aimed at evaluating motor neuron input to the muscle in question rather than gross muscle strength. Side-to-side MMT comparisons are useful for detecting subtle strength deficits. Particularly in well developed athletes, strength deficits are not observed with MMT; as much as 50% of muscle strength can be lost before MMT identifies weakness.[1] Therefore, MMT often must be augmented by more challenging muscle strength tests that usually employ athletes resisting their own body weight. For example, plantar flexion strength can be tested with repeated heel raises on the side in question compared to those of the contralateral side. The quadriceps can be tested with single-leg sit-to-stand testing and compared with results on the contralateral side.[2]

Table 4.1 Manual muscle testing

Grade	Description
0/5	No motor activity detected with patient effort
1/5	Flicker of muscle activity
2/5	Able to move primary joint through range of motion with gravity eliminated
3/5	Able to move primary joint through full range of motion against gravity
4/5	Muscle contraction greater than against gravity but less than full strength
5/5	Full strength through a full range of motion

Muscle Stretch Reflexes

Often termed "deep tendon reflexes," the reflex arc used in clinical practice to test the integrity of sensory and motor elements is more aptly termed "muscle stretch reflex" (MSR). This MSR terminology more closely reflects the anatomic reality of the arc that is generated by elements within the muscle and has little to do anatomically with the tendon (Fig. 4.1).[3]

The key to accurate MSR testing is relaxation. Thus, positioning the athlete in a comfortable position is crucial. Various facilitation techniques can also be employed to obtain reflexes including the following.

- Place the muscle/tendon in a slight stretch.
- Have the athlete look away from the reflex examination.
- Apply the Jendrassik maneuver, where the patient is asked to hook together the flexed fingers of the right and left hands and apply isometric force.[1]
- Use a weighted hammer with sufficient mass to load structures appropriately.

Wartenberg in 1944 described other reinforcements in his review of reflexes.[4] Common and uncommon reflexes can be tested.

When examining a patient for MSR, the clinician should observe for multiple characteristics of the

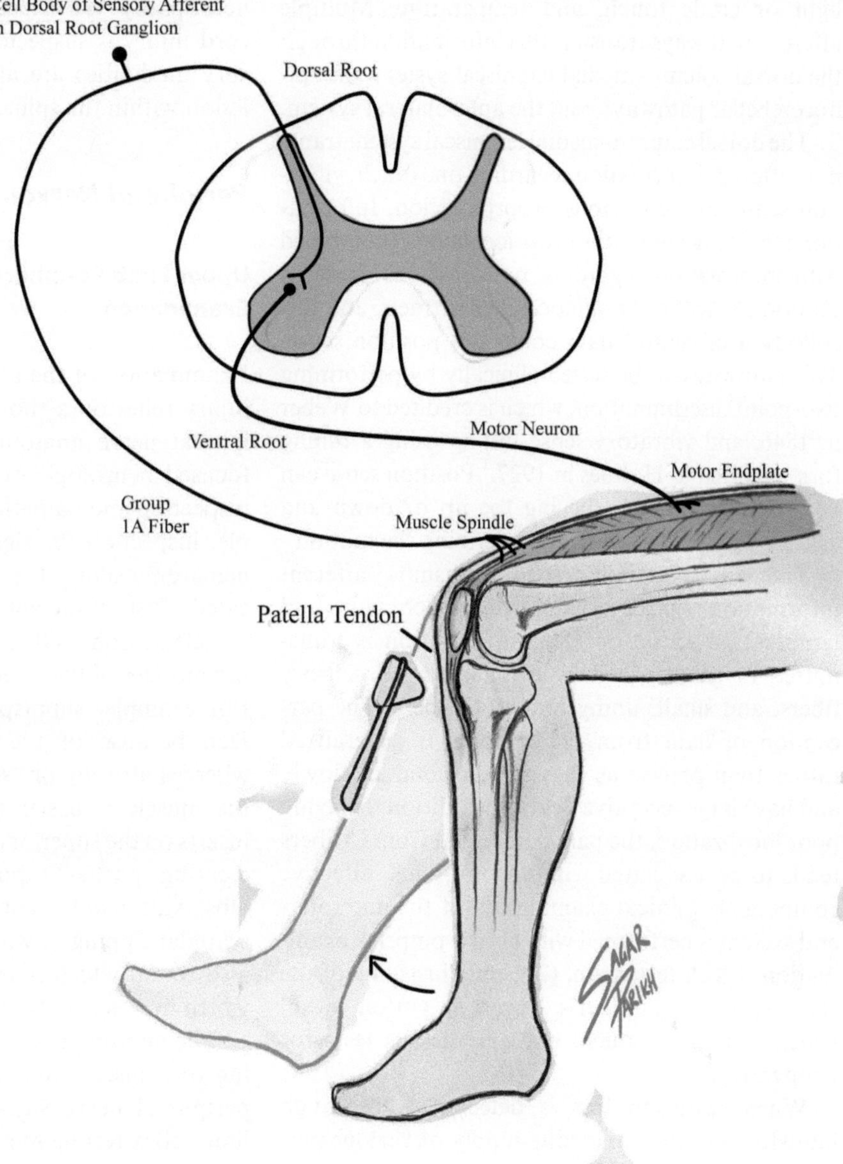

Fig. 4.1 Reflex loop, using knee jerk as an example

response, including the (1) threshold of elicitibility; (2) speed of antagonist response; and (3) spread to other muscles.[5]

In the setting of injury to the peripheral nerves (lower motor neuron injury), the expected clinical presentation is a decreased MSR response, usually seen as the lack of and/or a diminished asymmetrical response. If MSR demonstrates hyperreflexia, clonus, or spread to other muscles, it may be indicative of an upper motor neuron process. Reflex changes are rarely seen with athletic peripheral nerve injuries except in cases of radiculopathy and significant motor nerve injury.

Sensation Testing

Examination of sensation is complex as it is rather subjective and comprises various sensory pathways including modalities of discriminative touch, vibration sense, conscious proprioception, two-point discrimination, nonconscious proprioception, pain, light or crude touch, and temperature. Multiple afferent pathways transmit this information through the dorsal column–medial lemniscal system, the spinocerebellar pathways, and the anterolateral system.

The dorsal column–medial lemniscal system transmits afferent information regarding fine touch, vibration sense, and conscious proprioception. Information regarding conscious proprioception is combined with information regarding nonconscious proprioception carried in the spinocerebellar tracts, and this collection of central data comprises position sense. This pathway can be tested clinically by performing two-point discrimination, which is credited to Weber in 1846, and vibratory sense testing using a tuning fork, credited to Holmes in 1927.[1] Position sense can be tested by moving the big toe up or down and assessing patient accuracy in describing the motion.

The anterolateral system transmits afferent information regarding light/crude touch, pain, and temperature sensation. This information is transmitted in smaller, lightly myelinated Aδ sensory fibers, and small, unmyelinated C-fibers. The perception of data from these inputs is generalized rather than precise as these fibers conduct slowly and have large receptive fields. In addition to having poor localization, the pain perception from C-fibers tends to be associated with an emotional, affective component. Clinical examination of the anterolateral system is performed with (1) the pinprick examination, which tests pain; (2) gentle brushing of the skin with an examiner's finger or cotton swab, which tests light touch; and (3) various tests for temperature.[6]

When sensation loss is detected, a thorough knowledge of the cutaneous supply of various peripheral nerves and dermatomes is required to interpret accurately which nervous system structure is injured. For example, sensory loss in the lateral three digits suggests median nerve injury, whereas paresthesias in the medial two fingers suggest ulnar neuropathy. When a central process such as a spinal cord injury is suspected, distinguishing which sensory modalities are affected can help localize the lesion within the spinal cord.

Peripheral Nervous System Examination

Upper Limb Peripheral Nervous System Examination

Examination of the athlete with a suspected nerve injury relies on a thorough knowledge of the peripheral nerve anatomy. Prior to conducting the focused neurologic examination and special tests, inspection and palpation are performed. For example, inspection for signs of trauma, laceration, or hematoma along the course of the nerve is indicated. Inspection and palpation may also reveal muscle atrophy. Observing atrophy in certain deeper muscles of the upper limb and trunk is difficult. For example, supraspinatus atrophy may not be seen because of the overlying upper trapezius, whereas atrophy or "scalloping" of the infraspinatus muscle is easier to observe as the trapezius inserts on the superior aspect of the spine of scapula, creating partial exposure of the infraspinatus. Observation of the upper one-fourth can also reveal scapular tipping or winging. Careful inspection can also reveal which muscles are weak and therefore which nerves may be injured (Table 4.2).

The neurologic examination requires investigating the muscles and sensory supply served by the peripheral nerve suspected to be injured. Upper limb reflex testing may also be useful when investigating the central and peripheral nervous systems, particularly in cases of cervical myelopathy and radiculopathy. The Hoffman reflex, although its clinical significance is controversial,[7] is generally accepted as an upper motor neuron sign. It is

Table 4.2 Myotomes and peripheral nerves

Myotome	Peripheral nerve	Muscle	Action
C3/4	Spinal accessory	Upper trapezius	Shoulder shrug
C4-6	Axillary	Deltoid	Shoulder abduction
C6-8	Radial	Triceps	Arm extension
C6/7	Median	Pronator teres	Forearm pronation
C6/7	Radial	Extensor carpi radialis	Wrist extension
C8-T1	Ulnar	Abductor digitus minimus	Abduction of fifth digit

performed by grasping the middle finger of the patient and forcefully snapping the nail bed with the examiner's thumb. The presence of a positive response is quick flexion of the thumb and index finger. An incomplete response is seen when only the thumb flexes. There is a significant rate of false positives with this test. Sensitivity has been documented as 58% with a specificity of 78%.[8] Finally, special tests can be employed to detect upper limb muscle weakness and to provoke concordant symptoms through direct percussion, compression, and stretch testing.

Special Tests to Detect Upper Limb Muscle Weakness

Several special physical examination maneuvers can be utilized to reveal the weakness of specific muscles. An isolated injury to the anterior interosseous nerve, which can be involved in athletes with brachial neuritis, results in weakness of the flexor digitorum profundus, flexor pollicis longus, and pronator quadratus. This spectrum of muscle weakness results in the inability to make an "OK sign," which entails flexion of the first (thumb) and second digits distal to the interphalangeal joints (Fig. 4.2). When an injury is present, the patient compensates for the weakness by using ulnar-innervated muscles, the adductor pollicis, and thus collapsing or "beaking" the OK sign.

When a chronic or profound proximal median neuropathy is suspected, the active "Benediction test" can reveal long finger flexors and first and second lumbrical weakness. When the patient actively attempts to "make a fist," flexion at the fourth and fifth digits is normal (owing to an intact ulnar-innervated flexor digitorum profundus and superficialis and ulnar-innervated intrinsics), whereas the first and second digits do not flex (due to weakness of the flexor digitorum profundus and superficialis and first and second lumbricals). This creates the appearance of a hand giving a blessing (Fig. 4.3).

The passive "Benediction sign," on the other hand, is due to a severe ulnar nerve lesion often seen without provocation. This sign is a result of the loss of extension of the interphalangeal joints and unopposed hyperextension of the metacarpophalangeal (MCP) joint involving the fourth and fifth digits. The second and third digits are not involved owing to the first and second lumbricals' preserved innervation (they are innervated by the median nerve). On occasion, this sign is seen in bicyclists suffering ulnar neuropathy at the wrist (Guyon's canal).

The Wartenburg sign is another passive physical examination sign that provides clues to an ulnar nerve lesion. Clinically, this can result in atrophy of the intrinsic muscles, particularly the first dorsal

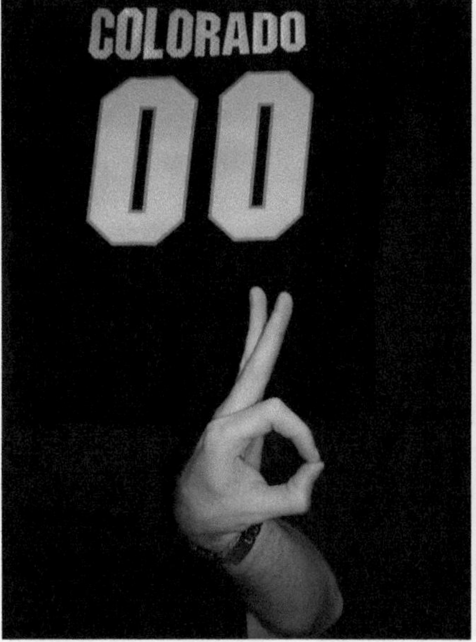

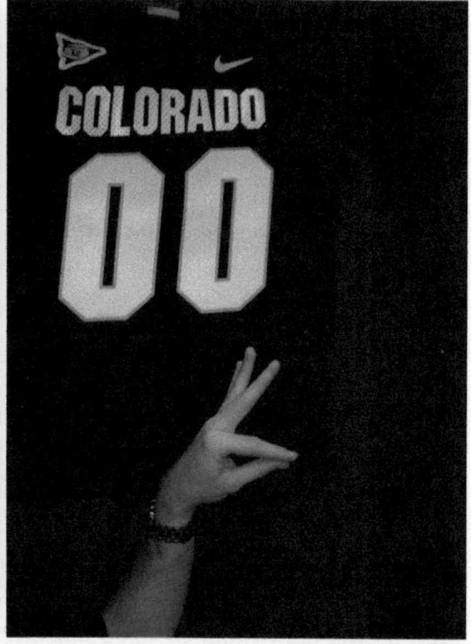

Fig. 4.2 (**a**) OK sign is used to detect anterior interosseous (median) nerve palsy. The OK sign is formed by contracting the pronator quadratus, flexor pollicis longus, and radial heads of the flexor digitorum profundus. (**b**) Example of beaking, which indicates weakness of anterior interosseous-innervated muscles

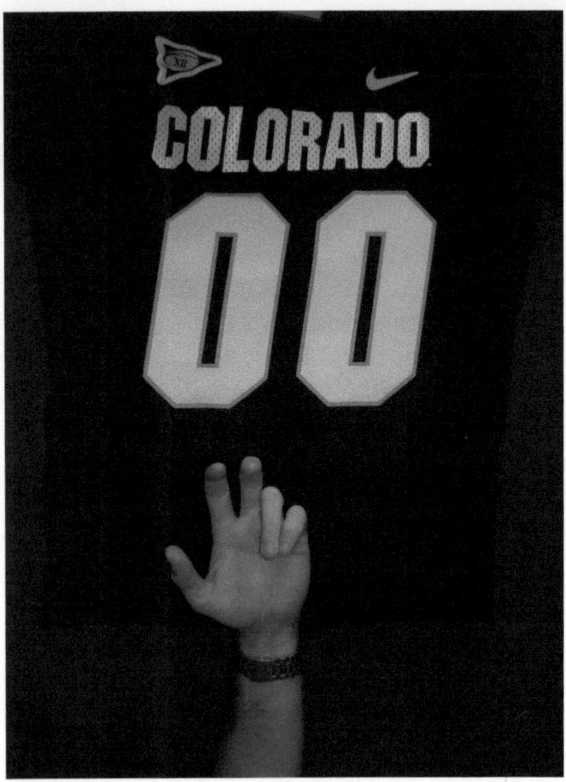

Fig. 4.3 Benediction sign

interosseous (FDI) and abductor digiti minimi (ADM) muscles. Weakness of the hand intrinsics is apparent when the patient complains of getting the fifth digit caught while placing the hand in a pocket. In athletics, a pitcher with an ulnar nerve injury at the elbow may note this finding as the initial manifestation of the injury.

A lesion at Guyon's canal affecting the deep branch of the ulnar nerve or a more proximal lesion affecting the fascicles to the adductor pollicis may result in a positive Froment sign. This finding is described as the inability of the patient to grasp a piece of paper when placed between the first (thumb) and second (index) digits without flexing the distal interphalangeal (DIP) joint of the thumb. This compensatory flexion of the thumb by the median-innervated flexor pollicis longus is a substitution for the weakness of the adductor pollicis.[9]

When severe and chronic ulnar and median neuropathy has been present, a so-called intrinsic-minus hand may result. Hopefully, deformities such as the *claw hand* or *ape hand* are not seen as they indicate nerve lesions that have been missed for a long time. The *claw hand* deformity describes the loss of extension at the interphalangeal (IP) joint and hyperextension of the MCP joint.[9] Hyperextension at the MCP joint is due to the unopposed action of the radial-innervated finger extensors. With mild lesions, extension at the MCP joints is the only abnormality on inspection.[10] Additionally, atrophy of the intrinsics and the FDI and ADM can be appreciated on inspection. The *ape hand* deformity results from an injury to the median nerve. It may involve the median nerve proximal to the hand but, more classically, involves a branch of the median nerve, the recurrent (thenar) motor branch, within the hand, resulting in weakness and atrophy of the thenar, median-innervated muscles. On inspection, the palm appears flattened owing to decreased thenar muscle bulk. The weakness results in loss of opposition and decreased abduction, limiting motion of the thumb to flexion and extension within the plane of the hand.

Volkmann ischemic contracture, originally described in 1881 by Richard von Volkmann, is an irreversible contracture of the forearm flexor muscles. These contractures result from vascular insufficiency, ischemia, and venous stasis from untreated elevated intracompartmental pressures. Contractures develop because of muscle necrosis affecting the flexor digitorum profundus and superfialis, flexor pollicis longus, and pronator teres. Contracture of these muscles cause a flexion deformity of the wrist, PIP, and DIP joints that mimics a neurogenic claw hand deformity. The nerves in the forearm are also susceptible to damage from elevated compartment pressures. When compartment syndromes develop in the forearm, emergent fasciotomy and median nerve decompression at potential entrapment sites is generally performed to avoid muscle necrosis and permanent nerve damage.[10]

There are no special tests or signs for radial nerve lesions. However, differing patterns of weakness on clinical examination are helpful in differentiating a proximal lesion involving the radial nerve from a distal lesion involving the posterior interosseous nerve. A lesion in the upper arm proximal to the spiral groove results in wrist drop and finger extensor weakness with intact IP joint extension. The latter is due to intact median and ulnar innervated intrinsic muscles. With more distal lesions involving the posterior interosseous nerve, the patient is able to extend and radially deviate at the wrist but is unable to extend at the MCP joints or abduct the thumb. These findings have been described as "finger drop with radial deviation."[10] Of note, if the triceps strength is significantly diminished from a radial nerve injury, the location may be assumed to be quite proximal along its course and within the axilla.

Upper Limb Provocation Tests: Nerve Tension Tests

The peripheral nerves and their respective roots have the ability to glide dynamically as the limb moves into different positions. Straight-leg raising is the prototypical nerve tension test; it is often referred to as a dural tension or adverse neurodynamic tension test. Accordingly, there are less well known nerve tension tests for the neck and upper limb. Upper limb tension testing (ULTT) is performed to elicit irritation of the upper limb neurologic structures. These tests are performed with subtle perturbation in limb position to isolate and stress the various nervous system structures.[11] Several variations have been described. Four common upper limb tension tests are outlined in Table 4.3. Testing is performed in sequential manner, altering the position of the shoulder first, then the forearm, wrist, and fingers and finally the elbow. Testing is done to reproduce or aggravate symptoms in the upper extremity.[11] Alterations of the cervical spine with contralateral flexion are used to sensitize the system further and elicit symptoms.

The "tethered" median nerve stress test, as described by LaBan, creates tension along the median nerve by simultaneous extension of the supinated wrist and DIP joint of the index finger. This position was held for 1 minute and was noted to result in proximal volar forearm pain in patients with chronic carpal tunnel syndrome.[12] Raudino has shown the sensitivity to be 42.8%.[13]

Upper Limb Provocation Tests: Compression Tests

The Tinel maneuver can be performed at various sites in the upper limb but classically at the wrist to elicit median nerve irritation. This test was originally developed during the American Civil War as a sign of nerve regeneration after injury, and its current use as a provocation test has a high false-positive rate (29%–45%).[10] A positive Tinel sign produces distal paresthesias along the nerve percussed. Wrist pain alone without parasthesias constitutes a negative Tinel maneuver at the wrist.

In the upper limb, these maneuvers are most commonly performed over the median nerve at the wrist for carpal tunnel syndrome and over the ulnar nerve at the elbow for cubital tunnel syndrome. However, such testing can be done at other superficial locations, such as the ulnar nerve at the wrist, median nerve in the forearm, radial nerve at the elbow, and the brachial plexus in the supraclavicular fossa. A positive Tinel sign with percussion over the brachial plexus is demonstrated with paresthesias in the distribution of the root, trunk, cord, or peripheral nerve of the plexus.[10,14]

Table 4.3 Upper limb tension tests

Region	ULTT1	ULTT2	ULTT3	ULTT4
Shoulder	Depress abduction (10)	Depress abduction (10)	Depress abduction (10), hand to ear	Depress abduction (10–90)
Elbow	Extension	Extension	Extension	Flexion
Forearm	Supination	Supination	Pronation	Supination
Wrist	Extension	Extension	Flexion, ulnar bias	Extension, radial bias
Fingers	Extension	Extension	Flexion	Extension
Shoulder		Lateral rotation	Medial rotation	Lateral rotation
Cervical spine	Contralateral flexion	Contralateral flexion	Contralateral flexion	Contralateral flexion
Nerve bias	Median n. Anterior interosseus n. C5-7 roots	Median n. Musculocutaneous n. Axillary n.	Radial n.	Ulnar n. C8-T1 roots

Adapted from Magee [11]
ULTT, upper limb tension test;

The brachial plexus compression test is performed by applying direct pressure over the plexus at the supraclavicular fossa between the scalene muscles. The test is positive if pain radiates into the ipsilateral shoulder and upper extremity. Pain at the site of compression is not diagnostic.[15]

The carpal compression test is performed when evaluating for carpal tunnel syndrome. It is performed by applying direct pressure over the median nerve at the carpal tunnel usually with both thumbs of the examiner. A positive test reproduces or exacerbates the patient's median nerve-derived symptoms with a brief duration of pressure (15 seconds to 2 minutes). The sensitivity and specificity have been found to be 87% and 90%, respectively.[16]

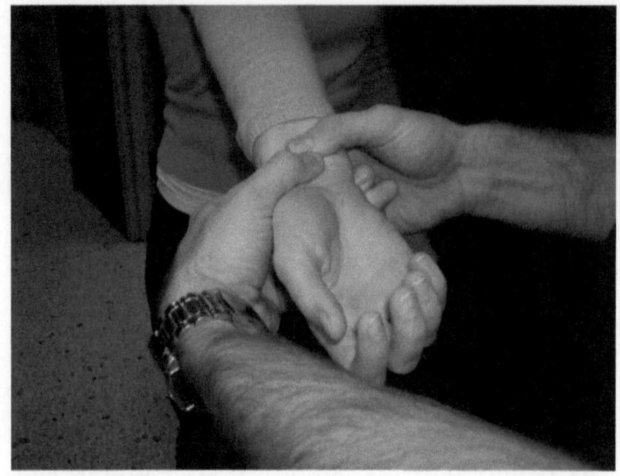

Fig. 4.5 Carpal compression test

Upper Limb Provocation Tests: Other Carpal Tunnel Syndrome Tests

The Phalen test is a compression test performed to assess for carpal tunnel syndrome. Carpal tunnel syndrome is generally thought of as an occupational injury but may occur with various athletic endeavors, such as long-distance cycling and mountain biking. The Phalen test (wrist flexion test) is performed by unforced complete flexion of both wrists. The patient maintains this position for 30–60 seconds. A positive test reproduces or aggravates the symptoms (paresthesias in a median nerve distribution). Sensitivity ranges from 71% to 80%[17–19] with a specificity ranging from 20% to 80%.[18,19] The Phalen and carpal compression tests may be arguably the best provocative tests for carpal tunnel syndrome (Figs. 4.4, 4.5).

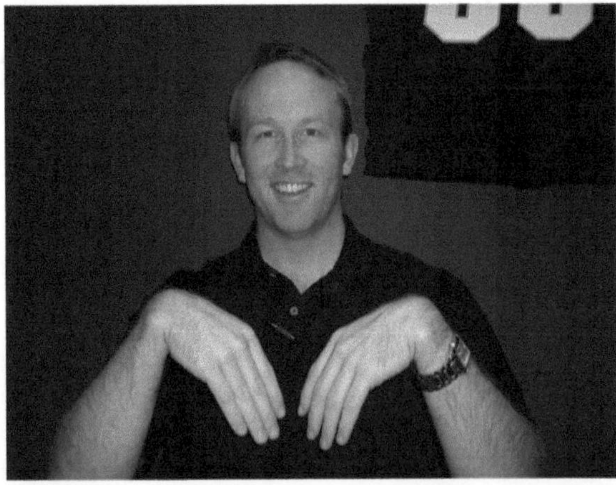

Fig. 4.4 Phalen maneuver

Tetro et al.[20] studied a combination test of wrist flexion, similar to the Phalen test, and median nerve compression, similar to carpal compression. Wrist flexion for the median nerve compression test is performed with the elbow extended, forearm supinated, and wrist flexed to 60°. Constant pressure with the examiner's thumb is applied over the median nerve at the carpal tunnel. The test is considered positive if symptoms (paresthesias or numbness) occur within 30 seconds. The sensitivity was 86% with a specificity of 95%.[20]

The reverse Phalen test is a variation of the Phalen test. This test compresses the median nerve and provokes symptoms through wrist extension, in contrast to wrist flexion. The patient is asked to place the palms of the hands together with fingers extended and the wrists in complete extension for 1 minute. A positive test results in pain and paresthesias in a median nerve distribution. The sensitivity and specificity have been found to be 43% and 74%, respectively.[21]

The lumbrical provocation test is performed by having the athlete make a fist forcefully for up to 60 seconds. This test may be particularly useful in exercise-induced carpal tunnel syndrome. A positive test reproduces the patient's symptoms. Yii and Elliot found the sensitivity to be 97% and the specificity 93%.[22]

Upper Limb Provocation Tests: Other Syndromes

Spinner described a group of examination maneuvers that may be helpful for identifying proximal median neuropathies. The Spinner test for pronator teres syndrome requires resisted wrist flexion and pronation, which reproduces symptoms. The Spinner test for lacertus fibrosis syndrome requires resisted pronation with the elbow in a flexed position, again reproducing symptoms. The Spinner test for flexor digitorum superficialis arch compression requires resisted finger PIP flexion, reproducing symptoms.[10]

Two provocation tests are used for diagnosing the radial tunnel syndrome. They were described by Eaton and Lister[23] to be used in conjunction with palpation over the radial tunnel at the elbow. The first test relies on increased pain with resisted forearm supination and is performed with the elbow extended to minimize the supination action of the biceps. The second test is performed by resisting middle finger extension with elbow extended, forearm pronated, wrist neutral, and finger extended. The presence of pain is a positive test. The former test is postulated to compress the radial nerve at the arcade of Frohse, and the latter test compresses the nerve at the radial tunnel. There is a degree of diagnostic ambiguity in differentiating the radial tunnel syndrome from lateral epicondylitis. Location of pain is often used to distinguish the two entities. Pain associated with lateral epicondylitis is proximal over the epicondyle, whereas pain from radial tunnel syndrome is located distally over the belly of the extensor muscle mass. Some consider worsening of pain with elbow extension, wrist flexion, and finger flexion to be indicative of lateral epicondylitis.[10] Although the posterior interosseous nerve is thought to be primarily a motor nerve, it has terminal branches that innervate the capsule and ligaments of the wrist joint. The distal posterior interosseous syndrome has been described as dull, aching pain along the dorsum of the wrist. Provocation of this pain can be attempted with extreme wrist dorsiflexion and pressure over the fourth compartment. No other clinical tests have been described.[10]

Lower Limb Peripheral Nervous System Examination

When considering neurologic injuries in the lower extremity, the inspection and palpation part of the examination may reveal important clues. For example, pain to palpation around the adductor hiatus and pes anserine tendon may indicate a saphenous nerve injury. Observation of an asymmetrically atrophied extensor digitorum brevis (EDB) muscle on the dorsum of the foot suggests peripheral nerve injury to the L5 nerve root, sciatic nerve, peroneal nerve, or localized trauma from shoe wear or ankle sprain. An example of a pertinent palpation clue is discovering fibrous tissue between the metatarsal bones. These masses correspond to Morton neuromas between the third and fourth toes[24] or second and third toes.[25]

Special Tests to Detect Lower Limb Muscle Weakness

Direct measurement of muscle girth can be undertaken, especially in the lower limb where limb dominance is not as big an issue. If quadriceps atrophy is suspected, the examiner can measure the thigh circumference 15 cm proximal to the superior border of the patella. Side-to-side comparison is then made.

The gluteal skyline test is performed with the patient prone and the examiner standing at the patient's feet. At rest an atrophied gluteus maximus will appear flat compared to the contralateral side. The patient is then asked to contract the gluteal muscles; the affected side may demonstrate less activation or less muscle bulk when compared directly with the other side. A positive test suggests pathology involving the inferior gluteal nerve, L5–S2 nerve roots, or gluteal inhibition.[10] This test may be done concurrently with manual muscle testing (MMT) of the gluteus maximus in the prone position as described above.

The Trendelenburg test, described in 1895, is performed by having the athlete stand on one leg. The test is considered positive if the contralateral hip is noted to drop, suggesting weakness of the gluteus medius and minimus on the ipsilateral side.[26] A study by Bird et al.[27] indicated 72% sensitivity and 77% specificity for a positive test result in women with a magnetic resonance imaging (MRI)-documented gluteus medius tear. The interobserver kappa coefficient was noted to be 0.676.

Single-leg squat testing is a valid, useful functional test that evaluates the strength of various lower limb muscles. In this test, athletes are asked to lower themselves as far as possible and then return to a standing position without losing their balance. Increased hip adduction or a "knee wobble" may be a sign of gluteal muscle weakness.[28]

Lower Limb Provocation Tests: Nerve Tension Tests

There are three basic nerve tension tests to perform in the lower limb: (1) straight-leg raising; (2) sit–slump test; and (3) femoral stretch test. A number of authors have described modifications and variations on these basic tests to enhance sensitivity for particular nerve roots or peripheral nerves. The tests are stated to be positive or negative for the purpose of research. A modification of the binary grading scale is proposed by the authors (Table 4.4) that takes into account the subtleties of nerve tension tests, including the added sensitivity of putting the peripheral nervous system on slack and tautness. This grading scale is also applicable in individuals who have disc herniations that do not produce pain past the knee.

The straight-leg raising (SLR) test, also known as the Lasegue test, is the classic nerve tension test and is most often used to detect lumbosacral radicular pathology. The test was named in honor of Charles Lasegue by his student J.J. Frost. To perform this test the patient is placed in a supine position with the examiner passively raising the athlete's leg off the table, performing passive range of motion into flexion at the hip. This test is considered to be unequivocally positive if this maneuver reproduces the patient's pain, particularly if pain is elicited between 20° and 70° of hip flexion. Early during the SLR, there is insufficient stress to increase root tension, but from 20° to 70° of hip flexion nerve tension increases. Pain elicited beyond 70° is more difficult to interpret as it may also be due to hamstring tightness or even sacroiliac joint pain.[10,29,30] Often in flexible athletes (e.g., dancers) this 70° cutoff may need to be adjusted upward, even up to 110° as the nerve tension may increase and hamstring length is not as important a factor.[10] The leg raising is thought to put particular nerve tension on the lower lumbosacral nerve roots from L4 to S1. Sensitivity of this test for lumbar disc herniation has been found in the literature to be 72%–97% with a specificity of 11%–66%.[29] Interrater reliability has also been examined using kappa coefficients. A coefficient of 1.0 indicates complete agreement between examiners, 0 indicates no agreement, and –1.0 indicates complete disagreement between examiners. For the SLR, kappa coefficients for the reproduction of patients' clinical symptoms was noted to be 0.36–0.81.[31] These authors defined a cutoff point of 0.4 as the lower limit of acceptable reliability for an examination.

Table 4.4 Grading nerve tension tests

Components of testing
1. Reproduction of concordant pain
2. Pain produced past knee or elbow
3. Pain worsening with nerve on stretch
4. Pain improving with nerve on slack
Grading
3 of 4 = positive
1 or 2 of 4 = equivocal
0 of 4 = negative
Grading Severity
note range of motion when pain occurs

Butler and colleagues have added sophistication to nerve tension tests with variations on testing depending on which nerve root or peripheral nerve is being examined. The Braggard test, a variation of the SLR, uses an increase in sciatic nerve tension to cause stress on symptomatic nerve roots and elicit radicular pain. This variation was also described by Fajersztajn. An SLR is performed as noted above; then, at the point in hip flexion where radiating pain is reproduced, the lower limb is lowered to a point where the patient reports relief of pain. At this angle of hip flexion, the examiner dorsiflexes the ankle on the tested limb. A positive Braggard sign is reproduction of the reported pain with this dorsiflexion due to increased tension in the sciatic nerve with the maneuver. If the common peroneal nerve is specifically examined, the SLR can be modified such that the end position is hip flexion to approximately 70°, hip internal rotation, and the ankle in plantar flexion and inversion.[10,32] This summation of positions should elicit pain in the sensory distribution of the common peroneal nerve. If the tibial nerve is specifically examined, the SLR can be modified by adding ankle dorsiflexion/eversion and toe extension to produce maximum stretch of that nerve. The focused stress placed on the tibial nerve distal to the knee may elicit an increase in the patient's sensory complaints in its distribution. The sural nerve can be maximally stretched in a similar way.[10]

The bowstring maneuver, described by Gower in 1888, is performed at the end of a traditional SLR test. When an SLR test is positive, the examiner maintains the position of the symptomatic lower extremity in hip flexion and then slightly flexes the knee. Pressure is then applied by the examiner's hands in the popliteal fossa over the tibial nerve, which increases the stretch on the sciatic nerve; a positive test is indicated by radiation of pain in the sciatic distribution with this maneuver. In patients with known disc herniation, a positive result was noted 71% of the time.[10,29] Interrater reliability was noted to be 0.11–0.49.[31]

Crossed SLR maneuver is a highly specific test described by Fajersztanjn in 1901 while performing cadaveric studies on nerve root tension, and occasionally referred to as the well leg-raising test of Fajersztanjn.[10,29] The test is performed similarly to the SLR, but the pain noted by the patient is in the contralateral lower limb. A positive result is thought to be due to a space-occupying mass, likely disc herniation, on the symptomatic side causing pain with the increase in root tension generated by flexion of the opposite limb. Specificity for disc herniation is high, with the literature indicating 88%–100%; however, the sensitivity is low at 23%–27%.[29] Interrater reliability was noted to be 0.02–0.74.[31]

The slump test, described in 1942 by Cyriax, is another basic nerve tension test that is thought to be more sensitive than the SLR because it broadly tenses the neuromeningeal tract (Fig. 4.6). There are several stages to this test. It begins with the patient in a seated position at the edge of an examination table with the knees freely in flexion. The examiner has the patient slump into a position of thoracic and lumbar flexion, and the examiner applies overpressure to the upper thoracic spine to augment the flexion component. Next, the patient is asked to flex the cervical spine and place the chin on the chest; again the examiner applies slight overpressure to the head to augment the flexion. Then, while maintaining flexion overpressure on the spinal segments, the examiner uses his or her other hand to extend the patient's knee, followed by dorsiflexion of the foot. Pain complaints may occur during any step of this process, and the patient must be monitored for development of symptoms during each phase. Given the summated stress on the posterior trunk and lower extremities, it is not uncommon for some discomfort to be generated in asymptomatic individuals. As such, this test is considered to be positive only if the patient's specific radicular complaints are reproduced.[10] Efforts to identify studies evaluating the sensitivity and specificity of this test for radiating pain with disc herniation did not identify any such studies.[29] However, Stankovic et al.[33] noted that 94% of patients with frank disc herniation had reproduction of their pain with the slump test compared to 78% of patients with disc bulges and 75% without pathology.

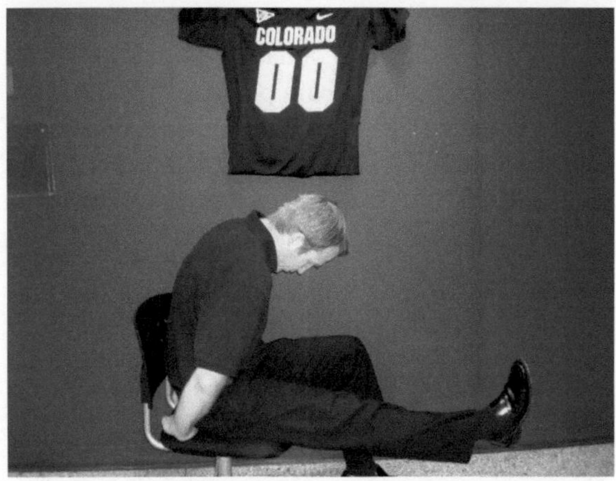

Fig. 4.6 Seated slump test

Another slump test, described by Pahor and Toppenberg,[34] is a modification of the previously described slump test to focus tension on the superficial peroneal nerve in the setting of an ankle sprain. The test is performed in the same manner as the Slump test with the addition of plantar flexion of the ankle and inversion of the foot. A positive test reproduces distal clinical symptoms in the superficial peroneal nerve sensory distribution and is suggestive of injury to that nerve that is often associated with a lateral ankle sprain.

The femoral stretch test (FST), credited to Wassermann in 1918, is the third basic lower limb nerve tension test; it allows testing of the upper lumbar roots and femoral nerve.[29] To perform the test the patient is placed in the prone (or side-lying) position with the examiner standing on the ipsilateral side of the examination table. The knee of the ipsilateral lower extremity is then flexed, moving the foot toward the buttock. A positive test produces pain in the anterior thigh and/or back in the same distribution as the patient's clinical complaint. This test primarily stresses the upper lumbar region and is thought to be most effective at testing the L2–4 nerve roots. The test may also be augmented with extension of the ipsilateral hip by the examiner once the knee is in a flexed position. This extension is achieved by lifting the knee off the examination table with one hand while stabilizing the patient's pelvis with the other. This testing position may also stretch the quadriceps and hip flexors. As with the SLR and slump tests, pain from muscle tightness must be excluded, perhaps through tightening and slackening the peripheral nerves, eliciting back pain in addition to thigh pain, and reproducing concordant pain. Review of the literature indicates that this is likely to be the best physical examination test available for upper lumbar nerve root pathology. It has been shown to be positive in 84%–95% of patients with a known high lumbar disc herniation.[29] Studies by Estridge et al.[35] and Christodoulides[36] noted a strong correlation between L3/4 disc herniation and a positive test, as well as, a positive test in 95% of patients with known lateral L4/5 disc protrusion involving the L4 nerve root. Interrater reliability was noted to be 0.27–0.77.[31] Other texts[10] have described a similar testing maneuver and called it the prone knee bending test or Nachlas test.

There are also numerous variations on the FST that attempt to evaluate individual peripheral nerves. A variation of the prone FST[10] attempts to localize the lateral femoral cutaneous nerve by placing maximal stretch on that nerve. The athlete is placed in a similar end position as with the FST, but hip adduction is also applied. A positive test is reproduction of the patient's clinical complaints in the anterior, lateral thigh. A saphenous nerve stretch variation has also been described by Butler[32] and others.[10] This variation adds hip abduction and internal rotation and, rather than mere knee flexion, knee extension, ankle dorsiflexion, and foot eversion is used to augment stretch on the entire course of the saphenous nerve. A positive test elicits the patient's clinical complaint in the sensory distribution of the saphenous nerve.

The crossed femoral stretch test, described by Cyriax in 1947,[29] is performed as described above for the femoral stretch test, except that the painful complaint correlating with the patient's clinical symptoms occurs on the contralateral thigh. A review of the literature failed to find any studies relating to the specificity and sensitivity of this test.

Lower Limb Provocation Tests: Piriformis Tests

Described by Pace and Nagle in 1976,[37] the Pace test is performed to evaluate the impact of the piriformis muscle on the sciatic nerve. With the patient sitting on the edge of the examination table with knees freely flexed, the examiner places his or her hands on the distal lateral thighs. The patient is then instructed to abduct and externally rotate the thighs forcefully against the examiner's hands. A positive sign is noted with pain and weakness on the ipsilateral side.

The FAIR test was described by Solheim et al. in 1981[38] as one that stresses the sciatic nerve as it passes by the piriformis muscle. The patient is placed with the examined lower extremity in a position of combined hip flexion/adduction/internal rotation (FAIR). Benson and Schutzer in 1999,[39] who examined 15 patients who underwent surgical release of the piriformis muscle, noted that 14 of the 15 had reproduction of their pain with the FAIR test preoperatively.

For the piriformis test, the subject is placed on his or her side with the lower extremity to be examined being uppermost and the contralateral extremity on the table. In this position, the examiner brings the examined hip to 60° of hip flexion and then applies an adducting force to move the knee toward the table. If the piriformis muscle itself is tight then, this movement elicits pain in the posterior gluteal region concordant with the location of the piriformis muscle. If the piriformis muscle is irritating the sciatic nerve, the test maneuver elicits pain in the buttock and radiating pain down the leg in the patient's clinical pain pattern.[11]

The Freiberg sign is described as an indication of piriformis muscle irritation of the sciatic nerve. It is pain elicited by passive internal rotation of an extended hip, an action that places the piriformis muscle on stretch.[11]

Lower Limb Provocation Tests: Compression Tests

The Tinel maneuver can be performed at various sites in the lower limb. As mentioned earlier, this test was originally developed as a sign of nerve regeneration after injury, and its current use as a provocation test has a high rate of false positives. Nerve percussion can be performed where peripheral nerves are superficial in the lower limb, such as tapping the peroneal nerve as it courses under the fibular head. A positive test reproduces the athlete's paresthesias in the leg or foot. Nerve percussion can also be performed at the anterior tarsal tunnel at the level of the extensor retinaculum, producing symptoms into the first web space.[11] Tapping over the tibial nerve at the (posterior) tarsal tunnel along the distal portion of the posterior aspect of the medial malleolus can reproduce sensory complaints in the plantar aspect of the foot.[11] The Valleix sign is a similar maneuver that requires the examiner to compress the posterior aspect of the medial malleolus and assesses for tenderness immediately distal or proximal to the tarsal tunnel. A positive test suggests impingement in the tarsal tunnel.

For the web space compression test, the patient is either seated comfortably at the edge of the examination table or in a supine position. The examiner cups the distal foot with one hand with the fingers on one border and the thumb on the opposite border and then squeezes the metatarsal heads together while at the same time palpating the intermetatarsal spaces with the other hand. This compression should elicit the patient's symptoms of pain between the palpated metatarsophalangeal (MTP) joints and possibly radiation of pain into the appropriate digits.[25] A similar examination has been described where the metatarsals are adducted with lateral stress placed on the first metatarsal and medial stress on the fifth metatarsal (metatarsal compression). This should elicit pain associated with a clicking sensation due shifting position of the neuroma in the interdigital space.[10]

Spine and Pudendal Examination

Examination of spinal disorders that present as upper or limb paresthesias and weakness can be quite involved. After inspection and palpation, range of motion testing of the neck or low back is crucial. The percentage of lost range should be recorded in all directions. Examiners should also note which directional range reproduces pain. A thorough neurologic examination, as discussed earlier, is necessary to rule out a neurologic deficit related to a potential spinal disorder. Lastly, special tests can be utilized.

Special Tests

The Spurling maneuver, cervical spine compression, or the foraminal compression test is the classic provocation test in the cervical spine. A positive test, indicated by concordant pain reproduction into the arm, is thought to represent cervical nerve root irritation from spondylitic changes or cervical herniated discs. The maneuver was initially described as lateral flexion toward the symptomatic side with downward pressure on the head worsening symptoms. However, modifications have been added to the original test where neck extension and ipsilateral rotation are also used. Conversely, lateral flexion away from the symptomatic side often reduces pain.[40] Some have suggested performing this test in three stages involving neutral compression, compression with extension of the neck, and compression with extension and rotation of the neck toward the symptomatic side.[41] We suggest a different sequence where the neck is initially extended, then ipsilaterally laterally flexed, then contralaterally rotated, and finally compression added. If arm or radicular pain is produced at any point, the test is ended and called positive. We advocate this sequencing as head compression has been, anecdotally, found to exacerbate radicular pain. It is important to note that neck pain alone is considered a negative response. Sensitivity and specificity studies show ranges of 40%–60% and 92%–100%, respectively.[42]

The shoulder abduction test-also known as the abduction relief or Bakody sign-was first observed by Spurling in 1956. This examination details the relief of upper extremity radicular symptoms with ipsilateral shoulder abduction as the patients bring the arm above their head. Some have postulated that abduction of the shoulder reduces traction on the mid-cervical nerve roots (C5/6), thus alleviating pain. More-current literature describes the test as passive or active shoulder abduction with resting of the hand on the top of the head.[43] This is thought to indicate cervical radicular pain from mid-cervical roots. The lower cervical roots may be put on tension with this maneuver. The sensitivity and specificity have been reported to be 43%–50% and 80%–100%, respectively.[42]

The neck distraction test-otherwise known as the axial manual traction test[7]-is another test designed to reduce symptoms, particular radicular symptoms from cervical pathology. This test is performed by placing one hand under the patient's chin and the other hand around the occiput, slowly lifting the patient's head.[11] A positive test is one in which pain is relieved when the head is distracted or lifted. This implies that pressure has been taken off the pain generators, the nerve roots.[11] The test could be performed in either the supine or seated position. One study using 10–15 kg of traction force found a sensitivity of 40%–43% and specificity of 100%.[42]

The Lhermitte sign is commonly sought when evaluating for cervical pathology involving the spinal cord. Such clinical conditions range from cervical spondylitic myelopathy to a spinal cord tumor to multiple sclerosis.[44–46] The test is performed as passive cervical flexion to end range with the patient in the sitting position.[7] It has also been described with positioning the patient in the long leg sitting position. The head and one hip is simultaneously flexed keeping the knees extended.[11] A positive test results in electric-like sensations down the spine and/or upper or lower extremities. Sensitivity and specificity testing results are conflicting.[15,47]

Pudendal Nerve

The pudendal nerve is derived from the ventral rami of S2–4 and represents the lowest branches of the anterior division of the sacral plexus. The nerve fibers enter the perineum through the lesser sciatic foramen medial to the ischial tuberosity and run through the Alcock canal with the pudendal vessels after which they divide into distal branches: the dorsal nerve of the clitoris/penis, perineal nerve, and inferior anal nerve.[48] The pudendal nerve is frequently injured chronically in cyclists from inappropriate pressure distribution in the region of the ischial tuberosities or acutely in a fall onto the groin. Injury to this nerve may result in dysesthesias in the sensory distribution.

Injury to the pudendal nerve would be expected to result in a decrease in sensation to the perineum and genitalia, especially posterior two-thirds of the scrotum and the analogous region of the labia majora. The pudendal nerve is the chief sensory nerve of the genitalia.[49] The pudendal nerve supplies motor fibers to the external anal sphincter and the external urethral sphincter, and it has branches to the perineal muscles.[49] Anal contraction may be noted either through visual inspection or by palpation with a digit. Bulbocavernosus reflex can also be performed. The dorsal nerve of the penis supplies the sensory afferent input of this reflex, and the inferior anal nerve supplies efferent motor output to a portion of the external anal sphincter. To perform this maneuver, the examiner placed a gloved second or third finger in the anus with the remaining fingers of the examination hand placed on the perineum to palpate for response. The glans of the penis is then pinched with forceps causing a reflexive contraction of the bulbocavernosus muscle. The afferent loop is via the S1 root and the efferent loop from L4/5 roots. Alternatively, this reflex may be obtained in a patient with an indwelling Foley catheter by tugging on the Foley catheter and observing the anus or palpating the perineum for response.

Vascular Examination

Athletes rarely have true "hard" findings of vascular injury, which include pulsatile bleeding, expanding pulsatile hematoma, cyanosis, decreased temperature, bruits, and thrills. The "five P's" of arterial insufficiency and compartment syndromes are also rare. These include *p*ain on passive extension of the muscle compartment involved, *p*ulselessness, *p*aresthesias, *p*allor, and *p*aralysis. Similar complaints are offered in the setting of significant venous congestion causing loss of arterial flow, a condition known as phlegmasia cerulea dolens. The prime clinical differentiator between arterial flow cessation due to direct arterial lesion and that due to venous obstruction is the presence of edema and a cyanotic, rather than pallor-like, appearance in the setting of severe venous obstruction.[50] Furthermore, arteriovenous fistulas, if they occur, can present with massive distension of distal superficial veins as arterial flow is directed into distensible veins. These hard findings require an emergent vascular surgery consult.[51]

"Soft" findings of vascular injury are more common in athletes. They include an asymmetrical pulse, isolated peripheral nerve injury, and a large nonpulsatile hematoma. Prolonged capillary refill is another soft sign of vascular injury that attempts to test distal perfusion but may be nonspecific and unreliable. The leg can be palpated for tenderness and tension that might suggest a compartment syndrome. Athletes suspected to have vascular injury need to be monitored and examined periodically as the injury may take time to manifest.

Palpation of pulses assesses for symmetry and strength. Pulses are graded on a 0–4 scale: 0, absent pulses; 2, normal pulses; 4, bounding (highly increased).[52] Some pulses, such as the dorsalis pedis and posterior tibial artery pulses, are not present in some healthy adults, in which case it is usually bilaterally absent.[49]

Given their low-pressure state, there is usually no palpable pulse in the venous system. Palpation should focus on identifying a possible hematoma or tenderness suggesting direct injury. In the event of thrombosis, the distal lower extremity may display a generalized tenderness to palpation. The venous system is a low-pressure system of thin-walled vessels that transport blood from the periphery back to the heart to complete the cardiac cycle. These vessels are often more superficial than their more thickly walled, high-pressure arterial counterparts; given their thin-walled, low-pressure nature, they are not readily palpated. However, their superficial location may make them more susceptible to injury during athletic injury; it also frequently makes them superficially visible in a lean athlete.

Palpation of hematomas may reveal pulsations. The examiner may palpate for tenderness, tissue fullness, compartment tightness, a palpable thrill, and especially pulses. However, he or she must be aware that the presence of a pulse does not ensure adequate blood flow as a pulse may be transmitted via multiple mechanisms including through a clot or a flap. Also a clot distal to the site of palpation may allow palpation of a pulse but may impede blood flow beyond that point.

Further auscultation of arteries can provide evidence of bruits. Finally, capillary refill can be performed by applying pressure to the nail bed or the hypothenar eminence. Refill is delayed or abnormal if the color (pink) does not return within 2 seconds after releasing the pressure.[11] With the patient supine, the distal phalanx of one of the toes is compressed for 5 seconds to cause local blanching. The normal color should return within 2 seconds for adult men and within 3 seconds for adult women.[53] Chronic vascular lesions may lead to chronic skin color changes, skin mottling and ulcerations, different hair patterns, and nail bed changes. Once again, comparison to the contralateral, asymptomatic side is crucial. Autonomic nervous system disorders, such as Raynaud phenomena, can be present in athletes, often associated with peripheral nerve disorders such as carpal tunnel syndrome. Vasoconstriction (often from exogenous cold temperature) can present as pallor, rubor, cyanosis, and excessive sweating of the hands. Chronic autonomic disorders, such as end-stage reflex sympathetic dystrophy (or complex regional pain syndrome) can manifest as dry skin, loss of skin rugal lines, and hand intrinsic muscle atrophy.[10]

The neurologic examination in the setting of arterial injury demonstrates a typical progressive pattern with light touch sensation being lost first, followed by complete anesthesia, and ultimately loss of motor function. However, if arterial structures are injured distally, the patient often has preserved distal motor function as the muscles responsible for this motion are located proximal to a distal lesion.[50]

Neurologic and vascular injuries may also demonstrate interplay between injuries to distinct structures. This relation may be seen with a concordant injury (e.g., laceration) that damages both structures as they run together in a neurovascular bundle or by a compressive injury to a nerve following the development of a space-occupying mass secondary to a vascular injury, such as a hematoma. The latter situation is also illustrated by a compartment syndrome in the setting of a vascular injury, as damage to vascular structures causes an increase in the pressure within a defined anatomic space and this pressure increase causes a neuropathic lesion in anatomically related neurologic structures. In addition to direct clinical examination by the physician, these structures can be visualized by use of duplex ultrasonography as well as venography, arteriography, and analysis of arterial Doppler waveforms.

Special Upper Limb Vascular Tests

Specialized tests are part of the vascular assessment of the upper extremity and may be integrated after the initial assessment is completed. These tests may be used for cervical spine pathology, brachial plexus lesions, or peripheral nerve injuries. Vascular assessment of the cervical spine region for sports injuries is limited to the carotid and vertebral arteries. Athletes can also suffer from vascular thoracic outlet syndrome, and a variety of tests can help diagnose this condition. Many of these tests, however, are hampered by a high rate of false positives. The popliteal artery is injured in up to 25% of knee dislocations,[54] so close attention must be paid to vascular injury in the setting of knee dislocation.

The vertebral artery can be assessed using the cervical quadrant test. For this test, the head and neck of the patient, who is supine, are passively extended and laterally flexed. The examiner then passively rotates the head in the same direction and holds it there for 30 seconds. A positive test provokes symptoms of dizziness or nystagmus, indicating compromise of the ipsilateral vertebral artery.[11] The DeKleyn-Nieuwenhuyse test, is a slightly modified variation of this test using extension and rotation without lateral flexion. Either of these tests may also compress the nerve roots of the lower cervical spine and assess for cervical radiculitis.[11]

The Allen test is commonly used to assess the arterial supply to the hand via the radial and ulnar arteries. The blood supply to the lateral hand is from the radial artery, and that to the medial hand is from the ulnar artery. If one supply is compromised, the blood supply is generally maintained by anastomotic connections. This can be clinically tested by obstructing one artery with external pressure and assessing vascular return through the other artery. If the unobstructed artery is competent, the blood flow and should return quite briskly. In contrast, if the unobstructed artery is occluded, return of blood is delayed or absent.

The Buerger test is designed to assess the integrity of arterial flow into the lower extremity. With the patient supine on the examination table, the examiner elevates the entire lower extremity to a 45° angle by flexing the hip. The leg, ankle, and foot are then monitored. If the foot blanches or prominent veins collapse shortly after elevation, the test is positive for reduced arterial flow. Next, the patient is moved into a seated position with the legs dangling over the side of the examination table; again, the distal portion of the lower extremity is monitored. If return of skin color and filling of veins takes longer than 1 minute, a positive result is confirmed.[11]

Special Vascular Tests for Thoracic Outlet Syndrome

The Adson maneuver, first described in 1927 by Adson and Coffey, reproduces compression of the subclavian artery between a cervical rib and the scalene arteries. This test is performed by first locating the radial pulse in the affected extremity, asking the patient to rotate his or her head toward the affected side. The patient extends the neck, and the examiner extends and externally rotates the shoulder while still palpating the radial pulse. The patient is asked to take a sustained deep breath while the examiner assesses for transient disappearance of the pulse.[11] A change in or loss of the pulse indicates a positive test. The sensitivity has been documented as ranging from 18% to 87% with a specificity of 94%.[55]

The Allen maneuver is a slight variation of the Adson maneuver and should not to be confused with the Allen *test* described earlier. The patient flexes the elbow of the affected upper extremity with the shoulder externally rotated and extended. The radial pulse is palpated in the affected limb, and the patient is asked to rotate his or her head contralaterally. Loss or alteration of the pulse is considered a positive test.

The Wright hyperabduction test was described in 1945 as a sign of neurovascular entrapment by the pectoralis minor muscle; the test is also used to assess the possibility of the thoracic outlet syndrome (TOS).[56] The test is performed with the affected arm elevated above 90° with the elbow flexed at 90° and the hand over the head (hyperabducted at the shoulder). The examiner palpates the radial pulse and assesses for any alteration. The validity of this test has been questioned as asymptomatic subjects have shown a loss or change in pulse.[57] No sensitivity or specificity data are known.[7]

The Halstead maneuver is performed similar to the above TOS maneuvers. The radial pulse is palpated, and the arm is extended at both the shoulder and the elbow. The patient's head is rotated to the opposite, asymptomatic side and extended. Downward traction is applied to the tested extremity. Disappearance of the radial pulse indicates a positive test.[11]

The costoclavicular test was originally noted in a study of patients with subclavian artery and vein compression. This maneuver assesses for loss of the radial pulse with retraction and depression of the shoulder and protrusion of the chest. No sensitivity or specificity was reported.[7]

The Roos test, first described in 1976 by Roos, is an elevated arm stress test (EAST). It is performed with the shoulder abducted to 90° and externally rotated with the elbow flexed to 90° (Fig. 4.7). The patient is instructed to open and close his or her fists at a moderate speed for 3 minutes. It should reproduce patient's symptoms: fatigue, heaviness, numbness and tingling, and possibly overt weakness.[57] The sensitivity and specificity are unknown.[7]

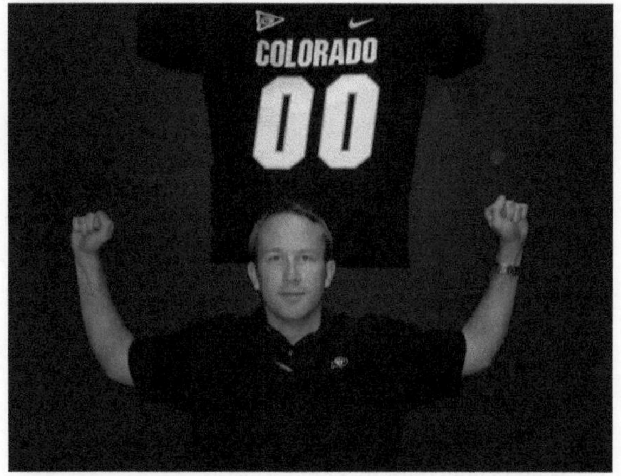

Fig. 4.7 Roos test

Special Vascular Tests for Venous Pathology

The Homans test was named for John Homans, a surgeon at Johns Hopkins who published a monograph on deep venous thrombosis (DVT) in 1939. The maneuver attempts to identify DVT by clinical physical examination. With the patient either seated or supine and the knees flexed, the examiner takes hold of the distal foot and rapidly dorsiflexes the ankle. If this produces pain in the calf, it is considered a positive Homan sign and suggests the presence of DVT in the calf. This examination is of marginal use in identifying the DVT. A clinical examination consisting of a positive Homan maneuver, swelling, calf tenderness to palpation, and rubor is noted to have a specificity of 30%–72% and a sensitivity of 60%–88%.[58]

The Trendelenburg-Brodie test was first described by Sir Benjamin Brodie in 1846 and later popularized by Friedrich Trendelenburg; it is occasionally referred to as the Trendelenburg test. The purpose of this test is to evaluate the function of the valves of the lower extremity veins, especially in patients with saphenous varicosities. With the patient supine, the examiner raises the leg above the heart by flexion at the hip. The lower extremity is held in this position by the examiner until the veins collapse. Next, a tourniquet is applied about the mid-thigh to compress the great saphenous vein, thus preventing it from draining blood back up to the torso. Then the examiner has the patient stand and observes the leg veins. In a normal person with intact venous valves, the greater saphenous vein should slowly fill from below within a minute, this filling is provided by intact arterial flow creating a positive displacement blood column up the greater saphenous vein. The tourniquet is removed after this 1-minute observation, and the lower extremity veins are again observed. The interpretation is in two parts. If the saphenous vein fills quickly during the first minute, while the tourniquet is in place, it suggests back-filling due to incompetent valves in communicating veins. If the saphenous vein fills rapidly after the tourniquet is removed, it suggests incompetent valves in the more proximal portions of the saphenous vein itself.[58]

A Trendelenburg test variation assesses for the presence of communicating veins and the competence of the deep venous system. The patient is supine with veins full and any varicosities engorged. In this position, a tourniquet is applied mid-thigh; then, once the greater saphenous vein is occluded, the lower extremity is elevated by the examiner. The veins in the lower extremity below the tourniquet are closely observed while the limb is elevated. If these veins gradually disappear, it suggests the presence of communicating veins between the superficial veins and the deep veins, that those veins have competent valves, and that the deep venous system is patent. Should the veins remain engorged, this suggests that either the deep venous system has become occluded, possibly due to DVT, or that there are no communicating veins between the deep and superficial venous systems.[58]

The lower limb may be also palpated to determine valve competence. To do so, the examiner places one finger over the distal saphenous vein, below the knee. The examiner then places a finger from his or her other hand over the saphenous vein proximal to the knee and imparts an impulse to the vein by "flicking" it with a finger. Incompetent veins allow retrograde transmission of this impulse down the leg, and this impulse can be palpated by the distal finger tip.[58]

The Perthes test is another way to evaluate for the presence of communicating veins, the patency of the deep venous system, and the integrity of the valves. For this test the patient is in a standing position with leg veins engorged. A tourniquet is placed about the mid-thigh, and the patient is instructed to walk for 5 minutes, after which time they are reexamined. If the distal veins have collapsed, it suggests that the deep venous system is patent, a communicating system is present, and the valves of the communicating system are functioning. This is due to the "milking" effect that the lower extremity muscles have on venous flow. The muscles force the blood from the saphenous system into the deep system, where it can flow back to the heart. If the distal veins remain unchanged and the patient notes leg pain, incompetence of the valves of both the saphenous and communicating veins is suggested. If the veins become more engorged and the patient notes pain, it suggests both occlusion of the deep venous system and incompetence of the communicating valves.[58]

References

1. Nadler SF, Rigolosi L, Kim D, Solomon J. Sensory, motor, and reflex examination. In: Malanga GA, ed. Musculoskeletal Physical Examination: An Evidence-Based Approach. 1st ed. Philadelphia: Elsevier Mosby; 2006:15–32.
2. Rainville J, Jouve C, Finno M, Limke J. Comparison of four tests of quadriceps strength in L3 or L4 radiculopathies. Spine 2003;28(21):2466–71.
3. Haines DE, Mihailoff GA, Yezierski RP. The spinal cord. In: Haines D, ed. Fundamental Neuroscience. 1st ed. Philadelphia: Churchill Livingstone; 1997: 129–41.
4. Wartenberg R. Studies in reflexes: history, physiology, synthesis and nomenclature: study I. Arch Neurol Psychiatr 1944;51(2).
5. Schwartzman R. Neurologic Examination. Malden, MA: Blackwell; 2006:189–206.
6. Warren S, Capra NF, Yezierski RP. The somatosensory system II: nondiscriminative touch, temperature, and nociception. In: Haines D, ed. Fundamental Neuroscience. 1st ed. Philadelphia: Churchill Livingstone; 1997:237–53.
7. Landes P, Malanga GA, Nadler SF, Farmer J. Physical examination of the cervical spine. In: Malanga GA, ed. Musculoskeletal Physical Examination: An Evidence-Based Approach. 1st ed. Philadelphia: Elsevier Mosby; 2006:33–57.
8. Glaser JA. Cervical cord compression and the Hoffman's sign. Presented at the 14th Annual Meeting of the North American Spine Society, 1999.
9. Agesen TA, Nadler SF, Wrightson J, Miller J. Physical examination of the elbow, wrist, and hand. In: Malanga GA, ed. Musculoskeletal Physical Examination: An Evidence-Based Approach. 1st ed. Philadelphia: Elsevier Mosby; 2006:119–87.
10. Dawson DM, Hallet M, Wilbourn AJ. Entrapment Neuropathies. 3rd ed. Philadelphia: Lippencott-Raven; 1999.
11. Magee DJ. Shoulder. In: Magee DJ, ed. Orthopedic Physical Assessment. 4th ed. St. Louis: Saunders Elsevier; 2006:207–319.
12. LaBan MM, Friedman NA, Zemenick GA. "Tethered" median nerve stress test in chronic carpal tunnel syndrome. Arch Phys Med Rehabil 1986;67(11):803–40.
13. Raudino F. Tethered median nerve stress test in the diagnosis of carpal tunnel syndrome. Electromyogr Clin Neurophysiol 2000;40(1):57–60.
14. Landi A, Copeland S. Value of the Tinel sign in brachial plexus lesions. Ann R Coll Surg Engl 1979;61:470–1.
15. Uchihara T, Furukawa T, Tsukagoshi H. Compression of brachial plexus as a diagnostic test of cervical cord lesion. Spine 1994;19:2170–3.
16. Durkan J. A new diagnostic test for carpal tunnel syndrome. J Bone Joint Surg Am 1991;73:535–8.
17. Gerr F, Letz R. The sensitivity and specificity of tests for carpal tunnel syndrome vary with the comparison subjects. J Hand Surg Br 1998;23(2):151–3.

18. Gellman H, Gelberman RH, Tan AM, Botte MJ. Carpal tunnel syndrome: an evaluation of the provocative diagnostic tests. J Bone Joint Surg Am 1986;68:735–7.
19. Phalen G. The carpal tunnel syndrome: clinical evaluation of 598 hands. Clin Orthop 1972;83:29–40.
20. Tetro AM, Evanoff BA, Hollstien SB, Gelberman RH. A new provocative test for carpal tunnel syndrome: assessment of wrist flexion and nerve compression. J Bone Joint Surg Br 1998;80(3):493–8.
21. Ghavanini MR, Haghighat M. Carpal tunnel syndrome: reappraisal of five clinical tests. Electromyogr Clin Neurophysiol 1998;38:437–41.
22. Yii NW, Elliot D. A study of the dynamic relationship of the lumbrical muscles and the carpal tunnel. J Hand Surg [Br] 1994;19(4):439–43.
23. Eaton CJ, Lister GD. Radial nerve compression. Hand Clin 1992;8:345.
24. Hoppenfeld S. Physical Examination of the Spine and Extremities. 1st ed. Upper Saddle River, NJ: Prentice Hall; 1976.
25. Krivickas L. Lower-extremity nerve injuries. In: Feinberg JH, ed. Peripheral Nerve Injuries in the Athlete. 1st ed. Champaign, IL: Human Kinetics; 2003.
26. Krabak BJ, Jarmain SJ, Prather H. Physical examination of the hip. In: Malanga GA, ed. Musculoskeletal Physical Examination. Philadelphia: Elsevier Mosby; 2006:251–78.
27. Bird PA, Oakley SP, Shnier R, Kirkham BW. Prospective evaluation of magnetic resonance imaging and physical examination findings in patients with greater trochanteric pain syndrome. Arthritis Rheum 2001;44(9):2138–45.
28. Plastaras CT, Rittenberg JD, Rittenberg KE, et al.. Comprehensive functional evaluation of the injured runner. Phys Med Rehabil Clin N Am 2005;16(3):623–49.
29. Solomon J, Nadler SF, Press J. Physical exam of the lumbar spine. In: Malanga GA, ed. Musculoskeletal Physical Examination: An Evidence-based Approach. 1st ed. Philadelphia: Elsevier Mosby; 2006:189–226.
30. Xin SQ, Shang QZ, Fan DH. Significance of the straight leg raise in the diagnosis and clinical evaluation of lower lumbar intervertebral disc protrusion. J Bone Joint Surg 1987;69A:517–22.
31. McCombe PF, Fairbank JC, Cockersole BC, Pynsent PB. Volvo award in clinical sciences: reproducibility of physical signs in low-back pain. Spine 1989;14:908–18.
32. Butler D. Mobilization of the Nervous System. Melbourne: Churchill Livingstone; 1991.
33. Stankovic R, Johnell O, Maly P, Willner S. Use of lumbar extension, slump test, physical and neurological examination in the evaluation of patients with suspected herniated nucleus pulposus: a prospective clinical study. Man Ther 1999;4(1):25–32.
34. Pahor S, Toppenberg R. An investigation of neural tissue involvement in ankle inversion sprains. Man Ther 1996;1:192–7.
35. Estridge MN, Rouhe SA, Johnson NG. The femoral stretching test: a valuable sign in diagnosing upper lumbar disc herniations. J Neurosurg 1982;57(6):813–7.
36. Christodoulides AN. Ipsilateral sciatica on the femoral nerve stretch test is pathognomic of an L4/5 disc protrusion. J Bone Joint Surg 1989;71:88–9.
37. Pace JB, Nagle D. Piriform syndrome. West J Med 1976;124:435–9.
38. Solheim LF, Siewers P, Paus B. The piriformis muscle syndrome: sciatic nerve entrapment treated with section of the piriformis muscle. Acta Orthop Scand 1981;52:73–5.
39. Benson ER, Schutzer SF. Posttraumatic piriformis syndrome: diagnosis and results of operative treatment. J Bone Joint Surg Am 1999;81:941–9.
40. Spurling RG, Scoville WB. Lateral rupture of the cervical intervertral discs: a common cause of shoulder and arm pain. Surg Gynecol Obstet 1944;78:350–8.
41. Bradley JP, Tibone JE, Watkins RG. History, physical examination, and diagnostic tests for neck and upper-extremity problems. In: Watkins RG, ed. The Spine in Sports. St. Louis: Mosby; 1996.
42. Viikari-Juntura E, Porras M, Laasonen EM. Validity of clinical tests in the diagnosis of root compression in cervical disease. Spine 1989;14:253–7.
43. Davidson RI, Dunn EJ, Metzmaker JN. The shoulder abduction tests in diagnosis of radicular pain in cervical extradural compressive monoradiculopathies. Spine 1981;6(5):441–6.
44. Ellenbery M, Honet, JC. Clinical pearls in cervical radiculopathy. Phys Med Rehabil Clin N Am 1996;7: 487–508.
45. Ellenberg M, Honet JC, Treanor WJ. Cervical radiculopathy. Arch Phys Med Rehabil 1994;75:342–52.
46. Malanga G. The diagnosis and treatment of cervical radiculopathy. Med Sci Sports Exerc 1997;29(7S):S236–45.
47. Sandmark H, Nisell R. Validity of five common manual neck provoking tests. Scand J Rehabil Med 1995;27:131–6.
48. Netter F. Atlas of Human Anatomy. 2nd ed. East Hanover, NJ: Novartis; 1997.
49. Moore KL, Dalley AF. Lower limb. In: Moore KL, Dalley AF, eds. Clinically Oriented Anatomy. 4th ed. Philapelphia: Lippincott Williams & Wilkins; 1997: 503–663.
50. Fleischer K. Vascular surgery. In: Blackbourne FK, ed. Advanced Surgical Recall. 1st ed. Philadelphia: Lippincott Williams & Wilkins; 1997:757–843.
51. Swartz M. Textbook of Physical Diagnosis: History and Examination. 3rd ed. Philadelphia: Saunders; 1998.
52. Mangione S. General appearance, facies, and body habitus. In: Mangione S, ed. Physical Diagnosis Secrets. 1st ed. Philadelphia: Hanley & Belfus; 2000:1–16.
54. Andrus A, Malanga, G., Stuart M. Physical examination of the knee. In: Malanga GA, ed. Musculoskeletal Physical Examination. An Evidence-Based Approach. 1st ed. Philadelphia: Elsevier Mosby; 2006:279–314.
55. Marx RG, Bombardier C, Wright JE. What do we know about reliability and validity of physical examination testes used to examine the upper extremity. J Hand Surg [Am] 1999;24(1):185–92.
56. Wright I. The neurovascular syndrome produced by abduction of the arms: the immediate changes produced in 150 normal controls and the effects on some persons of prolonged hyperabduction of the arms as in sleeping and some occupations. Am Heart J 1945;29:1–19.
57. Roos D. Congenital anomalies associated with thoracic outlet syndrome: anatomy, symptoms, diagnosis, and treatment. Am J Surg 1976; 132:771–8.
58. Mangione S. The extremities. In: Mangione S, ed. Physical Diagnosis Secrets. 1st ed. Philadelphia: Hanley & Belfus; 2000:479–93.

Chapter 5
Athletic Kinetic Chain Concepts in Nerve and Vascular Injuries

Mark A. Harrast and Nayna Patel

The kinetic chain concept originated in 1955 when Stendler described human kinesiology in terms of closed kinematic links.[1] In this theory, body segments are considered rigid, overlapping segments in series connected by movable joints. With this conceptual framework, Stendler noted differences in muscular recruitment patterns and joint motions when the distal segment (foot or hand) is fixed compared to when it is freely movable. In the closed chain (distal segment fixed), the movement of one joint is typical and thus predictable based on the movement of the other joints in series.

Clinically, closed kinetic chain rehabilitation began during the 1980s with new rehabilitation protocols after anterior cruciate ligament (ACL) reconstruction. Soon, kinetic chain assessment and rehabilitation/treatment programs were employed for many musculotendinous injuries, particularly in the athletic patient population. Although much of the biomechanical and clinical literature focuses on using kinetic chain rehabilitation for musculotendinous and joint injuries, the concepts are strong and broad enough to be adapted for the rehabilitation of almost any athletic injury, including neurovascular injury. This chapter presents the framework, theory, and practicalities of kinetic chain rehabilitation and assessment strategies and then demonstrates these concepts in the treatment of neurovascular injuries in athletes.

M.A. Harrast (✉)
Department of Rehabilitation Medicine, Department of Orthopaedics and Sports Medicine, University of Washington, Seattle, WA, USA

What is the Kinetic Chain?

The kinetic chain model employs a biomechanical approach to analyzing sporting activities and other complex movement patterns. It depicts the body as a linked system of interdependent segments, typically working in a proximal to distal sequence, to create a desired action at the distal segment.[2,3] An example is a pitcher who needs significant lower limb strength and flexibility as well as core/trunk strength to pitch competitively. The larger proximal musculature of the trunk and lower limbs helps generate enough force to execute a successful pitch. Toyoshima et al. demonstrated that the lower limbs and trunk contribute almost 50% of peak overhead throwing velocity.[4] The substantial forces that are transferred to the more distal segments of the shoulder and arm during pitching leave these segments vulnerable to injury.[5] Thus, the throwing athlete generates most of his or her throwing power through a complex sequence of muscle activation. Activation begins in the lower limb and translates through the hip and trunk into the arm, with eventual release of energy through the fingers and with the ball. Thus, a pitcher's elbow injury may have occurred as a result of overload of the most distal musculature in the kinetic chain (the upper limb in a pitcher) due to underlying core weakness and hip stiffness, resulting in improper throwing mechanics.

This kinetic chain model illustrates the contribution of the entire body during sporting activities rather than focusing on the action of individual segments. Normal, efficient motion and muscle

V. Akuthota, S.A. Herring (eds.), *Nerve and Vascular Injuries in Sports Medicine*,
DOI 10.1007/978-0-387-76600-3_5, © Springer Science+Business Media, LLC 2009

activation of the individual segments that form this kinetic chain occur in a proximal to distal sequence.[2,6] This proximal to distal sequencing must be considered in rehabilitation programs for athletic injury. It is an important sequence of activation as it provides an efficient, effective system to transfer force and produce greater velocity in the distal segement.[7] This is an effective means of energy transfer for most sports that rely on a high velocity force in the distal segment. This distal segment may be the hand of a pitcher or swimmer or the foot of a soccer player or runner.

General kinetic chain sequencing has been described for many sports. These sequences represent general patterns that are reproducible for the activity of the sport.[8–11] Table 5.1 lists the kinetic chain patterns of common sports.

tissue diagnosis is generally the easy part. It is the pathophysiology of the specific injured tissue (e.g., supraspinatus tendinopathy). The biomechanical diagnosis is formulated by understanding the athlete's specific functional anatomy and movement patterns that may be contributing to biomechanical "faults," creating stress on the specific tissue that eventually creates injury to that tissue. For example, a pitcher with dorsiflexion restriction has poor follow-through, which in turn creates more torque at the shoulder girdle (and rotator cuff).

Formulating a biomechanical diagnosis entails a thorough functional kinetic chain assessment. Evaluating the kinetic chain involves observing the athlete stationary and then functionally performing his or her sport. This entails evaluating the most proximal segment (in many land-based sports this is the

Table 5.1 Kinetic chain patterns in sports

Running: ground → leg → hip/trunk → opposite leg → ground
Kicking: ground → plant leg → trunk/opposite hip → kick leg → ball
Pitching: ground → leg → hip/trunk/opposite leg → shoulder → arm
Serving: ground → legs → trunk→shoulder → arm
Swimming: water → hand/wrist → arm/shoulder → trunk/legs → arm → water

Adapted from Kibler WB, Standaert CJ.[11] Copyright Elsevier 2007. Used with permission.

Likewise, the peripheral nervous system is part of the kinetic chain. The peripheral nerves have the capacity to move but also may have several tethering points, which can be common sites of injury. An example of kinetic chain issues within the peripheral nerve system is the *double crush syndrome,* which hypothesizes that a peripheral nerve injury along one site can indirectly lead to injury at another site (e.g., C6 radiculopathy and carpal tunnel syndrome). In sum, peripheral nerves, like muscle or tendon, can be victims of biomechanical issues elsewhere in the kinetic chain.

Kinetic Chain Assessment Techniques

For the clinical assessment of any sports-related injury it is imperative to formulate a biomechanical diagnosis in addition to the tissue diagnosis, particularly in overload or chronic injuries. Making the

foot planted on the ground) first and working upward to the most distal segment through the site of the pathologic/injured tissue. Creating the distinction between a local tissue diagnosis due to a distant tissue alteration promotes a "victim and culprits" approach to the assessment and management of sports-related injuries. This approach necessitates a broad perspective on the pathophysiology of the injured tissue causing symptoms and the biomechanical framework associated with the injury. The "victim" is the specific injured tissue and the "culprits" are the distant alterations in the biomechanical framework causing or exacerbating the tissue injury.[11] Thus, anterior knee pain (patellofemoral pain syndrome), the victim, may be associated with excessive hip internal rotation and femoral adduction and weakness of the gluteus medius, the culprits. An example in the upper limb is lateral epicondylitis secondary to posterior deltoid weakness. Much of this work from a kinetic chain perspective has been demonstrated in musculoskeletal and musculotendinous injuries; however, the same framework can be adapted to neurovascular injuries as well.

Using this approach in the assessment of sports-related injuries allows us to think more broadly in formulating management plans for such injuries. Many times, in particular with overload or chronic injuries, we need to abolish the mindset of just treating the clinical symptoms. It is important to emphasize restoration of function of all the physiologic and biomechanical alterations involved in the injury and not just be concerned about symptom resolution.

The medical history needs to be equally specific and broad. The answers to the typical questions about the specific injury or specific symptoms must be elucidated. However, the medical interviewing scope needs to be broadened to inquire about any previous injury either at the site of the current injury or at a distant site. The history of an athlete with knee pain needs to be questioned about prior ankle, hip, or low back injuries/symptoms as well. When evaluating shoulder pain, the clinician needs to inquire about prior hip, back, and elbow injuries/symptoms. The history then goes further than just determining if a prior injury was present; it should entail an understanding of the treatment and rehabilitation (if any) of the prior injury. It is important to realize that an inadequately rehabilitated prior injury may predispose to recurrent injury (e.g., ankle sprains, many running-related injuries). The runner who was previously immobilized in a walking boot for severe Achilles tendinopathy and then returns to running in a graduated fashion without rehabilitation of the biomechanical factors that may have predisposed him to the initial injury is at risk of creating the same stress that caused the initial overload of his Achilles tendon, creating a cyclical process of biomechanical overload leading to tissue failure.

The physical examination includes the standard peripheral joint and neurovascular examinations with appropriate provocative maneuvers in addition to a subsequent functional examination. The functional examination involves screening maneuvers for distant components of the kinetic chain to highlight any biomechanical faults that become more obvious during functional movement patterns. These screening tests include the following.[12,13]

- Coronal and sagittal standing posture
- Single-leg stability
- Standing—evaluate balance and pelvic and core stability
- Squatting—evaluate pelvic and core stability, hip mobility, femoral control, and knee, ankle, and foot motion
- Reach tests
- Sitting—evaluate lumbar flexibility
- Standing—evaluate balance and core stability
- Repetitive arm elevation and depression—evaluate scapular stability
- Glenohumeral rotation off a stabilized scapula—evaluate glenohumeral mobility

Rehabilitation Using Kinetic Chain Concepts

Once the biomechanical diagnosis is formulated, the tissue diagnosis is confirmed by other diagnostic tests (imaging as needed), and the athlete has been assessed through a functional kinetic chain approach, a treatment program is initiated. Typically, it involves a period of relative rest to allow injured tissue time to begin healing. It also generally involves a rehabilitation program, which entails correcting the biomechanical faults associated with the tissue injury (those that may have contributed to the cause of injury as well as those created by the injury); regaining flexibility, endurance, strength, and power; and eventual functional progression with sport-specific training.

A main component of a rehabilitation program for any athletic injury involves a focus on function. This functional emphasis necessitates knowledge of the sport and specific movement patterns the sport requires. The goal of most athletic rehabilitation is to return the athlete to the activity that caused the initial injury. Functional rehabilitation also requires working knowledge of the kinetic chain approach given the contribution of the underlying biomechanical faults distant to the site of injury to that initial injury. In kinetic chain functional rehabilitation programs, the legs and trunk are integrated into most exercises with the shoulders and arms to reinforce normal movement patterns and reduce the challenge of learning new movements during rehabilitation. The goal of this approach is to rehabilitate the entire neuromuscular system by integrating multiple body segments throughout the process rather than isolating a specific joint and gradually incorporating the rest of the body.[7]

Open Vs. Closed Chain Rehabilitation

Kinetic chain rehabilitation programs have been grouped into open and closed chains. Open kinetic chain activities involve free movement of the distal segment, whereas with closed chain activities the terminal segment is fixed. Open chain activities are also characterized by independence of joint motion (knee flexion is independent of ankle position), primarily concentric muscle contractions, and larger distraction and rotatory forces across the joints involved in the motion. Characteristics of closed chain activities include interdependence of joint motion (knee flexion depends on ankle joint dorsiflexion), and thus motion throughout the chain occurs in a predictable fashion. Initial muscle contractions are primarily eccentric; compressive forces across the joint are greater, which creates more joint stability and less shearing; and finally, closed chain motion in the lower limb is obviously more functional.

Closed kinetic chain (CKC) rehabilitation initially gained prominence in post-ACL reconstruction rehabilitation protocols to safely restore the quadriceps mechanism because cadaveric experiments documented anterior translation with open kinetic chain rehabilitation at knee extension.[14] Since then, CKC rehabilitation has been adapted to many athletic injuries from musculoskeletal to neurovascular injuries.

Principles of Closed Kinetic Chain Training

Understanding CKC function necessitates understanding the biomechanical factors contributing to joint stability as well as neuromuscular activation patterns. CKC exercises stimulate muscular co-contractions, which enhance stability in the weight-bearing position.[15,16] Returning to the example of rehabilitation after ACL reconstruction, CKC activities result in co-contraction of the quadriceps and hamstrings, which in turn reduce anterior shear and protect the ACL graft; thus co-contraction facilitates joint stability.

Biomechanical Factors

Biomechanically, CKC techniques emphasize the sequential movement and placement of functionally related joints and therefore require coordinated and sequential muscle activation patterns to control proper joint movement.[13] A primary principle of CKC function is that foot and ankle motion influences knee, hip, and pelvic motion and vice versa. Therefore, initiation of exercise in one segment of the kinetic chain results in predictable movements of the other segments. When analyzing kinetic chain motion, one can take a "bottom-up" approach or a "top-down" approach depending on the clinical scenario.

Understanding the influence of foot and ankle mechanics on the entire kinetic chain, as a "bottom-up" approach, is essential for accurate CKC rehabilitation prescription.[17] Pronation at the subtalar joint produces calcaneal eversion as well as talar plantar flexion and adduction. As the talus plantar flexes and adducts, tibial internal rotation ensues, resulting in knee flexion and genu valgum. This valgus moment at the knee encourages femoral adduction and internal rotation as the hip initiates flexion. With this tibial and femoral internal rotation, the pelvis also moves into internal rotation and an anterior tilt. For upright stability, the lumbar spine must extend and counter-rotate.

With this knowledge of kinetic chain motion, an example of posterior tibial tendonitis in a patient with obvious genu valgum can be analyzed from both the "bottom-up" and "top-down" approaches. Starting at the bottom, the culprit may be poor foot mechanics, anatomically or functionally, with excessive subtalar pronation during mid-stance, creating excessive forces up the kinetic chain as previously described. Evaluating this athlete from the top, the main causative issue may be at the hip girdle with gluteus medius weakness or inhibition allowing excessive femoral adduction and internal rotation, which sequentially produces increased tibial internal rotation and eventually increased subtalar pronation, increasing stress on the posterior tibialis tendon. The treating clinician may prescribe foot mobilization and in-shoe orthoses in one instance or prescribe a focus on core and hip girdle neuromuscular retraining and strengthening in the other instance.

Neurophysiologic Factors

Closed kinetic chain activities stimulate the proprioceptive system by emphasizing proprioceptive feedback to initiate and control muscle activation patterns.[18] Enhanced proprioception is especially important in athletic rehabilitation for injury prevention and performance.

Closed chain rehabilitation techniques facilitate functional restoration by reproducing patterned motions that, with continued practice, require less cognitive awareness so they become automatic and are performed with ease. Using functional CKC exercise enhances the nervous system's ability to recruit groups of muscles to work together.[17] This form of neuromuscular reeducation is an important step in any rehabilitation program, particularly for those athletes who have chronic overuse injuries with dysfunctional muscle activation patterns due to dysfunctional sustained postures and habitual movement patterns.

In summary, CKC rehabilitation is a key component of any athletic functional restoration program. Restoring appropriate athletic function requires a return of optimal biomechanical motions and neurophysiological muscle activation patterns. CKC training can replicate the imposed demands of sports to facilitate more natural muscular recruitment patterns and provide appropriate joint stability with the goal of decreasing stress on the injured tissue, preventing further injury or reinjury, and optimizing performance.

Neuromobilization

Neuromobilization is a technique used by clinicians as part of the nonsurgical treatment of peripheral nerve lesions. Butler and others have been advocates of gliding components of the peripheral nerve system to reduce scarring of nerves and to stretch surrounding soft tissue.[19] Whereas nerve stretching to end range may cause peripheral nerve injury, nerve glides (often akin to flossing) and nerve mobilization (avoiding end range) are thought to help with nerve healing and reducing nerve pain. Neuromobilization has been incorporated into rehabilitation of radiculopathies (particularly after lumbar surgery) as well as physical/occupational therapy treatment of carpal tunnel syndrome.[20,21] Athletes with various peripheral nerve injuries may benefit from neuromobilization, although limited evidence exists for its efficacy.

Case Scenarios

Sarah

Sarah is a 21-year-old undergraduate varsity swimmer with complaints of achy right shoulder pain with numbness and tingling along the medial aspect of the arm, forearm, and into the small finger.

Thoracic outlet syndrome (TOS) is a constellation of disorders that is related to compression or traction of neurovascular structures (brachial plexus 95%; subclavian vein 4%; subclavian artery 1%)[22] in the passageways located between the neck and axilla. The most proximal passageway is the interscalene triangle, which is bordered by the anterior scalene muscle anteriorly, the middle scalene muscle posteriorly, and the medial surface of the first rib inferiorly. The already small passageway can be further narrowed by fibrous bands, anomalous muscles, large transverse processes at C7, or a cervical rib. Entrapment underneath the pectoralis minor muscle can occur. Repetitive trauma and repetitive maneuvers are also implicated in the pathogenesis of TOS.[23]

Although the causes of TOS are diverse, pain is a common complaint. Pain can be located in the neck, shoulder, arm, forearm, wrist, and/or hand. Patients may experience paresthesias along the distribution of the ulnar nerve, as the lower trunk or medial cord of the brachial plexus is compressed in the axilla. A heavy sensation or coldness may be described. In more advanced cases, patients may exhibit loss of dexterity. Physical examination findings include a positive Roos or Adson test. Hand intrinsic muscle weakness and sensory deficits in the C8–T1 dermatomes may be present.

A review of TOS in the setting of the kinetic chain is important for several reasons. First, many biomechanical deficits exist in patients with TOS. Faulty upper body posture contributes to mechanical dysfunction seen in TOS. Inflexibility of anterior musculature (e.g., pectoralis minor and sternocleidomastoid muscles) contribute to compression and symptoms as well. First rib and upper thoracic dysfunction may aggravate compression of neurovascular structures. Scapular dyskinesis places abnormal loads on the rotator cuff and anterior chest wall muscles.[13] Second, conservative management of TOS should be the goal of treatment, as pain relief with surgical options are rarely a certainty and complications after surgery may be severe. For these reasons, a well designed conservative approach with evaluation of the kinetic chain is imperative for management of TOS.

A good rehabilitation program begins with basic rehabilitation principles. During the acute phase, the emphasis of rehabilitation should be on pain control through general modalities and overall flexibility.[24] Taping the scapula in an elevated position can reduce traction on the brachial plexus as well. Nerve gliding may be useful.

At first glance, rehabilitation of the swimmer's shoulder may appear to be an open kinetic chain issue, but Kibler argued well that the scapula and shoulder function in a CKC fashion.[13] Movements of the shoulder and scapula are coupled based on specific arm position. Strengthening the scapular stabilizing muscles, especially the serratus anterior and trapezius, is important to hold the scapula in more upward rotation. For this reason, rehabilitation of TOS in the swimmer should begin with CKC exercises, which provide greater proprioceptive feedback and protect joints via co-contraction, as previously described. Examples include clock exercises and modified press-ups,[13] which create scapular control without glenohumeral shear. Once appropriate scapular stability is obtained, the rotator cuff muscles can be strengthened via open chain exercises.

Correct muscle length is important for obtaining adequate scapular control. The posterior capsule, infraspinatous, and teres minor can contribute to scapular tilting and scapular protraction especially when the glenohumeral joint is internally rotated at 90°.[7]

A tight posterior capsule can be addressed through myofascial release and stretching. Stretching the upper trapezius, scalene, sternocleidomastoid, levator scapulae, and pectoral muscles should be incorporated in a rehabilitation program to improve muscle length. Activation of the scalene muscles has been shown to improve first rib dysfunction, decreasing compression of neurovascular structures.

The achievement of correct cervical spine posture, with head in a neutral position relative to the neck, is also important in the treatment of any patient with TOS. Diaphragmatic breathing activates the scalene and pectoralis minor muscles, elevating the first rib and pulling the scapula and thus the clavicle closer to the first rib, thereby reducing compression on the neurovascular plexus in the thoracic outlet. Good core strength and hip extension as well as flexibility in the lower extremities should also be incorporated into the rehabilitation program.[7,11,17]

Matthew

Matthew is a 24-year-old professional pitcher with complaints of elbow discomfort and numbness and tingling in the small and ring fingers.

Much of the force generated in anticipation of throwing a ball is absorbed at the medial aspect of the elbow. Overuse injuries at the elbow, including medial epicondylitis and avulsion fractures of the medial epicondyle, have been well described. In addition, throwing athletes can experience neurovascular injuries in the upper extremity secondary to the large transition of these forces. Ulnar neuropathy at the elbow, or cubital tunnel syndrome, is one example.

Injury to the ulnar nerve occurs via friction and volar subluxation of the ulnar nerve as it passes through the cubital tunnel.[25] Compression of the nerve or longitudinal traction results in ischemia.

Biomechanical factors associated with cubital tunnel syndrome are prolonged and/or repeated elbow flexion, which may compress or cause traction of the ulnar nerve. Cubital tunnel pressure has been shown to increase[26] as the elbow moves from an extended to a flexed position. Athletes, such as pitchers who repeatedly flex and extend the elbow, are at higher risk for cubital tunnel syndrome.

Athletes with cubital tunnel syndrome frequently experience pain and paresthesias at the small finger and medial aspect of the ring finger as well as the ulnar aspect of the hand. As the lesion is proximal to the takeoff of the dorsal ulnar cutaneous nerve, the dorsal hand is also affected. This is in contrast to ulnar neuropathy at Guyon's canal, which spares the dorsal ulnar cutaneous nerve. Patients may complain of the inability to put their small finger in their pocket and have a positive Wartenberg sign. Medial elbow pain is common. On examination, patients can have decreased sensation in the above dermatomal distribution. Weakness of the ulnar-innervated interossei is common and can result in claw hand if severe. Weakness of the more proximal ulnar innervated muscles—flexor digitorum profundus and flexor carpi ulnaris—is variable secondary to the less superficial location of these motor axons in the ulnar nerve as it crosses the elbow.[27] Patients may have a positive Finkelstein sign, indicating interossei weakness. Percussion over the cubital tunnel may yield a positive Tinel sign.

The rehabilitation of cubital tunnel syndrome begins with decreasing the compression or traction of the ulnar nerve. Protection of the cubital tunnel with an elbow pad or elbow orthosis to hold the elbow in 40°–60° of elbow flexion may help achieve this goal. Nerve gliding has been described as well and may be helpful in certain individuals.[28] Ergonomic evaluation may be indicated to evaluate for awkward postures that place stress on the ulnar nerve.

Beginning proximally, attention should again be paid to scapular control and glenohumeral stability, as shoulder and scapular stability are vital to the throwing athlete. The shoulder and scapula act in concert, coupling movements during throwing. The glenohumeral joint helps channel the forces generated by the trunk and lower extremity to the throwing arm.[7,13] Scapular retraction with control of scapular elevation and protraction is the primary goal. CKC exercises help develop proprioception, which is important for controlling the muscle patterns of co-contraction.

Stretching anterior thoracic wall muscles (e.g., pectoralis minor) is also important in these athletes. Glenohumeral internal rotation is often deficient in these athletes and can be addressed by the sleeper's stretch (Fig. 5.1). Postural exercises to correct any thoracic kyphosis is necessary to facilitate appropriate scapulothoracic and scapulohumeral rhythm.

As it is important to create a stable base, hip and trunk control over the planted leg is also vital in overall athletic performance. Poor posture should be addressed. Core and gluteal muscles should be strengthened as the forces involved in throwing are generated from them.

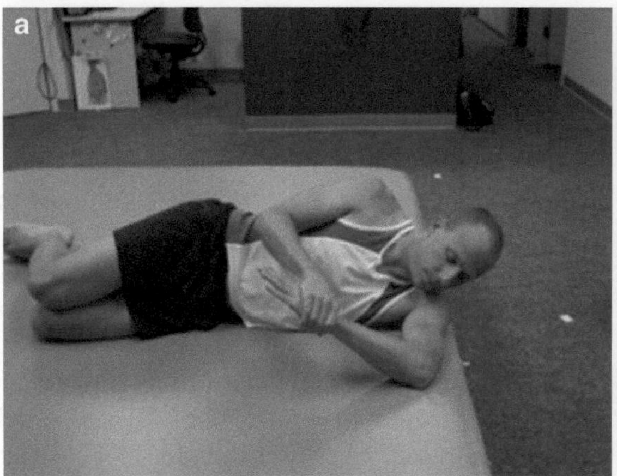

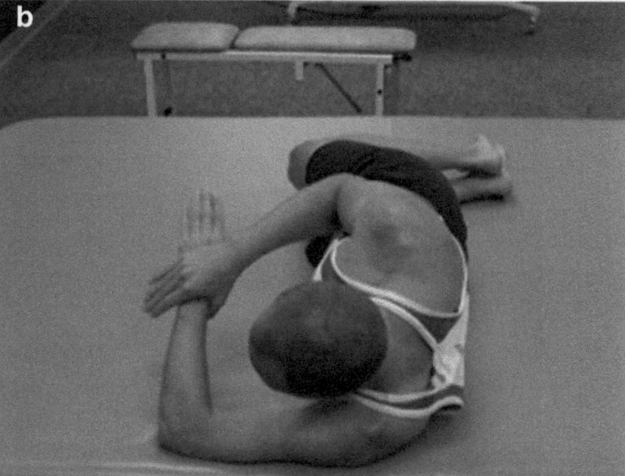

Fig. 5.1 Posterior capsule stretching with a stabilized scapula to improve glenohumeral internal rotation

More distally, attention should be paid to avoid aggressive elbow flexion, thus tractioning the ulnar nerve. The most distal sites of the kinetic chain can be addressed via strengthening the wrist and finger flexors and extensors, as well as the intrinsic musculature. An eccentric strengthening approach also addresses overuse injuries (e.g., medial epicondylitis) that are endemic in this population.

As athletes progress in their rehabilitation program, shoulder flexibility and strength should continue to be addressed, focusing on internal rotation range of motion and external rotation and scapular strength. Plyometrics and agility training should be added to a rehabilitation program to help prevent future injuries and achieve explosiveness in the athlete's specific sport. Modalities such as ice, heat, and ultrasound are usually not necessary, as little tissue change is expected during this period of time.

Jennifer

Jennifer is 17-year-old ballet dancer with medial ankle and foot pain and paresthesias along the plantar aspect of the foot.

Tarsal tunnel syndrome (TTS) is a condition that involves entrapment of the tibial nerve as it passes through the fibroosseus tunnel that lies posterior to the medial malleolus. The roof of the tarsal tunnel is the flexor retinaculum. The tibia forms the anterior border, and the calcaneus forms the lateral border. The tendons of the posterior tibialis, flexor digitorum longus, and flexor hallucis longus and the tibial artery and vein run through the tarsal tunnel as well. The tibial nerve is susceptible to injury because of the limited space within the tunnel. Both extrinsic factors (e.g., tight shoes and casts) and intrinsic factors (e.g., ganglion cysts and tenosynovitis) can be culprits in the development of TTS.[29] Activities such as running, dancing, and mountain climbing can predispose patients to the development of TTS.

Patients with TTS may present with vague symptoms. Paresthesias along the plantar aspect of the foot are frequent. Numbness in this distribution or along the medial heel is often present as well. Patients may complain of sharp, shooting pain in the medial heel radiating toward the foot. Cramps and achy sensation can occur. Walking and sports tend to aggravate these symptoms, and patients may complain of night pain as the syndrome progresses. Tenderness may be felt posterior and inferior to the medial malleoulus, and a Tinel sign may be present. Intrinsic foot weakness as well as sensory disturbances are variable depending on the degree of neuronal damage.

Biomechanical abnormalities can be observed in athletes with TTS. Overpronation places mechanical stretch on the tibial nerve in the tarsal tunnel. Excessive squatting associated with dorsiflexion may also predispose to the development of TTS. When examined, other deficiencies in the kinetic chain—e.g., poor core and trunk stability, poor femoral control, excessive knee valgus—may also be found. Poor femoral control may cause knee valgus, resulting in compensatory subtalar pronation. These biomechanical deficits should be addressed in the rehabilitation program.

A rehabilitation program for TTS begins with cessation of the activities that exacerbate the pain. A medial heel or sole wedge can help prevent excessive pronation. Taping and bracing has been described. Night splinting allows immobilization of the ankle to decrease tarsal tunnel pressures.[30]

Beginning at the site of pathology, muscle strength deficiencies and adequate flexibility of the forefoot and midfoot should be attained. Foot and ankle exercises help decrease edema within the tarsal tunnel and relieve compression of the posterior tibial nerve.[31] Specifically, the gastrocnemius and soleus muscles should be stretched, as they are often sites of inflexibility in dancers and can lead to overpronation. Insufficient tibialis posterior muscles should be strengthened.

The treatment of TTS must not stop at the foot; the entire kinetic chain must be addressed. Evaluating the knee and obtaining adequate femoral control are vital when treating TTS. Pronation of the subtalar joint results in obligatory tibial internal rotation,[32] which is followed by internal rotation and adduction of the femur and pelvis.[17] A kinetic chain rehabilitation program for TTS should focus on lateral hip rotators, gluteus medius, and gluteus maximus strength to control femoral and pelvic internal rotation. Specific examples include clam shell exercises and band walking (Fig. 5.2). Athletes can challenge the gluteal musculature with lunges in

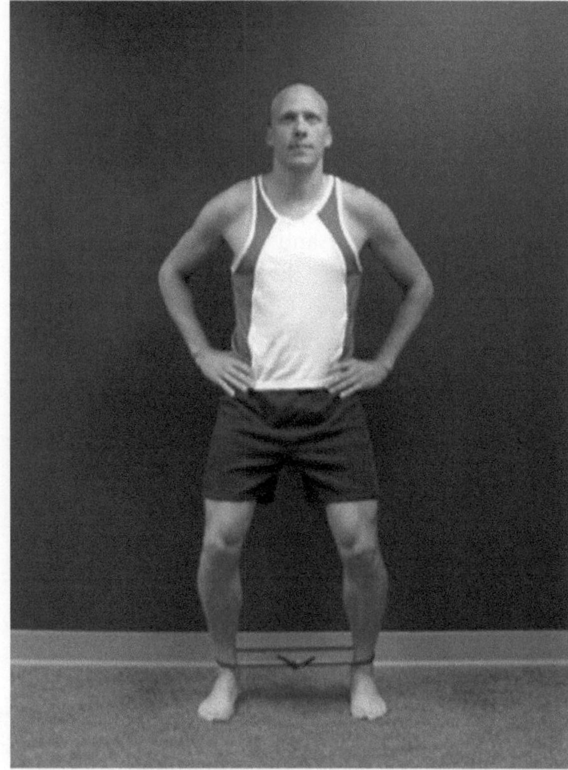

Fig. 5.2 Band walking for functional hip abductor strength

several planes of motion (Fig. 5.3). Appropriate femoral control can eliminate knee valgus, resulting in tibial external rotation and a more neutral or supinated position at the subtalar joint, thereby preventing compression of the tibial nerve in the tarsal tunnel.[17]

For continued functional progression to specific sports, the dancer should continue to work on overall conditioning of the kinetic chain, focusing on core strength and proper femoral control via hip girdle strengthening. General flexibility of the lower extremities, including the hamstrings and gastrocnemius, should be maintained. Plyometric training helps dancers regain explosiveness in their sport.

Evan

Evan is a 35-year-old recreational runner experiencing aching in the bilateral shins and tingling sensation in the web space between the first and second digits.

Chronic exertional compartment syndrome (CECS) is a cause of leg pain that results from elevated pressures within the fibroosseous compartments of the lower limbs. The most common compartment to be affected is the anterior compartment, which houses the tibialis anterior, extensor hallicus longus, extensor digitorum longus, and peroneus tertius muscles as well as the anterior tibial artery and vein and the deep fibular nerve. Although not the most common cause of leg pain in the athlete, chronic anterior compartment

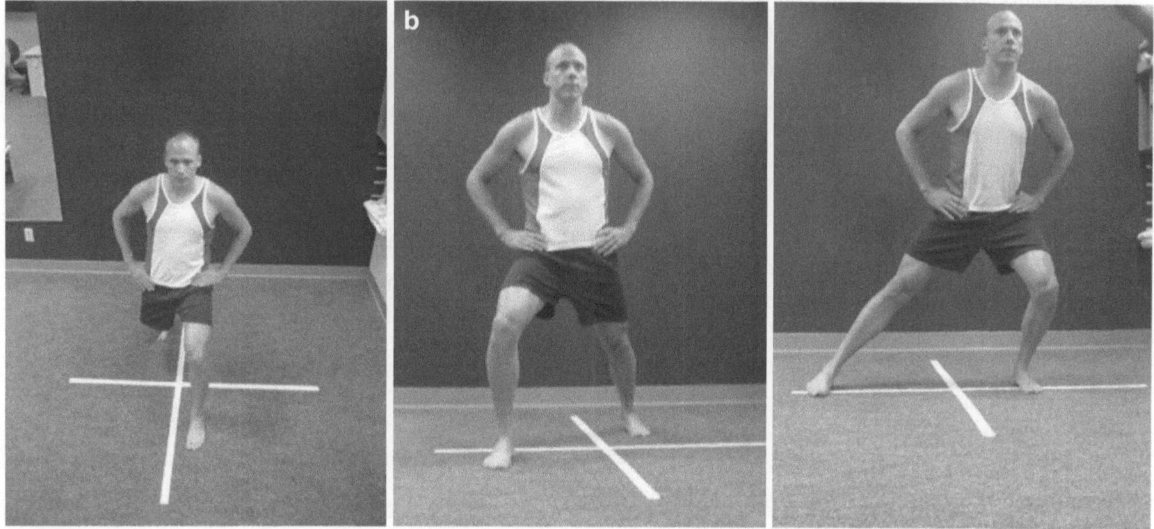

Fig. 5.3 Lunges in several planes of motion for gluteal strength (**a**) Standard lunge. (**b**) Diagonal lunge. (**c**) Side lunge

syndrome is implicated in 15%–33% of patients with exercise-induced leg pain.[33–35]

The hallmark of CECS is exercise-induced pain that is absent at rest. Athletes are usually involved in sports that involve a significant amount of running. Patients tend to describe the onset of pain after running a specific distance or within a certain time period, usually less than 30 minutes. As exercise continues, patients experience worsening pain that can be burning, aching, or cramping in the involved compartment. Radiation of pain to the foot may be present, as may associated muscle weakness and paresthesias. Termination of the activity results in cessation of the pain.

The physical examination of the patient at rest with CECS is usually unremarkable. At times, the involved compartment of the leg may appear brawny, or "woody," but the incidence of this appearance is variable. All patients with possible CECS should be examined after the specific exercise that provoked the symptoms whenever possible. After exercise, a firm compartment that is tender to palpation or with passive motion is evident. Fascial hernias are present in approximately half of all patients.[33] The neurologic examination can reveal weakness and paresthesias corresponding to the involved compartment. Patients with an anterior compartment syndrome may display weakness in dorsiflexion or decreased extensor hallucis longus strength. Paresthesias may be elicited between the first and second toes. A definitive diagnosis of CECS usually requires measurement of intracompartmental pressures.

The discussion of CECS in terms of the kinetic chain is important. Unless mild, CECS is often quite disabling, and athletes are often unable to participate in their sport.[34] Little attention is given to conservative management of CECS in the literature, and surgical options are often advocated prior to a trial of conservative therapy.[35] For some patients, a trial of rehabilitation is reasonable.

A rehabilitation program for CECS begins with relative rest and education. For most patients, cessation of the provocative activity for a period of time is mandatory. General aerobic activity can be maintained via open chain exercises, cycling, and deep water running. The terrain, type of athletic shoe, and training schedule should be addressed. Gentle stretching of the lower limb should be implemented to maintain overall flexibility, as should strengthening of weak muscles in the leg.

Decreased shock absorption in a supinated foot is well described in the literature.[17] It is reasonable to consider a rigid, supinated foot as a risk factor in the development of CECS, as the supinated foot is ill-equipped to absorb shock. Shock must then be absorbed in the lower leg. Subtalar supination results in compensatory tibial external rotation, which causes femoral and pelvic external rotation and abduction.[17] Thus, the kinetic chain approach to the rehabilitation to CECS can be similar, yet opposite to, the rehabilitation of TTS. Subtalar flexibility should be addressed but with the goal of obtaining subtalar neutral or subtalar pronation. Similarly, tibial and femoral control should be addressed. For CECS, rehabilitation should focus on increasing tibial internal rotation, femoral and pelvic internal rotation, and adduction.

The return to sport should be accomplished in a controlled, paced manner. Increased duration and intensity can be added as the athlete progresses. Continued flexibility and strength training should not be overlooked at this level. Plyometric training can help athletes maintain explosiveness while decreasing the incidence of overuse injury.

Summary

The rehabilitation of nerve and vascular injuries in athletes in many cases can be equated to the rehabilitation of musculoskeletal injuries in the same population. A kinetic chain approach can be used for both evaluation and rehabilitation, as the site of pathology and symptoms is typically distant from the actual culprit. The pathologic site is important and usually easy to delineate. However, the typically distant biomechanical deficits contributing to that pathology are even more important to discern in order to identify the targets of rehabilitation, successfully treat the symptoms, and return the athlete to his or her sport.

References

1. Steindler A. Kinesiology of the Human Body. Springfield, IL: Charles C Thomas; 1955.
2. Putman CA. Sequential motions of body segments in striking and throwing skills: description and explanations. J Biomechanics 1993;26:125–35.

3. Feltner ME, Dapena J. Three dimensional interactions in a two segment kinetic chain. Part I: General model. Int J Sport Biomech 1989;5:403–19.
4. Toyoshima S, Hoshikawa T, Miyashita M, et al. Contribution of the body parts to throwing performance. In: Biomechanics IV. Baltimore: University Park Press; 1974:169–74.
5. Fleisig GS, Barrentine SW, Escamilla RF, Andrews JR. Biomechanics of overhead throwing with implications for injury. Sports Med 1996;21:421–37.
6. Zattara M, Bouisset S. Posturo-kinetic organization during the early phase of voluntary upper limb movement. 1: Normal subjects. J Neurosurg Psychiatry 1988;51: 956–65.
7. McMullen J, Uhl TL. A kinetic chain approach for shoulder rehabilitation. J Athl Train 2000;35:329–37.
8. Hirashima M, Kadota H, Sakurai S, et al. Sequential muscle activity and its functional role in the upper extremity and trunk during overhead throwing. J Sports Sci 2002;20:301–10.
9. Marshall RN, Elliott BC. Long axis rotation: the missing link in proximal to distal segmental sequencing. J Sports Sci 2000;18:247–54.
10. Elliot B, Marshall R, Noffal G. The role of upper limb segment rotations in the development of racket head speed in the squash forehand. J Sports Sci 1996;14: 159–65.
11. Kibler WB, Standaert CJ. Functional restoration: return to training and competition. In: Frontera WR, Herring SA, Micheli LJ, Silver JK, eds. Clinical Sports Medicine: Medical Management and Rehabilitation. Philadelphia: Saunders; 2007:273–83.
12. Kibler WB, Livingston B. Closed kinetic chain rehabilitation for upper and lower extremities. J Am Acad Orthop Surg 2001;9:412–21.
13. Kibler WB. Closed kinetic chain rehabilitation for sports injuries. Phys Med Rehabil Clin N Am 2000;11:369–84.
14. Grood ES, Suntay WT, Noyes FR, Butler DL. Biomechanics of the knee-extension exercise: effect of cutting the ACL. J Bone Joint Surg Am 1984;66:725–34.
15. Wilk KE, Naiquan Z, Glenn SF, et al. Kinetic chain exercise: implications for the anterior cruciate ligament patient. J Sport Rehabil 1997;6:125–40.
16. Arms SW, Pope MH, Johnson RJ, et al. The biomechanics of the anterior cruciate ligament rehabilitation and reconstruction. Am J Sports Med 1984;12:8–18.
17. Lefever SL. Closed kinetic chain training. In: Hall CM, Brody LT, eds. Therapeutic Exercise: Moving Toward Function. Philadelphia: Lippincott Williams & Wilkins/ Walters Kluwer; 2005:283–307.
18. Hunt GC. Peripheral nerve biomechanics: application to neuromobilization approaches. Phys Ther Rev 2002; 7(2):111–21.
19. Butler D. Mobilisation of the Nervous System. Melbourne: Churchill Livingstone; 1991.
20. Kostopoulos D. Treatment of carpal tunnel syndrome: a review of the non-surgical approaches with emphasis in neural mobilization. J Bodyw Mov Ther 2004;8(1):2–8.
21. Devita P, Hortobagyi T, Barrier J. Gait biomechanics are not normal after ACL reconstruction and accelerated rehabilitation. Med Sci Sports Exerc 1998;30:1481–8.
22. Sanders RJ, Hammond SL, Rao NM. Diagnosis of thoracic outlet syndrome. J Vasc Surg 2007;46(3):601–4.
23. Kenal LA, Knapp LD. Rehabilitation of injuries in competitive swimmers. Sports Med 1996;22:337–4.
24. Lindgren KA. Conservative treatment of thoracic outlet syndrome: a 2-year follow-up. Arch Phys Med Rehabil 1997;78:373–8.
25. Aoki M, Takasaki H, Muraki T, et al. Strain on the ulnar nerve at the elbow and wrist during throwing motion. J Bone Joint Surg Am 2005;87:2508–14.
26. Wright TW, Glowczewskie F, Cowin D, Wheler DL. Ulnar nerve excursion and strain at the elbow and wrist associated with upper extremity motion. J Hand Surg [Am] 2001;26:655–62.
27. Kincaid JC. AAEE Minimonograph #31: the electrodiagnosis of ulnar neuropathy at the elbow. Muscle Nerve 1988;11(10):1005–15.
28. Akalin E, El O, Peker O, et al. Treatment of carpal tunnel syndrome with nerve and tendon gliding exercises. Am J Phys Med Rehabil 2002;81:108–13.
29. Kinoshita M, Okuda R, Abe M. Tarsal tunnel syndrome in athletes. Am J Sports Med 2006;34:1307–12.
30. Trepman E, Kadel NJ, Chisholm K, Razzano L. Effect of foot and ankle position on tarsal tunnel compartment pressure. Foot Ankle Int 1999;20:721–6.
31. Kibler WB, Herring SA, Press JM. Functional Rehabilitation of Sports and Musculoskeletal Injuries. Gaithersburg, MD: Aspen; 1998.
32. Sherman KP. The foot in sport. Br J Sports Med 1999; 33:6–13.
33. Touliopolous S, Hershman EB. Lower leg pain: diagnosis and treatment of compartment syndromes and other pain syndromes of the leg. Sports Med 1999;27:193–204.
34. Bong MR, Polatsch DB, Jazrawi LM, Rokito AS. Chronic exertional compartment syndrome: diagnosis and management. Bull Hosp Joint Dis 2005;62:77–84.
35. Blackman PG. A review of chronic exertional compartment syndrome in the lower leg. Med Sci Sports Exerc 2000;32:S4–10.

Part II
Upper Limb Syndromes

Chapter 6
Peripheral Nerve Injuries of the Elbow, Forearm, and Hand

Jacqueline J. Wertsch and Anne Zeni Hoch

Upper limb peripheral nerve problems are seen in both the "couch potato" and the athlete. Nerves are vulnerable to stretch, angulation, direct or indirect trauma, or chronic irritation from overuse or overload.[1] Nerve problems in the elbow, forearm, wrist, and hand region are not that surprising considering the complex biomechanics of the upper limb. There is increasing understanding of the importance of nerve movement during upper limb range of motion, which can involve various amounts of elbow flexion/extension, forearm pronation/supination, wrist ulnar/radial deviation, wrist flexion/extension, and finger movements. In addition to the complex movements that can occur in the distal upper limb, there are also many muscles with complex fascial structures. In view of the high level of muscular activity in the athlete, it is surprising that peripheral nerve injuries are reportedly relatively uncommon.[2] This chapter reviews peripheral nerve injuries and entrapments that have been recognized in the elbow, forearm, and hand for both athlete and nonathlete.

Median Nerve Syndromes

The median nerve contains nerve fibers from C5 to T1 spinal nerves with contributions from upper, middle, and lower trunks of the brachial plexus.[3] The most widely known median nerve problem is carpal tunnel syndrome (CTS). Because CTS is so commonly known, many are quick to assume that any numbness or weakness in the thumb or index finger is due to CTS.[4] Other potential sites of median nerve problems must be considered starting proximally from the neck level all the way distally to the hand (Fig. 6.1). Potential sites of nerve injury or entrapment in the neck or shoulder region are being covered in other chapters.

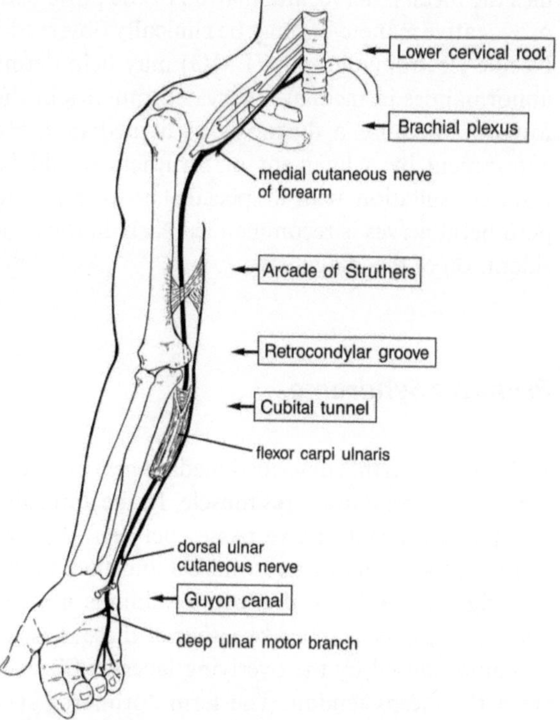

Fig. 6.1 Sites of entrapment for the median nerve

J.J. Wertsch (✉)
Department of Physical Medicine and Rehabilitation,
Medical College of Wisconsin, Milwaukee, WI, USA

V. Akuthota, S.A. Herring (eds.), *Nerve and Vascular Injuries in Sports Medicine*,
DOI 10.1007/978-0-387-76600-3_6, © Springer Science+Business Media, LLC 2009

In the antecubital region the most widely recognized anatomic sites of potential median nerve entrapment include the ligament of Struthers, lacertus fibrosus, pronator teres muscle, and sublimis arch of the flexor digitorum superficialis muscles.[4]

Ligament of Struthers

The ligament of Struthers is a rare anatomic structure, being noted in only 1% of upper limbs.[3] This ligament has been described as extending from an anomalous humeral bony spur to the medial epicondyle. The bony spur cannot always be seen on radiographs.[5] Most individuals who have a ligament of Struthers are asymptomatic, and median nerve compromise occurs only with some other contributing factor or trauma.[3,5–9] Diagnosis can be difficult. The patient may complain of pain in the wrist or medial forearm and paresthesias in the index or long finger.[5,10,11] The pain may be exacerbated with full extension of the elbow or supination of the forearm such as the follow-through phase of pitching.[9,11] Because the brachial artery accompanies the median nerve, attenuation of the pulse with provocative maneuvers may be clinically observed.[4] Needle electromyography (EMG) may help define abnormalities in median-innervated muscles in the forearm. Because a diagnosis of a median nerve entrapment by a ligament of Struthers would be rare, consultation with a specialist in upper limb peripheral nerves is recommended early in the consideration of this diagnosis.

Pronator Syndrome

In 1951, Seyffarth[12] described median nerve entrapment by the pronator teres muscle. In the antecubital area the median nerve passes between the two heads of the pronator teres muscle and then under the edge of the flexor digitorum sublimis muscle. The nerve can be trapped by either of these muscles or compromised by the overlying lacertus fibrosus from the biceps tendon. The term "pronator syndrome" has been used by many for a clinical picture of diffuse forearm pain and paresthesia in the distal median nerve distribution.[13] Unfortunately, variations in symptoms and signs are common,[14] and surgical outcomes are not convincing that the anatomic problem is the static relation of the median nerve and the pronator teres muscle.[15,16] Other structures in the area (e.g., lacertus fibrosus and sublimis arch of the flexor digitorum superficialis muscles) need to also be considered in the presence of antecubital median nerve problems.[16] Even an aberrant fibrous component of the flexor carpi radialis originating from the ulna can compromise the median nerve at this level.[7] Physical examination maneuvers to detect the pronator syndrome described by Spinner are discussed in a previous chapter.

Axonal changes should be evident on needle EMG if there is median nerve entrapment. A clear diagnosis of proximal forearm median nerve entrapment would then be preferred over the term nonspecific pronator syndrome. Other causes of proximal forearm symptoms (e.g., focal muscle or fascia injuries) should be specifically diagnosed and not lumped together as pronator syndrome. Use of the term pronator syndrome is discouraged in favor of a specific diagnosis including possible dynamic conditions in which the nerve is compressed only during sports activities. Clarity of diagnosis helps to guide management. In the athlete with possible dynamic proximal forearm median nerve compression, technique modification may be helpful along with rest and splinting.[13] This syndrome is seen in sports that require repetitive, forceful pronation and gripping.[17,18] Most commonly seen in throwers, pronator syndrome has been reported in weightlifting, archery, tennis, arm wrestling, and rowing.[19,20]

Anterior Interosseous Nerve

The anterior interosseous nerve (AIN), the largest branch of the median nerve, arises from the median nerve soon after it passes between the two heads of the pronator teres and under the flexor digitorum sublimis muscle. The AIN innervates three forearm muscles: the flexor pollicis longus, the radial part of the flexor digitorum profundus, and the pronator quadratus. Because the AIN does not have any cutaneous representation, it is often considered to be a pure motor nerve. This is technically not true because sensory fibers from the wrist radiocarpal, radioulnar, intercarpal, and carpometacarpal joints travel in the AIN.[21,22] Injury to the terminal branch of the AIN can be the source of persistent, dull aching volar wrist pain, which may be diagnosed by local block of the terminal AIN branch.

As early as 1918, Tinel recognized an isolated "neuritis" of the AIN branch of the median nerve.[23] Anterior interosseous nerve syndrome (AINS) was described in 1952 by Kiloh and Nevin.[24] They reported two cases that were spontaneous and recovered without treatment. Fearn and Goodfellow[25] reported the first case of surgically treated AIN with discovery of a fibrous band compressing the AIN in the region of the pronator teres. Although often described in earlier literature as idiopathic and spontaneous, AINS can have many causes including bone injuries, antecubital vascular procedures, metastasis, accessory muscles, and fibrous bands.[23] Consideration should always be given to the possibility of neuralgic amyotrophy or Parsonage Turner syndrome presenting with AIN weakness.[26,27] Careful clinical examination is needed to ensure there are no other sites of muscle weakness, such as serratus anterior scapular winging.

With AINS, the typical history is acute onset of thumb and index finger weakness. The patient may have noted difficulty using a fork, tearing out a check, or picking up a cup. There are no sensory complaints. Clinical examination reveals an inability to flex the terminal phalanges of the thumb and index finger. Because of this weakness, the patient is unable to form an "O" (Fig. 6.2), also called the OK sign. This abnormal pinch is quite constant and characteristic of the anterior interosseous nerve syndrome.[23] AINS can be confirmed on EMG examination. Needle EMG reveals abnormalities in the three muscles supplied by the AIN with normal examination results of other muscles. Sensory nerve conduction studies are normal. Clinical management depends on the etiology of the AINS.

Internal topography is an important issue for the AIN. Fascicular groups remain localized within the median nerve for long distances.[28,29] Because these fascicles are on the posterior aspect, a humeral supracondylar fracture may damage the AIN fibers of the median nerve.[30] Thus, this much

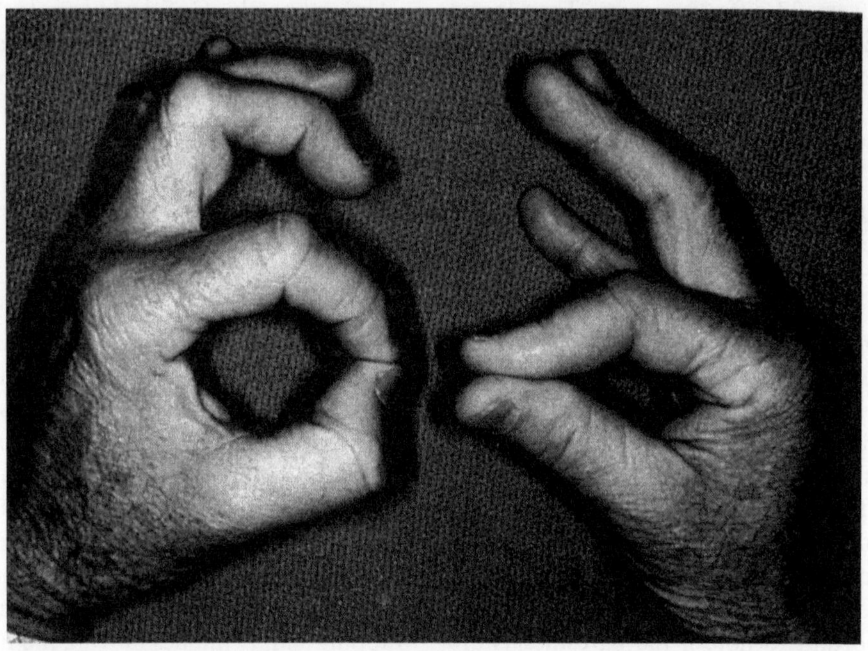

Fig. 6.2 Typical pinch sign with flattening of index pulp and classic palsy of the anterior interosseus nerve. From Plancher et al.[50] Copyright Elsevier 1996. Used with permission

more proximal partial median nerve injury may present just like an AIN problem with weakness confined to anterior interosseous innervated muscles.[31,32] A partial median nerve injury at the antecubital level presenting as pseudo-AINS has been reported.[33]

Carpal Tunnel Syndrome

The most frequently diagnosed peripheral nerve entrapment in the general population is carpal tunnel syndrome (CTS). In the athletic population, some believe that "the proximal forearm is the more usual anatomic location of median nerve impairment."[1] Sports involving repetitive wrist flexion and extension such as gymnastics or prolonged grip with cycling may cause more cases of CTS than other sports.[18,34] CTS is frequently noted in wheelchair athletes.[21] Krivickas and Wilbourn,[2] in a study of 333 athletes, found that 24 of the 28 median neuropathy cases were CTS. It is of interest that only 6 of their 24 patients with CTS were symptomatic. Collins et al.[35] reported CTS frequently in rowers and bicyclists secondary to hand position. In a separate retrospective review, Krivickas and Wilbourn[36] studied 180 athletes from 27 different sports. They found 43 athletes to have median neuropathies. 25 out of these 43 athletes were asymptomatic.

The carpal tunnel is an osseofibrous structure. The lunate, capitate, and trapezoid are the floor; the pisiform and hamate are medial; and the navicular and trapezium are lateral. The roof is the transverse carpal ligament, a portion of the volar carpal ligament (flexor retinaculum). Ten structures pass through the carpal tunnel: four flexor digitorum tendons, four flexor superficialis (or sublimes) tendons, the flexor pollicis longus tendon, and the median nerve.[3] CTS can be caused by anything that either decreases the size of the canal (e.g., thickening of the flexor retinaculum) or increases the volume of the contents (e.g., tendonitis).

Carpal tunnel syndrome is often described with the classic presentation of paresthesias in the thumb and index and long fingers that increases with activity. It is important to note if the paresthesias are episodic or constant, the exacerbating or remitting activities, and if there is nocturnal worsening. It is important to distinguish the individual describing nightly burning intense paresthesias (dysesthesias) from the individual reporting episodic hand tingling. The time course can also be revealing, with an acute presentation perhaps preceded by years of episodic symptoms. The patient may report that the hand feels clumsy, especially noting difficulty with fine motor activities such as buttoning a shirt. Proximal symptoms with discomfort and aching may be reported, especially in the extensor mass region.

Physical examination may reveal sensory changes in the median innervated digits. The motor examination may reveal weakness of palmar abduction, although this requires attention to common extrinsic substitution patterns that would be expected. During a careful clinical examination, abductor pollicis brevis weakness is quite sensitive in those with CTS.[3] A Phalen test can be quite helpful with details of how long the paresthesia lasts (less than 20 seconds would be expected) and what digit develops the paresthesias (most commonly the long finger). Tapping over the median nerve at the wrist to elicit a Tinel sign is commonly done. Because the carpal tunnel is tightest at its distal end, tapping in the palm at the distal end of the transverse ligament may increase the yield of the Tinel testing for CTS.[3]

Unfortunately, CTS has come to be associated with any hand numbness, and other causes of hand numbness may not be considered. Another unfortunate reality is that many physicians still believe that there is a high false-negative rate for nerve conduction studies in CTS. This was perhaps true in the early days before careful temperature control and short segment transcarpal studies.[29] Now, nerve conduction studies, including paired transcarpal studies, are considered by many to be the gold standard for CTS diagnosis. Nerve conduction studies for CTS would include both median and ulnar studies to make sure there is no diffuse slowing. Both sensory and motor studies should be done. The short segment paired transcarpal study would be considered the most sensitive test.[8] Paired digital sensory and paired motor studies would also be done. "Mapping" should be done when the motor studies are inconsistent with the sensory studies. Mapping simply implies moving the E1 (previously referred to as the active electrode) location and can be important for avoiding false-positive median motor studies.[37] Hsu et al. reported an isolated median mononeuropathy in the palm of an amateur golfer.[38]

Radial Nerve

The radial nerve is the largest peripheral branch of the brachial plexus. It receives contributions from the cervical roots C5–8 and is derived from the posterior cord of the brachial plexus. In the axilla, the radial nerve is posterior to the axillary artery and superficial to the subscapularis muscle and tendons of the latissimus dorsi and teres major. The radial nerve travels between the long and medial heads of the triceps, continuing to the spiral groove of the humerus.

Proximal Radial Nerve Entrapment

The term "high radial nerve lesions" has been used in the past for radial nerve lesions proximal to the division in the forearm into the posterior interosseous nerve and superficial radial sensory branch.[39] The classic "honeymooners" spiral groove radial neuropathies have wrist and finger extension weakness. Distal interphalangeal (DIP) joint extension is usually preserved owing to the mechanical effect of the intact median and ulnar innervated intrinsic muscles.[39] Compression of the radial nerve by the lateral head of the triceps muscles following strenuous muscular effort has been described.[1,21,32,34] This site is distal to the branches innervating the triceps and anconeus muscles, both of which would be expected to be spared clinically and on needle EMG studies. Compression of the radial nerve by the long head of the triceps has also been reported.[22,32,34] Compression or injury in the spiral groove may be seen in activities that require forceful adduction of the shoulder, as seen in gymnastics[17] and wrestling.[40] Activities that require forceful extension of the elbow against resistance, such as throwing (e.g., discus, javelin, baseball) are associated with high radial nerve entrapment.[18,19,41] "Runner's radial palsy," an unusual and distinct entity that presents with numbness in the distal forearm and dorsum of the hand of runners who keep their elbow acutely flexed while running, is another example of a high radial nerve lesion. The nerve in this injury is compressed between the humerus and triceps. Treatment is altering the running position, resulting in complete resolution of symptoms.[42]

Forearm Radial Nerve Entrapment

The radial nerve innervates the brachioradialis and extensor carpi radialis longus distal to the spiral groove. In the lateral antecubital region, the radial nerve lies between the brachialis and brachioradialis muscles and passes over the annular ligament of the radius. In the proximal forearm, the radial nerve bifurcates into a sensory branch and a motor branch, the posterior interosseous nerve (PIN). The PIN usually innervates the extensor carpi radialis brevis and sends several branches to the supinator prior to going through the arcade of Frohse. As the PIN emerges from the supinator, it supplies the muscles in the extensor forearm, including the extensor digitorum communis, extensor digiti quinti, extensor carpi ulnaris and the deeper muscles (abductor pollicis longus, extensor pollicis longus and brevis, extensor indicis proprius). Similar to the AIN, the PIN terminates at the wrist, with several sensory branches innervating the carpal joints.[43]

Historically, radial tunnel syndrome and supinator syndrome have both been described.[44] The radial tunnel syndrome remains a somewhat controversial disorder, while the supinator syndrome is currently more clearly called posterior interosseous nerve syndrome (PINS). They differ in their clinical presentations, with the radial tunnel syndrome often described as "resistant tennis elbow" because it presents with pain as its primary feature whereas PINS characteristically has painless weakness.

Radial Tunnel Syndrome

In 1972, Roles and Maudsley[45] introduced the term "radial tunnel syndrome." The radial tunnel was described as extending from where the radial nerve pierces the lateral intermuscular septum to where the PIN enters the supinator muscle. Radial tunnel syndrome presents with lateral elbow pain. Objective motor or sensory loss in the distribution of the radial nerve would not be expected.

When evaluating a patient for radial tunnel syndrome, the main differential diagnosis to consider is lateral epicondylitis, or "tennis elbow." Physical examination findings may help differentiate the two. With radial tunnel syndrome there is pain upon palpation of the extensor forearm muscle mass a few centimeters distal to the lateral epicondyle, whereas with lateral epicondylitis the point of maximum tenderness is at the lateral epicondyle.[10] Resisted supination is more painful with radial tunnel syndrome.[10] Three characteristic findings are described for radial tunnel syndrome: pain upon palpation of the extensor forearm muscle mass about the radial head; pain in the forearm upon resisted supination; and lateral elbow pain with resisted elbow, wrist, and long finger extension.[39] The initial treatment is rest for both radial tunnel and lateral epicondylitis, followed by stretching and strengthening.[46]

Radial tunnel syndrome is often seen in those athletes who repetitively pronate and supinate and in those who are stressed in wrist extension, as in weightlifting, bowling, rowing, discus, racquet sports, swimming, and golf.[18,19,47] Roles and Maudsley thought that radial tunnel syndrome mimics and may coexist with lateral epicondylitis in up to 10% of patients.[45] Werner found an 8% coincident lesion in 203 patients.[48]

Posterior Interosseous Nerve Syndrome

The classic presentation of PINS is painless weakness of the wrist and finger extensors without sensory impairment. Wrist extension weakness generally is not complete owing to sparing of the extensor carpi radialis longus (ECRL), which receives innervation from the main radial nerve before the PIN branch. The characteristic radial deviation during attempted wrist extension is explained by the imbalance of a strong direct radial-innervated ECRL with weak PIN-innervated extensor carpi ulnaris (ECU). Weakness of finger extension would also be expected. Weakness of the brachioradialis and superficial radial sensory impairment would not support a PINS but, instead, suggests a higher radial nerve lesion. Electrodiagnostic studies should be done to confirm and grade the PINS. Denervation, motor unit changes, and recruitment abnormalities would be expected proportional to the clinical weakness. Surgical treatment is often necessary.[39]

Cheiralgia paresthetica refers to isolated injury of the superficial sensory branch of the radial nerve. Numerous etiologies have been described, including direct trauma, fibrosis from hemorrhage, handcuffs, and pressure (from tight watchbands, a cast, tight wristbands, tape, archery guards, gloves).[17,49] Direct trauma may be responsible for this syndrome in contact sports such as hockey, football, and lacrosse.[50]

Ulnar Nerve

The ulnar nerve receives contributions from C8 and T1 nerve roots and is the distal continuation of the medial cord of the brachial plexus (Fig. 6.3). No branches arise from the ulnar nerve in the arm. The ulnar nerve goes under the arcade of Struthers, which is the mid-arm band of fascia connecting the deep investing fascia of the anterior and posterior compartments of the arm. Proximal to the arcade of Struthers the nerve is freely mobile. In the area of the arcade, the nerve travels from the anterior to posterior compartments of the arm.

At the elbow, the ulnar nerve travels between the medial epicondyle and the olecranon in the retrocondylar groove. The superior edge of the medial epicondyle is an interesting site where the ulnar nerve has a fairly tight curve as it comes posteriorly toward the retrocondylar groove. This site should be carefully examined with inching nerve conduction studies when evaluating idiopathic ulnar neuropathies. Continuing distally, the nerve passes between the two heads of the flexor carpi ulnaris (FCU), passing under the humeroulnar aponeurotic arcade, which along with the underlying bone and ligaments form the cubital tunnel. The ulnar nerve continues in the forearm resting on the flexor digitorum profundus (FDP) and covered by the FCU.

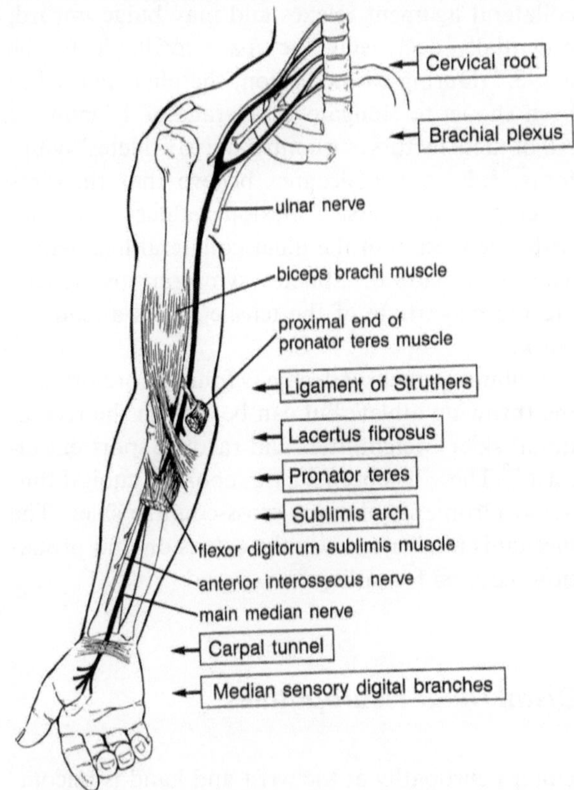

Fig. 6.3 Sites of entrapment of the ulnar nerve

At the wrist, the ulnar nerve enters the hand through Guyon's canal, which is bound medially by the pisiform and laterally by the hook of the hamate. In the hand, the ulnar nerve divides into a superficial branch and a deep branch. The superficial branch innervates the palmaris brevis and divides into the palmar digital sensory branches. The deep ulnar motor branch supplies all other ulnar innervated hand muscles. The dorsal ulnar cutaneous (DUC) nerve branch comes off the main ulnar nerve 5–10 cm proximal to the wrist, but the DUC can be identified as an independent bundle for some distance proximal.[28] This anatomic feature explains the clinical observation that the DUC nerve is quite sensitive to proximal ulnar problems.

The ulnar nerve exists in a dynamic relation with anatomic structures in the elbow region.[51] With extension, the nerve becomes redundant within the retrocondylar groove; with flexion, the medial ligament of the elbow bulges into the floor of the retrocondylar groove. Elbow flexion tightens the humeral ulnar arcuate ligament over the ulnar nerve, decreases the volume in the cubital tunnel, and elongates the ulnar nerve from its previously slack position. With extreme elbow flexion, the medial head of the triceps can exert a posterior force on the nerve. Partial or complete subluxation of the ulnar nerve occurs in up to 16% of the population.[52] A subluxing ulnar nerve is rarely of any clinical significance.

Proximal Ulnar Neuropathies

Episodic paresthesias in the ring and little fingers are a common human experience, similar to leg paresthesia noted with leg crossing. The dynamic nature of ulnar paresthesias is vastly underappreciated and in need of much more research. The patient with a proximal ulnar neuropathy has a persistent sense of decreased sensation in the ulnar digits, hypothenar region, and dorsal ulnar hand. The forearm should not have any numbness. There is no elbow pain. There may be a sense of weakness in the hand. Patients may report difficulty getting objects out of their pockets because their little finger gets caught on the pocket edge (Wartenberg sign).

On clinical examination there may be impaired sensation in the ulnar nerve distribution. The motor examination may reveal ulnar intrinsic muscle weakness with preserved median intrinsic muscle strength. The ulnar innervated palmaris brevis muscle can be important to examine by looking for the presence or absence of palmaris brevis hypothenar skin wrinkling. This is a fairly reliable physical finding in significant ulnar neuropathies and should always be included as either a pertinent positive or negative finding. A positive Froment sign is seen with ulnar neuropathies owing to the median innervated flexor pollicis longus attempting to compensate for the weak ulnar intrinsic muscles. The Wartenberg sign with the little finger hanging out in an abducted position can also been seen in ulnar neuropathies, reflecting the misbalance of the weak ulnar interossei muscles and the intact radial innervated extensor muscles.[53] Although both the Froment sign and the Wartenberg sign are indicative of ulnar neuropathy, neither identifies the site of the lesion.[54] The Tinel sign over the ulnar nerve should be interpreted with caution because it has been noted to be present in more than 80% of asymptomatic normal people.[6,54]

Although an ulnar neuropathy at the elbow is frequently considered first in patients presenting with "ulnar" sensory symptoms, a broad differential diagnosis must be considered, including cervical radiculopathy, medial cord brachial plexopathy, or even vascular or visceral problems.[55] It is widely recognized clinically that even patients with CTS may present with "ulnar" sensory symptoms.[56]

The role of electrophysiologic data in the evaluation of suspected ulnar neuropathies has been the subject of many publications. Parameters that have been utilized have included motor, mixed nerve, and sensory conduction velocity of the elbow segment; comparison of the elbow segment velocity to that of an adjacent nerve segment; inching; change in the size or configuration of the compound muscle action potential or sensory nerve action potentials; and the pattern of needle examination abnormalities in ulnar-supplied muscles.[57] When interpreting ulnar nerve conduction studies, it should be remembered that the exact site where the cubital begins can be extremely variable. In a patient in whom the ulnar amplitude may appear to drop at the "below elbow" site, this may simply reflect a proximal origin of the cubital tunnel and should not be misinterpreted as a conduction block. Further work is needed on all ulnar techniques to examine repeatability, correlation to clinical features, and outcomes. Current research efforts are exploring refinements of inching, the usefulness of including the dorsal ulnar cutaneous study, and the role of E2 (previously referred to as the reference electrode).[57,58]

The act of throwing is often responsible for ulnar nerve involvement at the elbow in athletes. Tremendous forces develop at the elbow with angular velocities up to 7000°/s.[18] Studies have shown that the position of elbow flexion and wrist extension creates a threefold increase in ulnar nerve pressure in the cubital tunnel; when the upper extremity is placed in the cocking position of a throw, the pressure increases to six times the resting pressure.[59] Biomechanically, several processes cause an elevation of pressure. The arcuate ligament lengthens with elbow flexion until the proximal edge becomes taut at 90° of flexion. At the same time, the ulnar collateral ligament relaxes and may bulge inward, potentially decreasing the space available to the nerve.[60] During elbow flexion, the ulnar nerve has been shown to elongate an average of 4.7 mm.[1,51] All of these factors can contribute to athletes' symptoms. Jobe and colleagues believe that throwers develop a progressive flexion valgus deformity with attenuation of the ulnar collateral ligament.[61] This exacerbates the athletes' symptoms by increasing the magnitude of the tensile forces already at work.

Cubital tunnel syndrome is found more often in the throwing athlete but can be seen in the recreational skier, weightlifter, and racquet sport enthusiast.[62] There has been a case report of cubital tunnel syndrome involving a cross-country skier. The mechanism of injury was the extension and pronation required for poling.[63]

Distal Ulnar Neuropathies

Ulnar neuropathy at the wrist and hand is uncommon.[31,64,65] Reported etiologies have included ganglion cysts, ulnar artery thrombosis, carpal fractures (especially the hamate), anomalous muscles, and repetitive trauma or direct pressure.[1,65] In the athlete, the most widely known cause is pressure from handlebars seen in bicyclists (Fig. 6.4). [1,66]

The Guyon canal, or ulnar tunnel, is the depression between the pisiform and the hook of the hamate. It is different from the carpal tunnel in that the roof is quite thin, there are no tendons in the Guyon canal, and there are vascular structures including the ulnar artery and its associated veins.[67] Problems that can occur with the ulnar nerve distally in the wrist have been classified by Shea amd McClain.[31] Type I has involvement of all parts of the nerve including the hypothenar muscles, the deep ulnar motor branch to the ulnar intrinsic muscles, and the ulnar digital sensory fibers. Type II involves only the deep ulnar motor branch. Type III involves only the superficial ulnar sensory branches. Unfortunately, this classification scheme does not include the branch to the palmaris brevis muscle. This motor branch initially travels with the ulnar digital sensory fibers as the superficial branch of the ulnar nerve. Clinicians are increasingly aware of this

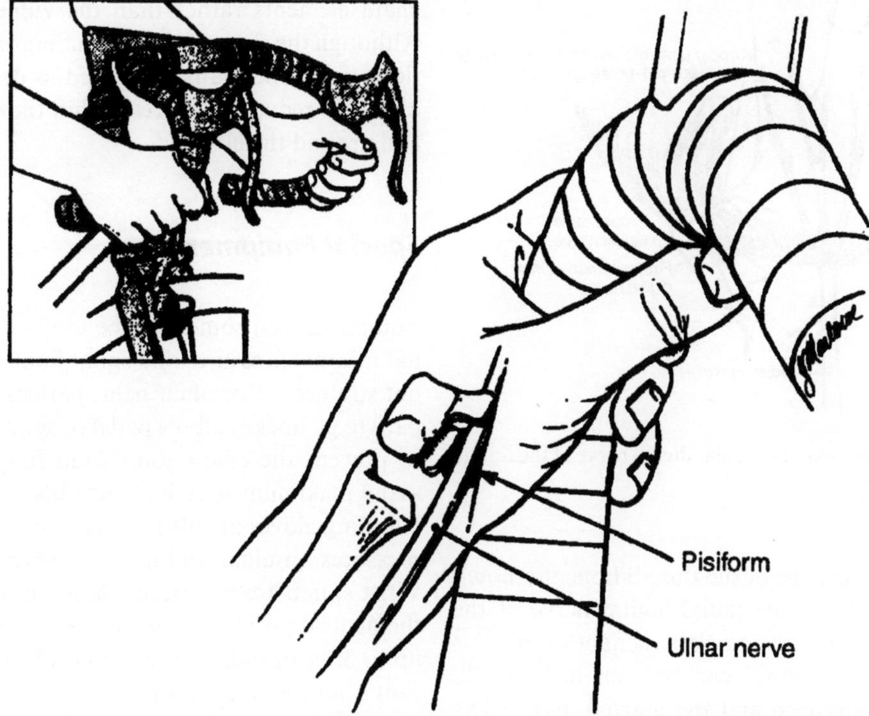

Fig. 6.4 Mechanism of injury for cyclist's palsy. From Plancher et al.[50] Copyright Elsevier 1996. Used with permission

unusual anatomy and finding it useful to check for palmaris brevis wrinkling with little finger abduction in all cases of suspected ulnar neuropathy[65]

To evaluate possible distal ulnar nerve problems beyond a detailed history and physical examination, electrodiagnostic studies can be helpful. An initial paired transcarpal study should be done to rule out a possible CTS presentation with ulnar sensory symptoms.[56] Ulnar digital sensory studies should be done both orthodromically and antidromically to avoid misinterpretation of an interosseous far field motor response as a prolonged digital sensory response. Ulnar motor studies can be done by recording over the hypothenar muscles or any of the ulnar intrinsic muscles.[57] Caution is urged during interpretation of ulnar motor studies, however, as the E2 is always active and is a significant factor that can affect not only amplitude and waveform shape but even latency.[58] Needle EMG of many ulnar intrinsic muscles, including both volar and dorsal interossei, are often needed to localize a true distal ulnar neuropathy.[65]

Isolated entrapment of the DUC nerve has been reported[68] and should be considered in any patient presenting with ulnar hand sensory symptoms. The DUC passes between the flexor carpi ulnaris and the ulna to pierce the fascia in the distal forearm. It appears vulnerable to irritation by fast repetitive forearm pronation and concomitant wrist flexion. Isolated entrapment of the DUC was initially reported in a grocery store clerk who had to pass objects over a static universal product code (UPC) reader; the disorder was thus named "pricer palsy."[68] The technology improvement to wand-type UPC readers makes this less likely to occur currently, but isolated DUC entrapment should still be considered in those involved in sports activities with a lot of forearm/wrist repetitive movements.

Digital Nerves

Injury to the digital nerves is often the result of repetitive trauma over the palm or digits. The most common example, described by Dobyns et al.[69] in 1972, is the bowler's thumb. The term bowler's thumb describes an injury to the ulnar digital sensory nerve to the thumb caused by direct

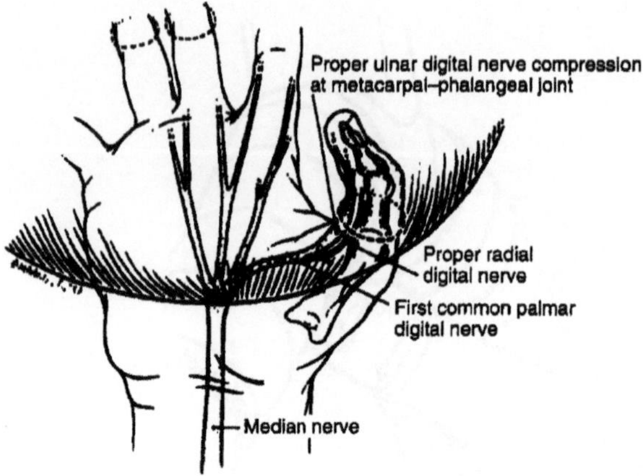

Fig. 6.5 Compression of the ulnar digital nerve of the thumb in bowler's thumb

trauma from the edge of the thumb hole of a bowling ball (Fig. 6.5). The radial digital nerve of the index finger is similarly at risk in racquet sports.[70,71] Digital nerve symptoms can be seen in baseball, handball, gymnastics, and the martial arts.[17] The chronic nature of the injury was demonstrated by Buckhout and Warner, who showed that digital nerve involvement in handball players occur in those with more than 2 years or 200 hours of play.[72]

Treatment

Focal neuropathies of the elbow, forearm, and hand can all be treated similarly. After diagnosis and severity of neuropathy is elucidated and underlying conditions are addressed, a typical treatment algorithm can be applied.

Activity Modification

First, activity modification should be considered. For example, in bicyclists experiencing ulnar neuropathy at the wrist or carpal tunnel syndrome, the hand/wrist position should be modified so excessive pressure does not occur. Reducing repetitive loads on nerves at their tethering points has also been advised. Overhead athletes can be rehabilitated to generate kinetic forces through proximal kinetic chain elements rather than the vulnerable elbow. Although the evidence is unclear, ergonomic corrections in the individuals engaged in desk work may also help reduce pressures within the carpal tunnel and around the elbow.

Special Equipment

Equipment can sometimes be used to reduce external/internal pressures and splint joints so nerves are not stretched. For ulnar neuropathies at the elbow, pads (e.g., hockey elbow pads) or splints can be used to prevent the elbow joint from fully flexing and avoid maximum stretch of the ulnar nerve. Padded bicycling gloves are also thought to reduce external pressures on ulnar and median nerves at the wrist. Wrist splints (carpal tunnel braces), particularly in the neutral position, have also been shown to help up to 30% of individuals with CTS achieve significant symptom reduction.[73]

Medication

Medications have been used empirically to treat various neuropathies. Antiinflammatory drugs, neuropathic medications, diuretics, and various analgesics have been used with mixed success. There is no good literature on the use of nonsteroidal antiinflammatories as monotherapy for CTS and little literature for other neuropathies. Vitamin B_6 (pyridoxine) has been used for CTS, but theoretically it should only help individuals with concomitant peripheral neuropathy. Injected corticosteroids are relatively frequently used for CTS but not other neuropathies. Bland concluded that 70% of CTS patients significantly improve with carpal tunnel corticosteroid injection, but 50% relapse within 1 year.[73]

Surgery

Surgical release can be utilized to treat various neuropathies. Carpal tunnel release surgery is common and appears to "cure" CTS in at least 75% of individuals.[73] Open and endoscopic carpal tunnel release can be performed for recalcitrant and severe CTS cases. Endoscopic surgery may be appealing to athletes as it offers a faster recovery time. However, individuals should be cautioned that endoscopic methods are not as well studied as others, and complication profiles are not as clear owing to incomplete exposure and transection of the transverse carpal ligament. Ulnar nerve surgery about the elbow is also frequently performed for recalcitrant ulnar neuropathies. Surgery may include release and decompression (e.g., in cases where the ulnar nerve appears to be entrapped distal to the elbow at the humeroulnar aponeurotic arcade) or an anterior transposition and medial epicondylectomy (e.g., in cases where ulnar neuropathy occurs at the ulnar groove). According to a study by Bartels et al., ulnar nerve surgery at the elbow works about two-thirds of the time using either technique.[74] The authors advocated for simple decompression rather than transposition, as decompression engendered less cost and fewer complications. In athletes, ulnar nerve surgery at the elbow is often accompanied by repair of an injured ulnar collateral ligament (via palmaris longus tendon transfer).

References

1. Weinstein SM, Herring SA. Nerve problems and compartment syndromes in the hand, wrist, and forearm. Clin Sports Med 1992;11(1):161–88.
2. Krivickas LS, Wilbourn AJ. Sports and peripheral nerve injuries: report of 190 injuries evaluated in a single electromyography laboratory. Muscle Nerve 1998;21(8):1092–94.
3. Wertsch JJ, Melvin J. Median nerve anatomy and entrapment syndromes: a review. Arch Phys Med Rehabil 1982;63(12):623–7.
4. Wertsch JJ. Median neuropathies at the elbow. In: American Association of Electrodiagnostic Medicine (AAEM) Course: Unusual Mononeuropathies. Rochester, MN: AAEM; 2000:7–10.
5. Laha RK, Dujovny M, DeCastro SC. Entrapment of median nerve by supracondylar process of the humerus: case report. J Neurosurg 1977;46(2):252–5.
6. Alfonso MI, Rioja LN, Wang S, et al. Tinel's sign of the ulnar nerve at the elbow. Muscle Nerve 1998;21:1571.
7. Johnson RK, Spinner M, Shrewsbury MM. Median nerve entrapment syndrome in the proximal forearm. J Hand Surg [Am] 1979;4(1):48–51.
8. Mills KR. Orthodromic sensory action potentials from palmar stimulation in the diagnosis of carpal tunnel syndrome. J Neurol Neurosurg Psychiatry 1985;48(3):250–5.
9. Symeonides PP. The humerus supracondylar process syndrome. Clin Orthop 1972;82:141–3.
10. Kessel L, Rang M. Supracondylar spur of the humerus. J Bone Joint Surg Br 1966;48(4):765–9.
11. Smith RV, Fisher RG. Struthers ligament: a source of median nerve compression above the elbow: case report. J Neurosurg 1973;38(6):778–9.
12. Seyffarth H. Primary myoses in the M. pronator teres as cause of lesion of the N. medianus (the pronator syndrome). Acta Psychiatr Neurol Scand Suppl 1951;74:251–4.
13. Rettig AC, Shelbourne KD, McCarroll JR, et al. The natural history and treatment of delayed union stress fractures of the anterior cortex of the tibia. Am J Sports Med 1988;16(3):250–5.
14. Eversmann WW Jr. Compression and entrapment neuropathies of the upper extremity. J Hand Surg [Am] 1983;8(5 Pt 2):759–66.
15. Werner CO, Rosen I, Thorngren KG. Clinical and neurophysiologic characteristics of the pronator syndrome. Clin Orthop 1985;(197):231–6.
16. Mackinnon SE, Dellon AL, ed. Surgery of the Peripheral Nerve. New York: Thieme; 1988.
17. Long RR. Nerve anatomy and diagnostic principles. In: Pappas M, editor. Upper Extremity Injuries in the Athlete. New York: Churchill Livingstone; 1995:53–4.
18. Sicuranza MJ, McCue FC III. Compressive neuropathies in the upper extremity of athletes. Hand Clin 1992;8(2):263–73.
19. Cabrera JM, McCue FC III. Nonosseous athletic injuries of the elbow, forearm, and hand. Clin Sports Med 1986;5(4):681–700.
20. Whitaker JH. Compressive neuropathies. In: Strickland JW, Rettig AC, eds. Hand Injuries in Athletes. Philadelphia: Saunders; 1992:209–28.
21. Burnham RS, Steadward RD. Upper extremity peripheral nerve entrapments among wheelchair athletes: prevalence, location, and risk factors. Arch Phys Med Rehabil 1994;75(5):519–24.
22. Wertsch JJ, Sanger J. Thumb extension in radial nerve injuries. Arch Phys Med Rehabil 1986;67:678–9.
23. Wertsch JJ. AAEM case report #25: anterior interosseous nerve syndrome. Muscle Nerve 1992;15(9):977–83.
24. Kiloh LG, Nevin S. Isolated neuritis of the anterior interosseous nerve. BMJ 1952;1(4763):850–1.
25. Fearn CB, Goodfellow JW. Anterior interosseous nerve palsy. J Bone Joint Surg Br 1965;47:91–3.
26. Rennels GD, Ochoa J. Neuralgic amyotrophy manifesting as anterior interosseous nerve palsy. Muscle Nerve 1980;3(2):160–4.
27. England JD, Sumner AJ. Neuralgic amyotrophy: an increasingly diverse entity. Muscle Nerve 1987;10(1):60–8.
28. Jabaley ME, Wallace WH, Heckler FR. Internal topography of major nerves of the forearm and hand: a current view. J Hand Surg [Am] 1980;5(1):1–18.
29. Watchmaker GP, Gumucio CA, Crandall RE, et al. Fascicular topography of the median nerve: a computer based study to identify branching patterns. J Hand Surg [Am] 1991;16(1):53–9.
30. Jones ET, Louis DS. Median nerve injuries associated with supracondylar fractures of the humerus in children. Clin Orthop 1980;(150):181–6.
31. Shea JD, McClain EJ. Ulnar-nerve compression syndromes at and below the wrist. J Bone Joint Surg Am 1969;51(6):1095–103.

32. Steward JD. Anatomy of nerve fascicles and their relevance in focal peripheral neuropathies. In: American Association of Electrodiagnostic Medicine (AAEM) Course D: Focal Peripheral Neuropathies. Rochester, MN: AAEM; 1991:43–8.
33. Wertsch JJ, Sanger JR, Matloub HS. Pseudo-anterior interosseous nerve syndrome. Muscle Nerve 1985;8:68–70.
34. Szabo RM, Madison M. Carpal tunnel syndrome. Orthop Clin North Am 1992;23(1):103–9.
35. Collins K, Storey M, Peterson K. Nerve injuries in athletes. Physician Sports Med 1988;16:92–6.
36. Krivickas LS, Wilbourn AJ. Peripheral nerve injuries in athletes: a case series of over 200 injuries. Semin Neurol 2000;20(2):225–32.
37. Ferdjallah M, Wertsch JJ, Ahad MA, et al. Nerve conduction topography in geriatric hand assessment. J Rehabil Res Dev 2005;42(6):821–8.
38. Hsu WC, Chen WH, Oware A, et al. Unusual entrapment neuropathy in a golf player. Neurology 2002;59(4):646–7.
39. Dawson EM, Hallett M, Wilbourn AJ, eds. Entrapment Neuropathies, 3rd ed. Philadelphia: Lippincott-Raven; 1999.
40. Mackinnon SE, Dellon AL. The overlap pattern of the lateral antebrachial cutaneous nerve and the superficial branch of the radial nerve. J Hand Surg [Am] 1985;10(4):522–6.
41. Mitsunga MM, Nakano K. High radial nerve palsy following strenuous muscular activity. Clin Orthop 1988;234:39.
42. Pickering TG. Runner's radial palsy. N Engl J Med 1981;305(13):768.
43. Spinner M, ed. Injuries to the Major Branches of the Peripheral Nerves of the Forearm. 2nd ed. Philadelphia: Saunders; 1978.
44. Khanna P, Zeni AI, Niedfeldt M, et al. Scapular winging in a professional ballet dancer. Med Sci Sports Exerc 1999;31(5):S98.
45. Roles NC, Maudsley RH. Radial tunnel syndrome: resistant tennis elbow as a nerve entrapment. J Bone Joint Surg Br 1972;54(3):499–508.
46. Simmons BP, Wyman ET. Occupational injuries of the elbow. In: Millender LH, Louis DS, Simmons BP, eds. Occupational Disorders of the Upper Extremity. New York: Churchill Livingstone; 1992:157–60.
47. Regan WD, Morrey BF. Entrapment neuropathies above the elbow. In: DeLee JC, Drez D Jr, eds. Orthopaedic Sports Medicine. Philadelphia: Saunders; 1994:844–59.
48. Werner CO. Lateral elbow pain and posterior interosseous nerve entrapment. Acta Orthop Scand Suppl 1979;174:1–62.
49. Spinner M. The arcade of Frohse and its relationship to posterior interosseus nerve paralysis. J Bone Joint Surg Br 1968;50:809–12.
50. Plancher KD, Peterson RK, Steichen JB. Compressive neuropathies and tendinopathies in the athletic elbow and wrist. Clin Sports Med 1996;15(2):331–71.
51. Apfelberg DB, Larson SJ. Dynamic anatomy of the ulnar nerve at the elbow. Plast Reconstr Surg 1973;51(1):79–81.
52. Childress HM. Recurrent ulnar-nerve dislocation at the elbow. Clin Orthop 1975 May;(108):168–73.
53. Wartenberg R. A sign of ulnar palsy. JAMA 1939;112: 1688.
54. Mackinnon SE, Dellon AL, eds. Surgery of the Peripheral Nerve. New York: Thieme; 1988.
55. Wertsch JJ. Hand numbness: ulnar. In: American Association of Electrodiagnostic Medicine (AAEM) Course A. Rochester, MN: AAEM; 1997:27–33.
56. Wertsch JJ, Oswald TA, Vennix MJ, et al. Ulnar paresthesias as a presenting symptom of carpal tunnel "syndrome." Muscle Nerve 1994;17:1082.
57. Wertsch JJ, Oswald TA, Kincaid J. Ulnar techniques (workshop handout). Rochester, MN: American Association of Electrodiagnostic Medicine, 1994.
58. Phongsamart G, Wertsch JJ, Ferdjallah M, et al. Effect of reference electrode position on the compound muscle action potential (CMAP) onset latency. Muscle Nerve 2002;25(6):816–21.
59. Pechan J, Julis I. The pressure measurement in the ulnar nerve: a contribution to the pathophysiology of the cubital tunnel syndrome. J Biomech 1975;8(1):75–9.
60. Butters KP, Singer KM. Nerve lesions of the arm and elbow. In: Deter JC, Drez DJ, eds. Orthopaedic Sports Medicine: Principles and Practice. Philadelphia: Saunders; 1994:802–71.
61. Jobe FW, Stark H, Lombardo SJ. Reconstruction of the ulnar collateral ligament in athletes. J Bone Joint Surg Am 1986;68(8):1158–63.
62. Glousman RE. Ulnar nerve problems in the athlete's elbow. Clin Sports Med 1990;9(2):365–77.
63. Fulkerson JP. Transient ulnar neuropathy from Nordic skiing. Clin Orthop 1980;(153):230–1.
64. Olney RK, Hanson M. AAEE case report #15: ulnar neuropathy at or distal to the wrist. Muscle Nerve 1988;11(8):828–32.
65. Wertsch JJ. Neuropathies at the wrist and hand. In: American Association of Electrodiagnostic Medicine (AAEM) Course: Unusual Mononeuropathies. Rochester, MN: AAEM; 2000:11–6.
66. Burke ER. Ulnar neuropathy in bicyclists. Physician Sportsmed 1981;9:53–6.
67. Sunderland S. Ulnar Nerve Lesions. Nerve and Nerve Injuries. New York: Churchill Livingstone; 1978:760–72.
68. Wertsch JJ. Pricer palsy. N Engl J Med 1985;312(25):1645.
69. Dobyns JH, O'Brien ET, Linscheid RL, et al. Bowler's thumb: diagnosis and treatment; a review of seventeen cases. J Bone Joint Surg Am 1972;54(4):751–5.
70. Dobyns JH, Sim FH, Linscheid RL. Sports stress syndromes of the hand and wrist. Am J Sports Med 1978;6(5):236–54.
71. Osterman AL, Moskow L, Low DW. Soft-tissue injuries of the hand and wrist in racquet sports. Clin Sports Med 1988;7(2):329–48.
72. Buckhout BC, Warner MA. Digital perfusion of handball players: effects of repeated ball impact on structures of the hand. Am J Sports Med 1980;8(3):206–7.
73. Bland JD. Treatment of carpal tunnel syndrome. Muscle Nerve 2007;36:161–71.
74. Bartels R, Verhagen W, van der Wilt GJ, et al. Prospective randomized controlled study comparing simple decompression versus anterior subcutaneous transposition for idiopathic neuropathy of the ulnar nerve at the elbow: Part 1. Neurosurgery 2005;56:522–30.

Chapter 7
Peripheral Nerve Injuries of the Shoulder and Upper Arm

Kelly C. McInnis and Lisa S. Krivickas

Introduction

Nerve injuries about the shoulder and proximal upper limb are uncommon but important causes of pain and dysfunction in athletes. In general, athletes involved in overhead sports appear to be at increased risk for nerve injuries in the shoulder region, which can be challenging for the clinician to identify and treat. This chapter takes a comprehensive look at the peripheral nerves in the upper arm that are susceptible to injury and gives a detailed approach to the evaluation and management of the disorders that result.

Suprascapular Nerve Injury

Suprascapular nerveinjury is one of the more common upper limb peripheral nerve injuries in athletes. This injury represents about 1%–2% of all shoulder disorders that cause pain.[1] On the other hand, 28% of full-thickness rotator cuff tears have been noted to be associated with peripheral nerve lesions, particularly suprascapular neuropathies. Among athletes, suprascapular nerve entrapment is most often reported in those who play overhead repetitive sports. It primarily affects patients younger than 40 years of age.[2]

The suprascapular nerve originates from the proximal upper trunk of the brachial plexus at Erb's point. It has contributions from the fifth and sixth anterior cervical roots and occasionally from the fourth root.[3] As the nerve traverses laterally, it crosses the posterior triangle of the neck, deep to the omohyoid muscle and the anterior border of the trapezius muscle, to reach the superior scapular border. It then travels anterior to posterior through the scapular notch and into the suprascapular fossa. The transverse scapular ligament bridges the notch over the nerve. The corresponding artery and vein travel superior to the ligament, outside the notch. In the suprascapular fossa, the nerve gives off two motor branches to the supraspinatus muscle while receiving sensory branches from the posterior glenohumeral capsule, acromioclavicular joint, and coracohumeral ligament. In 15% of patients, the suprascapular nerve receives cutaneous sensory fibers from the upper lateral arm (deltoid patch).[4] The nerve then travels obliquely under the supraspinatus muscle to the base of the lateral supraspinatus fossa and the rim of the glenoid. It enters the infraspinatous fossa through the spinoglenoid notch. A spinoglenoid ligament covers the spinoglenoid notch in about 50% of individuals.[5] It then divides and terminates into two or more branches to supply the infraspinatus muscle. Figure 7.1 illustrates the anatomy of the suprascapular nerve.

There are many causes of suprascapular neuropathy. The nerve may be injured as a result of instability, compression, traction, repetitive microtrauma, or direct trauma. Additionally, it may be part of a generalized brachial plexus disorder or neuralgic amyotrophy. Injury can occur at various sites along the course of the suprascapular nerve,

K.C. McInnis (✉)
Department of Physical Medicine and Rehabilitation, Harvard Medical School, Boston, MA, USA

V. Akuthota, S.A. Herring (eds.), *Nerve and Vascular Injuries in Sports Medicine*,
DOI 10.1007/978-0-387-76600-3_7, © Springer Science+Business Media, LLC 2009

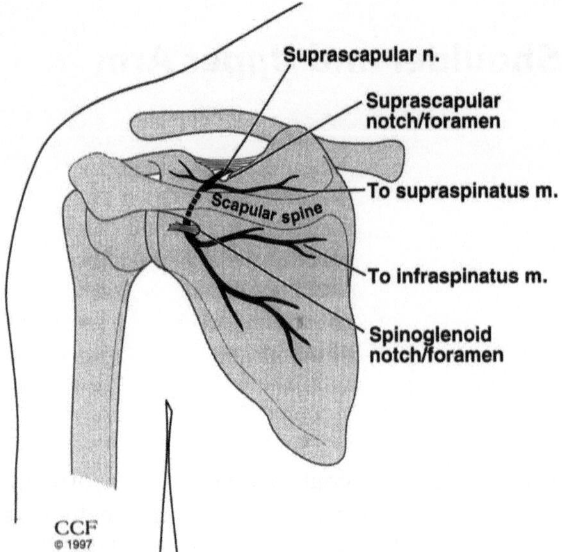

Fig. 7.1 Posterior view of the termination of the suprascapular nerve, showing the two principal sites of injury: suprascapular notch and spinoglenoid notch. From Dawson M, Hallett M, Wilbourn A. Entrapment Neuropathies. 3rd ed. Philadelphia: Lippincott-Raven; 1999:353. Used with permission

but it is most often compromised at the suprascapular notch, the spinoglenoid notch, or at its origin, Erb's point. Each region of injury results in a clinically distinct syndrome. In athletes, the spinoglenoid notch appears to be the most common site of entrapment.

Injury to the nerve as it passes through the suprascapular notch may be caused by compression of the overlying transverse scapular ligament. The literature reports several anatomic variations that can contribute to entrapment at this site, including a narrow notch, a bifid or calcified transverse scapular ligament, or an adjacent bony fracture.[6–9] A mechanical stretch or traction injury can also occur at the suprascapular notch and has been reported as the *sling effect*.[10,11] This term refers to the close adherence of the nerve to the inferior surface of the transverse scapular ligament with extremes of scapular motion. Rapid stretching of the nerve can occur with cross-body adduction, forward flexion, and external rotation.[12] Damage to the blood vessels supplying the suprascapular nerve can be affected by a similar traction mechanism. Microvascular trauma can result in ischemic injury to the nerve.[13] This decrease in blood flow in the vasa nervorum is thought to occur most commonly at the suprascapular notch.

Injury to the nerve as it courses through the spinoglenoid notch may be a result of compression by a space-occupying lesion (e.g., a ganglion cyst) or enlarged notch veins.[14] Ganglion cysts are thought to be sequelae of abnormalities within the shoulder joint where there is intraarticular disruption such as a capsular or labral tear created by instability. The synovial fluid produced in response to this pathology may be forced into the notch tissues by a one-way valve mechanism, resulting in fluid collection in a cyst. Ganglia have been implicated in both suprascapular and spinoglenoid notch impingement. However, because of the proximity of the posterior shoulder capsule to the glenohumeral joint, they are more likely to cause spinoglenoid notch compromise.[15,16] In addition, Sandow and Ilic[17] described impingement of the infraspinatus branch of the suprascapular nerve against the lateral edge of the scapular spine by the tendinous margin of the infraspinatus and supraspinatus with extreme abduction and full external rotation of the shoulder. The spinoglenoid notch is also a potential site of traction and repetitive trauma injury as the nerve takes a sharp turn through this landmark, with potential fixation by an overlying spinoglenoid ligament.[11] Spinoglenoid notch suprascapular nerve lesions are thought to be relatively painless with infraspinatus weakness because the sensory fibers from the glenohumeral joint is received proximal to the notch. However, studies have shown that pain occurs regardless of whether the injury is at the suprascapular or spinoglenoid notch.[15]

A less common site of injury to the suprascapular nerve is at its origin from the upper trunk of the brachial plexus-Erb's point. The mechanism may be a traction injury incurred during a fall onto the acromion of the shoulder with a resultant distraction force generated between the neck and the shoulder, similar to the mechanism of burner or stinger brachial plexus injury.[18] Erb's point may also be an area of potential nerve fixation where the nerve takes a sharp turn and can be stretched and irritated by repetitive overhead shoulder activities.

The suprascapular nerve may be susceptible to direct trauma by dislocation of the glenohumeral joint, fracture of the proximal humerus or scapula, or penetrating trauma.[19] It can be injured iatrogenically during a distal clavicle resection procedure, arthroscopic shoulder stabilization, open rotator cuff repair, or during positioning for spine surgery.[4,20–23] In addition, it can be injured as part of a more complex or generalized brachial plexus disorder. The suprascapular nerve is one of the peripheral nerves of the shoulder girdle often affected by neuralgic amyotrophy (Parsonage-Turner syndrome).

Mechanism of Injury in Sport

Given the pathogenesis of suprascapular nerve injury, it is not surprising that it occurs most often in athletes involved in overhead repetitive sports with shoulder instability. Compression at the spinoglenoid notch has been reported in volleyball players, racquet-sport players, weightlifters, baseball pitchers, a football player, a gymnast, and a dancer.[24–31] Injury during the volleyball float serve and the overhead motion in the various other sports are thought to occur from compression at the spinoglenoid notch as the infraspinatus eccentrically contracts to decelerate the internal rotation of the shoulder during the follow-through.[28]

During the volleyball float serve, the goal is not maximum speed of the arm, as with other throwing motions, but rather to impart a *floating* or *knuckleball* trajectory to the ball. To achieve this, the athlete must strike the ball sharply so the arm is suddenly retracted just after striking it. This requires much more intense shoulder stabilization than that provided by the external rotators.[32] Therefore, as documented by dynamic electromyography (EMG) analysis, the infraspinatus muscle is much more intensely activated during the float serve than with throwing actions such as pitching, in which deceleration is more progressive.[33] This eccentric contraction of the infraspinatus muscle required to slow the arm and stabilize the shoulder increases the distance between the points of origin and termination of the nerve, and the nerve may be stretched across the lateral edge of the spine of the scapula.[32]

Ferretti et al.[28] identified suprascapular neuropathy isolated to the infraspinatus muscle, demonstrated by EMG, in 12 of 96 asymptomatic elite volleyball players. Moreover, Holzgraefe et al.[34] reported suprascapular neuropathy in 33% of elite volleyball players on their serving side. Time spent training was thought to be the most important contributing factor, suggesting repetitive stretch of the nerve as the mechanism of injury.

Entrapment of the suprascapular nerve has been reported in various other sports. In baseball pitchers, suprascapular nerve injury may occur at the suprascapular or the spinoglenoid notch and is thought to be due to repetitive, rapid stretching of the nerve with the extreme scapular throwing motions, especially during the follow-through phase.[26] In dancers, suprascapular neuropathy has been reported and postulated to be due to entrapment at the spinoglenoid notch secondary to repetitive, forceful movements of the arm in external rotation and abduction.[29] Injury at the suprascapular notch has also been reported in weightlifters and hikers.[35,36] Bodybuilders are at risk because of the repetitive activity of the shoulder required for upper extremity weightlifting. The mechanism of isolated suprascapular nerve injury in hikers is likely due to excessive shoulder traction and improper waist support for the backpack.[37] A single report of a suprascapular nerve lesion without a history of trauma has been reported in a basketball player, perhaps due to the repeated nerve traction over the coracoid notch while dunking the basketball.[38] The action of blocking or tackling by football players can cause direct trauma to the shoulder and scapular regions, which can lead to suprascapular neuropathy. In a similar respect, the excessive shoulder and scapular manipulation that occurs while wrestling, such as with the hammerlock maneuver, can lead to nerve injury.[39]

Physical Examination and Diagnostic Tests

The clinical evaluation of suprascapular nerve injury begins with the history and physical examination. Patients often report the insidious onset of poorly localized pain over the posterolateral aspect of the shoulder that is worsened by overhead activity. They may describe the pain as a dull ache, burning, or deep and diffuse. The pain pattern may be similar to that of a C5 or C6 radiculopathy. The clinician may appreciate atrophy of the infraspinatus (injury likely at the spinoglenoid notch) or atrophy of both supraspinatus and infraspinatus (injury likely at the suprascapular notch or more proximally). Infraspinatus atrophy is more obvious than supraspinatus atrophy because the trapezius covers the supraspinatus muscle. Atrophy is best evaluated with shoulders in forward flexion or viewed from above the shoulder girdle.

The clinician may elicit tenderness upon palpation over the notch sites or over the acromioclavicular joint. Pain may be reproduced with extreme shoulder extension or internal rotation, placing a stretch on the nerve. Manual muscle testing may reveal weakness of shoulder external rotation greater than abduction. However, the athlete may not complain of weakness during sporting-specific activities because of adequate compensation of the posterior deltoid and teres minor muscles.[28] The examiner should perform a thorough shoulder examination to rule out other shoulder pathology. Provocative maneuvers that may help identify rotator cuff, labral, and instability pathology should be included. The main differential diagnosis for suprascapular neuropathy is rotator cuff pathology, so a thorough shoulder examination for impingement should be performed.

Diagnostic evaluation may include needle EMG with nerve conduction studies (NCSs), various imaging studies, and possibly a diagnostic nerve block at the suprascapular notch. Electrodiagnostic tests may confirm the diagnosis and localize the lesion. Positive findings on NCSs occasionally include prolonged distal motor latencies when the suprascapular nerve is stimulated at Erb's point; and compound muscle action potentials (CMAPs) are recorded from both the supraspinatus and infraspinatus muscles. However, NCS are technically limited by the necessity of recording CMAPs with a needle electrode, which invalidates the utility of the amplitude measurement. Suprascapular neuropathy may exist with normal NCSs.[1,40] Two-channel recording sites at both spinati muscles are sometimes useful for detecting conduction slowing (rather than axonal or conduction block injury) if latencies measurements are profoundly different from those on the normal side. Positive findings on needle EMG examinations may include fibrillation potentials or other abnormal spontaneous activity, large and/or polyphasic motor units, and decreased recruitment in the infraspinatus muscle with or without similar findings in the supraspinatus muscle. Other differential diagnoses such as C5/6 radiculopathy and upper brachial plexus lesions can often be ruled out by electrodiagnostics.

A variety of imaging techniques may be helpful for evaluating suprascapular nerve injury. Plain radiographs are usually unremarkable. A notch view radiograph may be used to assess the shape of the suprascapular notch and visualize a calcified transverse scapular ligament. Computed tomography (CT) may also reveal osseous abnormalities that may be impinging on the nerve. Magnetic resonance imaging (MRI) of the shoulder region can be useful for assessing suprascapular nerve injury. It can depict space-occupying lesions, which may be a source of compression. A ganglion cyst appears as low signal intensity on T1-weighted images and high signal on T2-weighted images (Fig. 7.2).

If a ganglion cyst is identified, various sequences can illustrate concurrent labral or posterior capsule defects in the shoulder joint. MRI can also identify soft tissue masses, osseous tumors, and vascular malformations that can compress the nerve. Acute entrapment of the suprascapular nerve is depicted on water-sensitive T2-weighted or short-inversion-time inversion recovery (STIR) sequences as hyperintensity involving the affected supraspinatus or infraspinatus muscles, whereas chronic compression produces atrophy and fatty infiltration of the involved muscles.[41] Thus, different muscle edema patterns can help distinguish the location and duration of the lesion. In addition, some medical centers have high-field 3 T (tesla) MRI scanners that have the capacity to demonstrate the course of the nerve. MRI can also be valuable for ruling out other potential shoulder pathology, such as a rotator cuff tear.

Another useful test may be a diagnostic nerve block. Relief of shoulder pain after an injection of 1% lidocaine into the suprascapular notch from a posterosuperior approach is consistent with suprascapular nerve injury at this site.[42–44] Sensitivity and specificity have not been well tested for either blind or image-guided injection for suprascapular neuropathy.

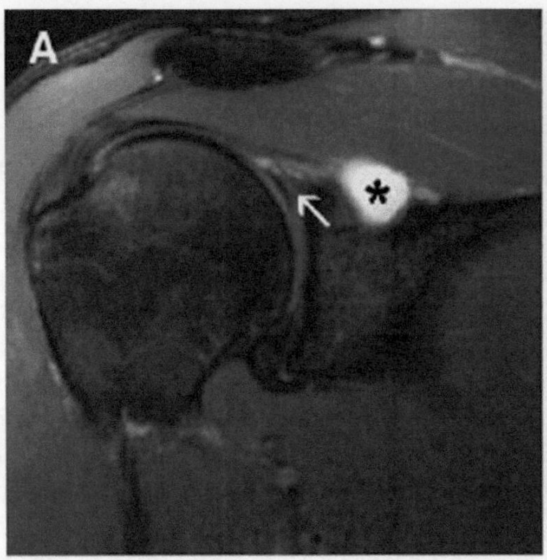

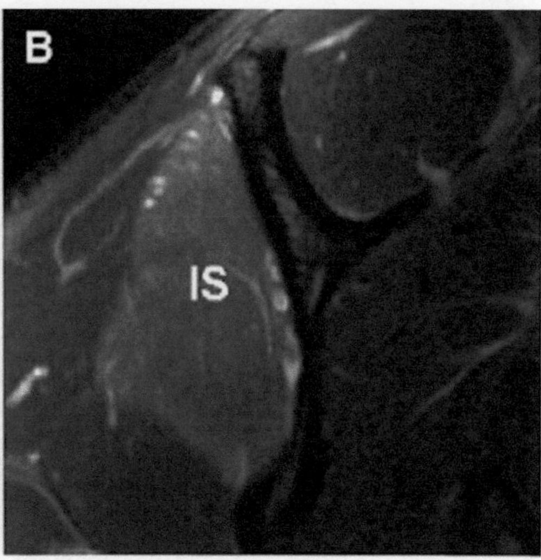

Fig. 7.2 Suprascapular nerve syndrome. Oblique coronal (**A**) and oblique sagittal (**B**) fat-suppressed, T2-weighted magnetic resonance (MR) images depict a ganglion cyst (*asterisk*) within the suprascapular notch associated with a tear of the superior labrum (*arrow*). Denervation edema of the infraspinatus (IS) muscle is noted. This figure was published in: Bencardino and Rosenberg,[41] Copyright Elsevier 2006. Used with permission

Treatment

The initial management of most suprascapular nerve injuries is nonoperative care, particularly if there is no evidence of a space-occupying lesion (e.g., a ganglion cyst). Previous reports have suggested that nonoperative care is as efficacious as operative care.[15] A conservative treatment program begins with relative rest and pain management. All of the peripheral nerve injuries discussed in this chapter are treated with a similar protocol for pain management. Neuropathic medications (e.g., antiepileptic agents, tricyclic antidepressants) may be helpful if neuropathic pain is a major symptom. Antiinflammatory agents may also be used to provide pain relief. Modalities that can be used to reduce pain include ice, heat, and transcutaneous electrical nerve stimulation. Nerve blocks and acupuncture have also been described to help to alleviate pain.

Therapeutic exercises include shoulder range of motion in all planes, with emphasis on maintaining full motion of the posterior capsule. Stretching the posterior capsule is particularly important because it theoretically decreases tension of the spinoglenoid ligament. Postural modifications and proprioceptive exercises may improve scapular stabilization. Controlled strengthening exercises of the shoulder girdle muscles should focus on the rotator cuff, deltoid, and periscapular muscles, particularly the serratus anterior, trapezius, and rhomboid muscles. The goal is to enhance compensatory muscle strength and thus regain muscular balance about the shoulder.[45] This conservative treatment program is based on intuitive concepts and anecdotal experience. There is currently no scientific evidence to prove the efficacy of any or all components of the above-suggested rehabilitation program. In the absence of a space-occupying lesion such as a cyst, most cases of suprascapular nerve palsy resolve completely within 6–12 months after diagnosis.[12,25]

If there is confirmed evidence of a ganglion cyst or other lesion, surgical intervention may be warranted. Percutaneous cyst decompression or open excision can be performed to remove the source of compression. Shoulder arthroscopy may be the procedure of choice to perform cyst decompression if there is concurrent intraarticular pathology, such as a labral tear, that can be débrided or repaired. It has been shown that ganglion cysts that cause suprascapular nerve compression at the spinoglenoid notch are associated with labral tears, seen arthroscopically or by MRI, in nearly 90% of cases.[46–48] Often, correcting the intraarticular lesion alone removes the one-way valve and allows the cyst to decompress.[15,46,47,49,50]

If there is not a mass compressing the nerve, surgery may be indicated when the patient has persistent symptoms despite 6–12 months of nonoperative management and/or no improvement of EMG findings.[45] The degree of axon loss can help determine whether surgery will be successful. If there is evidence of complete axonal loss that has persisted for at least 1 year, surgery is unlikely to restore full strength of the shoulder, but it may be effective in relieving pain. In fact, in 49% of individuals, atrophy remains despite surgery. Thus, the goals and expectations of the patient should be discussed prior to surgical intervention.

If the lesion is at the transverse scapular ligament or the spinoglenoid ligament, a surgical procedure may be performed to section the ligament and release the nerve. A notchplasty can also be performed, in either location, if there is a narrow or sharp (V-shaped) notch. There are reports of arthroscopic visualization and release of the transverse scapular ligament.[51,52] Most surgical outcomes are positive, with relief of pain and nearly full recovery of strength despite potentially persistent atrophy. With appropriate rehabilitation, muscle function can be maximized to provide the balance needed for overhead sports and return to full athletic activity.

Axillary Nerve Injury

Axillary nerve injury is relatively uncommon in the general population, representing fewer than 1% of all nerve injuries,[53] but relatively common in sports. In one case series of more than 200 sports-related peripheral nerve injuries, axillary neuropathy was the third most common mononeuropathy reported.[54] The main sources of axillary nerve injury in sports are anterior shoulder dislocation and proximal humeral fracture. Direct contusion, quadrilateral space syndrome, and iatrogenic injury during surgery are less common causes.

The axillary nerve originates from the fifth and sixth cervical nerve roots, with occasional contribution from the fourth root in a prefixed brachial plexus. It is a terminal branch of the brachial plexus, derived from the posterior cord. It passes under the coracoid process, anterior to the subscapularis muscle and posterior to the axillary artery. It courses posteriorly at the inferior border of the subscapularis muscle, medial to the musculotendinous junction. It receives a sensory branch from the anterior articular capsule at this point. It continues posteriorly, adjacent to the inferomedial capsule; and, joined by the posterior circumflex artery, it enters the quadrilateral space. The quadrilateral space is bordered by the teres minor muscle superiorly, the teres major and latissimus dorsi muscles inferiorly, the long head of the triceps tendon medially, the subscapularis muscle anteriorly, and the humeral shaft laterally. At this point, the axillary nerve gives off branches to the inferomedial aspect of the glenohumeral capsule.[55] It then tracks around the surgical neck of the humerus and divides into two branches, one to the anterior and middle deltoid and the other to the posterior deltoid. The posterior branch gives off a small branch to the teres minor and terminates as the upper lateral brachial cutaneous nerve to supply skin sensation overlying the deltoid muscle (deltoid patch). The posterior branch of the axillary nerve is closest to the glenoid rim and may be the most susceptible to injury. Occasionally, the deltoid patch is supplied by the suprascapular nerve. Figure 7.3 illustrates the anatomy of the axillary nerve.

Injury to the axillary nerve is most commonly the result of a traumatic event causing traction to the nerve at the shoulder. This is usually associated with glenohumeral dislocation or humeral fracture. Stretching of the nerve over the humeral head occurs when the humeral head dislocates from the glenoid fossa in an anteroinferior direction. The incidence of axillary nerve injury has been reported to be 19%–55% of anterior shoulder dislocations.[56–59] Luxatio erecta, or inferior glenohumeral dislocation, is a rare shoulder dislocation usually caused by a hyperabduction injury to the arm. This type of injury has an even greater rate of axillary nerve injury, reported to be as high as 60%.[60] The risk of nerve injury via dislocation increases with the following factors.[58,61,62]

- Age (older than 50 years)
- Time to reduction (left unreduced for more than 12 hours)

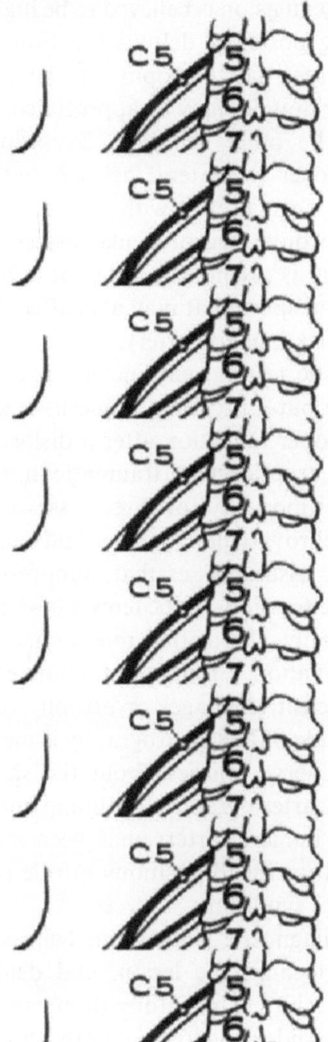

Fig. 7.3 Axillary nerve course and cutaneous invervation. From Dawson M, Hallett M, Wilbourn A. Entrapment Neuropathies. 3rd ed. Philadelphia: Lippincott-Raven; 1999:335. Used with permission

- Degree of injury (greater trauma and greater hematoma)

Axillary nerve injury can occur in as many as 58% of proximal humeral fractures.[63] The lateral cutaneous innervation and the branch to the teres minor muscle are closest to the glenoid rim, so they are most vulnerable to posttraumatic injuries.[64] Injury to the nerve can also be the result of blunt trauma to the shoulder. An impact to the anterolateral shoulder or posterior shoulder, in the region of the quadrilateral space, can directly damage the axillary nerve.

Quadrilateral space syndrome is a nebulous cause of axillary nerve injury. This syndrome is thought to be the result of chronic compression of the posterior humeral circumflex axillary artery, often accompanied by axillary nerve entrapment.

With its close proximity to the glenohumeral joint, the axillary nerve is susceptible to injury during any surgical procedure near the shoulder (e.g., arthroscopy, stabilization, rotator cuff repair). The nerve is vulnerable during routine arthroscopic procedures as it lies 2 cm inferior to the standard posterior portal. Depending on the procedure, the nerve may be injured in 1%–8% of patients undergoing shoulder surgery.[65] Finally, as is the case with the suprascapular nerve, the axillary nerve is one of the peripheral nerves of the shoulder girdle often affected by neuralgic amyotrophy (Parsonage-Turner syndrome).

Mechanism of Injury in Sport

Axillary nerve injury most commonly occurs after anterior shoulder dislocation, a fairly frequent athletic injury. There is a risk of shoulder dislocation in any sport where there is potential for falls or collisions, such as football or hockey.[39,66] Axillary nerve injuries may also be the result of blunt trauma to the anterolateral shoulder. This mechanism of injury has been described in football players after a hard tackle or block, where there is compression of the nerve as it travels on the deep surface of the deltoid between the hard helmet or ground and the humerus.[67,68] This type of direct impact injury has also been reported in boxing, hockey, rugby, martial arts, wrestling, and gymnastics.[62,69–71]

Acute entrapment of the axillary nerve in the quadrilateral space has been described in a wrestler secondary to violent contraction of the muscles surrounding the quadrilateral space.[24] The same author reported an arm wrestler with axillary nerve injury likely due to compression by hypertrophied shoulder girdle and arm muscles.[24] Axillary nerve injury has also been observed without trauma in two volleyball players in their dominant arms, likely from repeated microtrauma and stretching of the nerve with extreme shoulder motions.[72] Chronic irritation of the nerve by osteophytes at the posterior inferior glenoid margin has been reported in professional baseball players.[73] Rucksack paralysis in hikers has also occasionally presented as an isolated axillary neuropathy, presumably due to excessive traction from a backpack without proper waist support.[37,74]

Quadrilateral space syndrome with axillary nerve entrapment has been reported in athletes, attributed to fibrous bands or hypertrophied muscles chronically constricting the artery and nerve as they course through the quadrilateral space. This nebulous and controversial syndrome is thought to occur when the axillary nerve becomes further constricted by having the shoulder in a repetitive overhead position, specifically shoulder flexion, abduction, and external rotation. Obvious deltoid weakness is not usually apparent in quadrilateral space syndrome.

Physical Examination and Diagnostic Tests

The clinical diagnosis of axillary nerve injury may be difficult because the signs and symptoms are often vague. Initially, these injuries may be subclinical as the symptoms may be masked by concurrent shoulder dislocation or fracture. Furthermore, some athletes with mild injuries are entirely asymptomatic, regardless of the mechanism of injury to the nerve. The patient may note early fatigue with overhead activity or heavy lifting. They may also report weakness of their shoulder or numbness of the lateral arm.

Physical examination should include passive and active range of motion and strength testing in all shoulder planes. The patient may exhibit weakness with shoulder abduction, forward flexion, extension, and external rotation. It is important to assess external rotation strength as 45% of this strength is from the teres minor muscle.[75] The patient may exhibit weakness in both the deltoid and teres minor muscles, depending on the site of the lesion. Hertel et al. proposed the *extension lag sign* as a specific diagnostic test for axillary nerve injury.[76] The arm is brought passively into full extension, and the patient actively attempts to hold the arm in this position. If deltoid function is impaired, the arm drops, which is considered a positive test. This position of extension is believed to be highly specific to isolating posterior deltoid function. When the patient is seen late, atrophy of the deltoid and teres minor muscles may be appreciated when compared to the other shoulder. Sensation may be decreased over the lateral deltoid, but it can be completely normal even with a severe motor deficit.[77] A thorough neurovascular assessment of the affected arm is essential to rule out a lesion in the quadrilateral space that may also affect the posterior circumflex humeral artery.

Diagnostic testing may include plain radiography to rule out a proximal humerus fracture or to confirm proper reduction after a dislocation if the athlete has experienced a traumatic injury. MRI is the optimal modality for direct assessment of the axillary neurovascular bundle and quadrilateral space. Soft tissue masses that compress the nerve and signal alterations of the teres minor muscle and, less commonly, the deltoid muscle may be identified. Denervation can manifest as increased signal on water-sensitive images or atrophy of the muscle.[41] The role of MR neurography is under investigation for nerve injuries about the shoulder.[45,78] Subclavian arteriography, outlining the posterior circumflex humeral artery, has been suggested in resting and overhead positions to rule out quadrilateral space syndrome.

Electrodiagnostic studies can help confirm the diagnosis, localize the lesion, and determine the severity of injury. This information can establish a baseline to guide prognosis and predict an expected timeline of recovery. Reinnervation of the deltoid muscle occurs first in the posterior deltoid. Thus, it is important to sample all three regions of the deltoid muscle (anterior, middle, posterior) as well as the teres minor with needle examination to assess the status of nerve damage as well as nerve recovery. Axillary nerve motor NCSs can also be performed with stimulation over Erb's point and surface electrode recording over the deltoid muscle. Latency measurement is not as helpful because of the technical difficulties in distance measurement with proximal NCSs and because axillary nerve lesions rarely cause merely conduction *slowing*. Because axillary nerve lesions are either a conduction block or axonal loss, amplitude measurements of the created CMAP can reveal a decrease when compared that of the other side.

Treatment

Nonsurgical management consisting of relative rest, observation, and physical therapy is successful in managing most axillary nerve injuries in athletes.[70,71] The rehabilitation program consists of shoulder range of motion exercises and periscapular muscle strengthening as the nerve recovers. Physical therapy may need to be modified for initial protection of the anterior labrum and capsule in the case of axillary nerve injury after shoulder dislocation. Progressive resistance exercises should focus on maximizing rotator cuff and deltoid strength.

The prognosis depends largely on the mechanism and severity of injury to the nerve. Incomplete axillary nerve injury, by clinical examination and EMG testing, has a favorable prognosis. A good prognosis can be expected if the NCS demonstrates an axillary nerve CMAP amplitude on the symptomatic side that is at least 15% of the amplitude measured in the contralateral axillary nerve. In most cases of incomplete axillary nerve injury, gradual improvement can be expected with excellent functional recovery.

Complete axillary nerve lesion, demonstrated by EMG, warrants that the athlete be clinically reevaluated at about 2-month intervals for signs of nerve recovery based on the physical examination. Because the axillary nerve is relatively short, recovery should be seen in most axonal lesions between the third and fourth months after the injury.[71] Generally, axillary nerve injury due to traumatic dislocation or fracture has a better prognosis than injury due to a direct blow. In both cases, return to sport is possible and quite likely. In general, recovery of at least 80% of deltoid muscle strength is recommended to permit a return to play.[79]

Surgical exploration may be indicated if the athlete has persistent symptoms with no clinical or electrodiagnostic evidence of nerve recovery within 3–6 months.[80,81] Surgical intervention 1 year or more after the injury is associated with a poorer prognosis for functional recovery.[81] Surgical options include neurolysis, neurorrhaphy, nerve grafting, nerve transfer, and neurotization. In a case series by Kline and Kim, 66 patients with isolated axillary neuropathy underwent nerve graft repair leading to good recovery of deltoid muscle strength and adequate function of the involved shoulder.[82] The study did not comment on the athletic activity of the patient population and therefore could not draw conclusions regarding return to sport. Tendon transfers are usually salvage procedures, and the patient should be informed that the procedure is unlikely to allow a return to play.

Long Thoracic Nerve Injury

Long thoracic nerve injury is uncommon in sports. When this nerve is damaged, however, it can be quite disabling to athletes. It has been injured during many sporting activities. The common scenario for long thoracic nerve palsy in sports appears to be traction of the nerve during tennis.

The long thoracic nerve is a pure motor nerve that arises from the fifth, sixth, and seventh cervical nerve roots. There is a contribution from C8 in about 8% of patients and from the intercostal nerves in about 20% of patients.[83] The C5 and C6 nerve root contributions unite with the C7 nerve root distal to the scalene muscles to form the long thoracic nerve. The nerve travels within the axillary sheath posterior to the trunks of the brachial plexus. It traverses distally and laterally below the clavicle and under the first and second ribs. It then courses along the chest wall in the mid-axillary line to the border of the serratus anterior muscle, supplying branches to all digitations (Fig. 7.4).

The serratus anterior muscle originates from the first through the ninth ribs and inserts on the costomedial border of the scapula. The upper fibers insert onto the superior angle of the scapula and stabilize it during the initial stages of abduction. The middle fibers insert onto the vertebral border of the scapula and are instrumental in protraction of the scapula. The lower fibers of the serratus anterior insert onto the inferior angle of the scapula and are primary upward rotators of the scapula during abduction.[84] Serratus anterior is an important component of the force couple that stabilizes the scapula.

Acute or recurrent trauma has been identified as the most frequent mechanism of long thoracic nerve injury.[85–88] Repetitive microtrauma is a common cause of injury to this nerve, especially when sports-related. It is thought to occur owing to traction or stretching of the nerve while the arm is in an

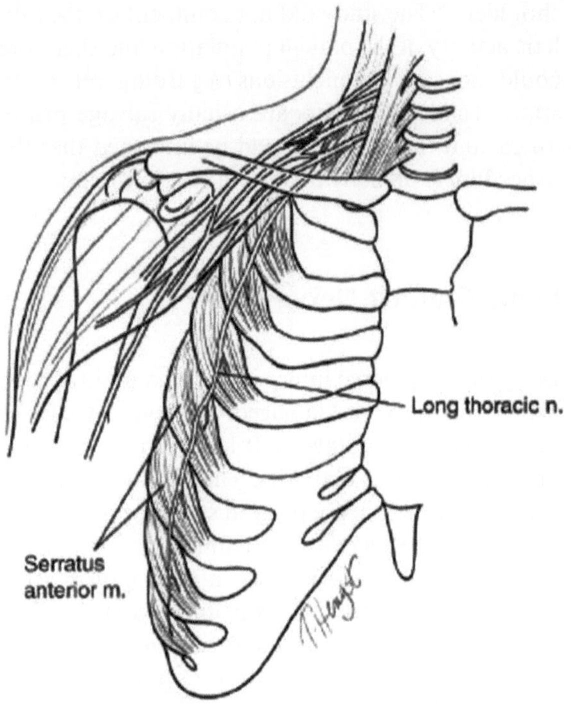

Fig. 7.4 Anatomy of the long thoracic nerve. Note the long thoracic nerve branching off before the brachial plexus and becoming subcutaneous about the level of the first or second rib, sending off branches to the digitations of the serratus anterior muscle. From Safran.[84] Copyright 2004 by The American Orthopaedic Society for Sports Medicine. Reprinted by permission of SAGE Publications, Inc.

overhead position and the neck is turned or tilted to the contralateral side.[89] The nerve is susceptible to traction injury between its two points of relative fixation-the scalenus medius muscle at the base of the neck and the superior aspect of the serratus anterior muscle.[86] In fact, with a severe stretch, the nerve may double in length between points of fixation, resulting in a neurapraxic lesion or more severe axonal damage.[90] The nerve may also be stretched over the rough prominence of the second rib.[91] The long thoracic nerve is susceptible to direct trauma. Although it is well protected along the superior chest wall down to the level of the inferior portion of the pectoralis major muscle, it becomes subcutaneous as it exits the pectoralis major, where it is at risk for injury.

Nontraumatic causes of long thoracic nerve injury include compression and neuralgic amyotrophy. The nerve can be compressed at numerous locations. It can be compressed between the scalene muscles, by a cervical rib, between the clavicle and second rib, between the second rib and the coracoid, by the inferior angle of the scapula, or by inflamed bursae or aberrant calcifications.[83,86,92,93] There are many bursae along the course of the nerve-including the subscapular, accessory subscapular, subcoracoid, supracoracoid-that can potentially compress the nerve.[93] Additionally, long thoracic nerve injury can be a consequence of neuralgic amyotrophy (Parsonage-Turner syndrome), which can be idiopathic, associated with viral infection, or appear after surgery. Neuralgic amyotrophy has a predilection for pure motor nerves, such as the long thoracic nerve.

Mechanism of Injury In Sport

Isolated serratus anterior muscle paralysis in the athlete may result from acute injury or, more insidiously, from repetitive motions, positioning, or strain. A wide variety of sports have been implicated in injury to the long thoracic nerve. The position of maximum traction of the long thoracic nerve, with the athlete's head turned away from the elevated arm, occurs commonly when throwing a baseball, football, or javelin and when spiking or serving a volleyball or tennis ball. A ballet dancer stretching during a warm-up and certain yoga positions have also been reported to cause this injury.[94]

Traction injury to the nerve may be secondary to asynchronous motion of the arm and scapula, which can occur with a missed shot or follow-through motion in golf, handball, or tennis or in contact sports in which the arm is jerked into an abnormal position.[95] This type of injury has also been reported in a boxer missing a punching bag, placing the scapula in a maximally protracted position.[96] Traction injuries have also resulted from repetitive motion such as swimming, prolonged positioning of the arm while shooting a rifle,[97,98] and extreme shoulder motions in basketball and football.[96,99] Long thoracic injury has been reported in an archer repetitively drawing back a bow[85] and in a racecar driver repetitively pulling back on the hand clutch.[86] It has also been described in a gymnast doing exercises on the rings and in a ten-pin bowler.[86] Fatigue of the periscapular muscles, as seen in backpackers, rope skippers, and weight lifters, allows abnormal scapular motion on the chest wall, resulting in a traction injury to the long thoracic nerve. Weightlifting exercises most commonly associated with long thoracic nerve palsy include behind-the-neck French curls and the bench press.[86,97] All of these exercises can produce marked translation of the scapula on the chest wall.

Direct trauma to the long thoracic nerve has been described in football after blocking or tackling with the impact directed at the shoulder and axillary region.[39] This injury can potentially occur with a blow to the thorax in the area of the fourth and fifth ribs in any contact sport. There is a case report of long thoracic nerve palsy in a judo competitor after shoulder dislocation.[100] This nerve injury can also be caused iatrogenically by surgical intervention to the chest wall in the region of the serratus anterior muscle.

Physical Examination and Diagnostic Tests

Patients presenting with long thoracic nerve injury often complain of pain in the shoulder and periscapular region that can radiate down the arm and up into the neck. Muscle pain is often posterior secondary to rhomboid and levator scapula spasm due to overactivity and compensation for a weakened serratus anterior muscle. The patient may report that the symptoms are worsened by overhead activity or by tilting the head away from the elevated, ipsilateral arm. There may be painful popping or clicking of the scapula with shoulder motion. The patient may also complain of the insidious onset of shoulder weakness and loss of throwing power.

Physical examination reveals decreased active shoulder-forward flexion and dysfunction of scapulohumeral rhythm compared to the asymptomatic side. The clinician may also appreciate the scapular winging that is classically associated with long thoracic nerve injury and serratus anterior muscle paralysis. Winging at the inferior scapular border can be elicited with shoulder-forward flexion or wall push-up at 90° of shoulder flexion with internal rotation. Scapular winging may not be present until 2 weeks after the injury. At rest, the clinician may observe elevation and retraction of the scapula such that the inferior pole of the scapula appears closer to the midline and slightly more elevated than the contralateral scapula. It is an important skill on physical examination to be able to distinguish the scapular winging patterns and the associated clinical features that occur with various neuromuscular disorders, including facioscapulohumeral dystrophy (FSH) and limb girdle muscular dystrophy (Table 7.1).

Electrodiagnostic studies are used to confirm the diagnosis. The needle EMG examination is helpful for documenting the severity of the nerve injury and for following recovery. The spinal accessory nerve and the trapezius muscle should also be evaluated in the study as spinal accessory nerve injury is in the differential diagnosis of scapular winging. Furthermore, concomitant trapezius weakness may compromise the results of surgical intervention for long thoracic nerve injury. Plain radiographs are usually unremarkable but should be obtained to assess for a cervical rib or calcifications, which may be causes of long thoracic nerve injury. Other imaging studies, such as CT and MRI scans are not particularly helpful.

Treatment

Nonsurgical treatment is initially indicated for all patients. A treatment plan in athletes includes activity modification to avoid putting the nerve at risk for stretch and further injury. Athletes should avoid lifting heavy objects or participating in activities that exacerbate symptoms. They should avoid lying with their hand behind their head in the abducted, externally rotated position for prolonged periods of time as this maneuver results in protraction of the scapula and traction on the recovering long thoracic nerve.[86] The pain management protocol for peripheral nerve injuries discussed above for suprascapular nerve injury may be utilized to alleviate pain.

Therapeutic exercise consists of maintaining full range of motion of the glenohumeral and scapulothoracic joints to prevent stiffness and contracture. The stretching program should focus on

Table 7.1 Clinical features of common neuromuscular causes of scapular winging

Neuromuscular cause	Pain	Deformity at rest	Winging provocation	Scapular displacement	Associated features
Long thoracic nerve (serratus anterior weakness)	Minimal, localized to scapular region	Minimal winging inferior scapula, lower medial border closer to spine	Shoulder forward flexion, wall push-up with elbows extended	Inferior angle farther from midline	
Spinal accessory nerve (trapezius weakness)	Mild to moderately severe, supraclavicular fossa and shoulder	Shoulder droop, suprascapular fossa atrophy from trapezius wasting, minimal winging; inferior angle closer to spine	Shoulder abduction	Inferior angle toward midline	
Dorsal scapular nerve (rhomboid weakness)	Predominant complaint, medial border of scapular	Minimal winging, subtle rhomboidal atrophy if chronic	Slowly lower arms from forward flexed position	Shifted laterally and dorsally, especially inferior portion	
Facioscapulohumeral dystrophy (FSH) (lower trapezius, rhomboid, serratus anterior weakness)	Minimal	Mild to severe winging depending on stage of disease	Abduction or forward flexion	Upward giving a scalloped appearance to the shoulder girdle; patients often unable to go > 90°	Often asymmetrical; facial muscle weakness; preservation of deltoid bulk with weakness/atrophy of biceps and triceps; normal or mildly elevated CK
Limb girdle muscular dystrophy 2A (calpain deficiency) or 2I (FKRP deficiency)	Minimal	Mild to severe winging depending on stage of disease	Abduction or forward flexion	Protrusion of medial border; variable	Pelvic girdle weakness; normal facial muscle strength; very high CK

FKRP, fukutin-related protein; CK, creatine kinase

passive range of motion exercises to stretch the rhomboid and pectoralis minor muscles, avoiding a fixed, retracted position of the scapula on the chest wall. A strengthening program should focus on the scapular stabilizers including the trapezius, rhomboid, and levator scapula muscles. Muscular compensation is difficult in this injury as no other muscle can adequately substitute for the function of the serratus anterior. Bracing to maintain the scapular position has been suggested by some authors to attempt to limit further winging of the scapula and decrease stretch on the nerve during recovery,[83,86] but the brace is cumbersome and generally poorly accepted by the athlete.

Athletes should be informed that most cases of atraumatic long thoracic nerve injury improve within 6–9 months, and almost all cases resolve satisfactorily within 1 year.[85,86] However, maximum recovery may take as long as 2 years, and mild residual winging may persist.[101] Return to sporting activity can occur once the athlete's symptoms have resolved, even if early fatigue of the serratus anterior muscle is noted on physical examination.

The indications for surgery for patients with long thoracic nerve injury are symptoms persisting beyond 1–2 years despite nonoperative management and no improvement of electrodiagnostic studies. The goal of surgery is to provide a scapula that is stable and pain-free, especially during overhead activities. Surgical options include dynamic muscle transfer, fascial sling suspension, scapulothoracic fusion, and nerve transfer. Muscle transfer options include using the pectoralis major, pectoral minor, rhomboids, or teres minor muscle as donor. Dynamic muscle transfer is thought to provide control of the scapula and some scapulothoracic motion. Currently, pectoralis major muscle transfer appears to have the best results. The sternal head of the pectoralis major tendon is transferred to the inferior angle of the scapula and is augmented with a fascia lata autograft. Favorable results have been reported, with notable improvement in function, pain relief, and resolution of winging.[102–104]

Scapulothoracic fusion may be done as a salvage procedure after other procedures have failed. However, approximately one-third of total shoulder elevation is lost with scapulothoracic fusion, and complications such as pneumothorax and pseudarthrosis occur in up to one-half of patients.[101] Scapulothoracic fusion often has a prolonged recovery as the arm must be immobilized for about 3 months, followed by an extensive physical therapy program to regain range of motion and strength. With all of the surgical options, patients are able to return to performing all functional activities of daily living, but their return to sports is unlikely. Residual dysfunction and asymptomatic scapular winging are common.

Spinal Accessory Nerve Injury

The spinal accessory nerve (cranial nerve XI) is not a true peripheral nerve; however, it can be included in the discussion of nerve injuries about the shoulder because it supplies the trapezius muscle. The trapezius muscle is an important muscle for shoulder and scapular stability and function. Spinal accessory nerve injury is rare in athletes. It is more commonly injured during surgery in the neck region.

The spinal accessory nerve is a pure motor nerve that exits the base of the skull at the jugular foramen and picks up contributions from the nerve roots of C2–4. It then innervates and passes obliquely through the upper third of the sternocleidomastoid muscle. It courses subcutaneously at the floor of the posterior cervical triangle as it travels to supply the trapezius muscle. The nerve traverses on the deep surface of the trapezius muscle, on the medial border of the scapula (Fig. 7.5).

The trapezius has three main groups of muscle fibers that allow shoulder and scapular motion and stability. Specifically, the upper fibers elevate the scapula; the middle fibers stabilize and retract the scapula, pulling it midline; and the lower fibers depress the scapula.[105] The most important functions of the trapezius are to resist drooping of the shoulder and assist in abduction of the arm, allowing overhead activities.

The most common pathogeneses of spinal accessory nerve injury are related to its subcutaneous location in the neck. It is most often injured at the upper border of the trapezius, about 1 inch above the clavicle.[70] It can be injured iatrogenically by various surgical procedures in the neck region. It may be inadvertently sectioned during cervical

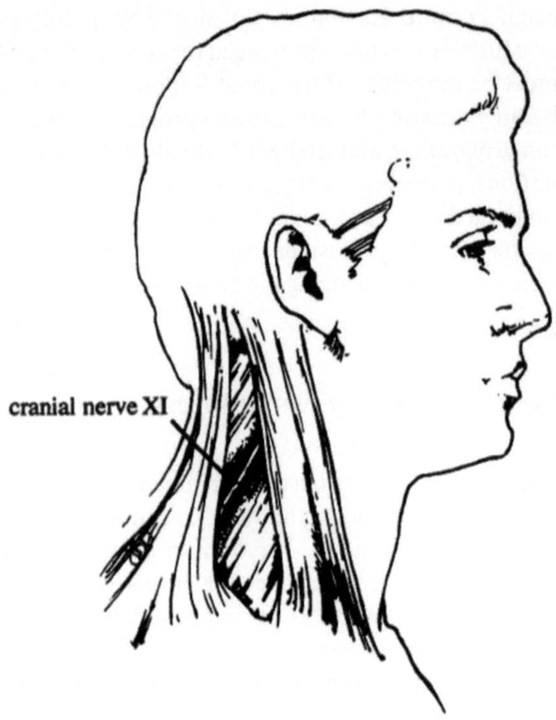

Fig. 7.5 Lateral view of the neck showing the spinal accessory nerve (cranial nerve XI). The spinal accessory nerve's location in the neck in close proximity to the deep lateral chain of lymph nodes render it susceptible to injury by both a direct blow to the neck and biopsy of lymph nodes in this area. From Duralde.[79] Used with permission

lymph node biopsy, subcutaneous mass or cyst excision, radical neck dissection for a tumor, or during carotid endarterectomy. Isolated injuries to the spinal accessory nerve have also been reported with penetrating trauma to the base of the neck and direct blows to the neck as well as traction injuries after a fall on the shoulder where there is forced increase in acromiomastoid distance.[70]

Mechanism of Injury in Sport

In athletes, spinal accessory nerve injury may be the result of a direct blow across the neck with an ice hockey, lacrosse, or field hockey stick.[70,106] The nerve is susceptible to a direct blow at the upper border of the trapezius from an opposing football player's helmet. There have been similar reports of direct trauma to the nerve in judo, karate, and kickboxing.[107] Traction injuries have also been reported in athletes after a fall on the acromion.[70] There are reports of spinal accessory nerve injury during the wrestling cross-face maneuver, in which the head is forcefully rotated toward the opposite shoulder.[77,108] Stretch injury of the spinal accessory nerve has also been reported with heavy weightlifting.[77]

Physical Examination and Diagnostic Tests

Athletes with spinal accessory nerve injury may complain of pain that ranges from mild and aching to severe and disabling. The pain localizes to the posterior shoulder and medial scapula and may radiate down the arm. It may be gradual in onset and represent straining and spasm of the remaining scapular muscles, impingement syndrome secondary to forward rotation of the scapula, or stretching of the brachial plexus.[108,109] Patients may complain of a heavy feeling about the shoulder. Female athletes may notice difficulty keeping the bra strap on the affected shoulder. The patient should be examined from behind with the shoulders exposed. The athlete with trapezius muscle paralysis may demonstrate drooping of the shoulder and an asymmetrical neckline.[108,109] The normal contour of the trapezius between the neck and lateral shoulder is lost, and the distal clavicle and acromion may appear more prominent secondary to atrophy of the overlying trapezius. With trapezius muscle dysfunction, the scapula lowers and moves farther from the midline and the inferior angle is drawn upward by the rhomboid muscles.

Muscle strength testing may reveal an abnormal shrug test where the athlete is not able to shrug symmetrically. The shoulder shrug test may not be reliable, however, as an intact levator scapulae muscle can compensate to perform this function. Thus, trapezius muscle function is best tested in abduction with the shoulder internally rotated (same position as for the *empty can* test). Full abduction is impossible in this position without an intact trapezius.[79] The athlete may also have weakness in forward flexion above the horizontal plane as well as loss of normal scapulohumeral rhythm throughout shoulder range of motion. The Neer weight duration test, in which the patient holds a heavy object at arm's length, may be helpful to identify early fatigue pain.[110]

Scapular winging may occur, but it is typically not as dramatic as that seen with long thoracic nerve injury. At rest, winging due to a spinal accessory nerve injury may be minimal, typically with the inferior angle of the scapula closer to the midline. It tends to be most pronounced in the plane of abduction, in contrast to long thoracic nerve palsy. The scapula moves upward and laterally on abduction, with the superior angle more displaced from the midline than the inferior angle. With forward flexion of the shoulder, the flaring of the inferior angle of the scapula corrects because of the intact action of the serratus anterior muscle, holding the scapula to the thorax (Table 7.1).[111]

Electrodiagnostic testing can help confirm the diagnosis of spinal accessory nerve injury, provide insight into the prognosis, and track recovery of the nerve. The function of the trapezius, sternocleidomastoid, and potentially transferable muscles (levator scapulae, rhomboid major and minor) are typically assessed. As for the other nerve injuries discussed, needle EMG can demonstrate specific signs of acute or chronic denervation of involved muscles. Serial electrodiagnostic tests to follow the recovery of the injured nerve can help in the decision regarding nerve exploration versus muscle transfer. Plain radiography of the cervical spine, shoulder, and chest is indicated to rule out other pathology. CT and MRI scans are not necessary unless other diagnoses, such as mass lesions or disc disease, are suspected.

Treatment

Nonsurgical treatment is initially implemented for spinal accessory nerve injury consisting of activity modification and medications to manage symptoms. Patients are encouraged to avoid overhead activities. Slings and braces have been used to support the scapula against the chest wall, but often this is of little use, particularly in the long term.[112]

Therapeutic exercise focuses on attempting to strengthen the compensatory muscles to eliminate pain and alleviate drooping of the shoulder and weakness of elevation. As with the serratus anterior muscle, no muscles about the scapula can adequately substitute for the function of the trapezius muscle.[79] Thus, strengthening exercises for the remaining scapular muscles are of limited benefit. These forms of conservative management are generally unsuccessful, especially in active patients who wish to return to their prior level of competition.[112,113]

There are several surgical options in cases of spinal accessory nerve injury, including neurolysis, nerve repair (direct repair or with a graft), and static and dynamic scapular stabilization procedures. Good results can be expected from repair of the spinal accessory nerve if it is performed within 20 months after the injury, as the nerve is basically a purely motor nerve and the distance from the injury to the motor end plates is short.[114] Surgery for cases of closed trauma to the spinal accessory nerve, where the continuity of the nerve remains intact, is indicated if adequate muscle function has not returned and symptoms persist for approximately 1 year despite an adequate conservative treatment program or when previous nerve surgery has failed.[115] Static stabilization procedures for trapezius paralysis include scapulothoracic fusion, fasciodesis, and stabilization of the scapula to the vertebral spinous processes with fascial grafts.[115] Although favorable results are seen early with static procedures, they generally deteriorate over time because the grafts tend to stretch.

Dynamic procedures include transfer of the levator scapulae with or without transfer of the rhomboid muscles. The Eden-Lange procedure involves lateral transfer of the levator scapulae and both rhomboids to new locations on the scapula, allowing them to substitute for the function of the upper, middle, and lower trapezius muscle.[116] Bigliani and colleagues[109] demonstrated favorable results at early and intermediate follow-up visits in patients who underwent the Eden-Lange procedure for persistent trapezius weakness. In a more recent study by Romero and Gerber,[117] the Eden-Lange procedure resulted in highly satisfactory long-term outcomes. In general, surgery for spinal accessory nerve injury is useful for restoring functional activities of daily living but is usually not adequate to return the athlete to sports activity.

Dorsal Scapular Nerve Injury

There are rare reports of isolated dorsal scapular nerve injury in the literature. The dorsal scapular nerve is a pure motor nerve; it originates from the fifth cervical spinal nerve root immediately after it exits the neural foramen, within the posterior cervical triangle, deep to the prevertebral fascia.[118] It can share a common trunk with the long thoracic nerve. It pierces the middle scalene muscle and travels between the posterior scalene muscle and the serratus posterior superior and levator scapulae muscles to innervate the rhomboid major and minor muscles and occasionally the levator scapulae muscle (Fig. 7.6).

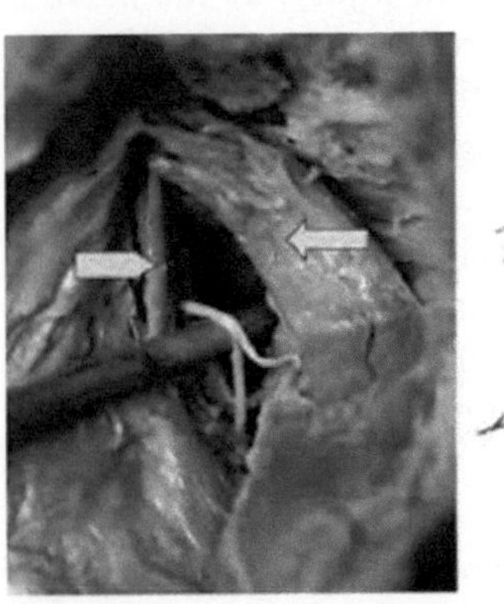
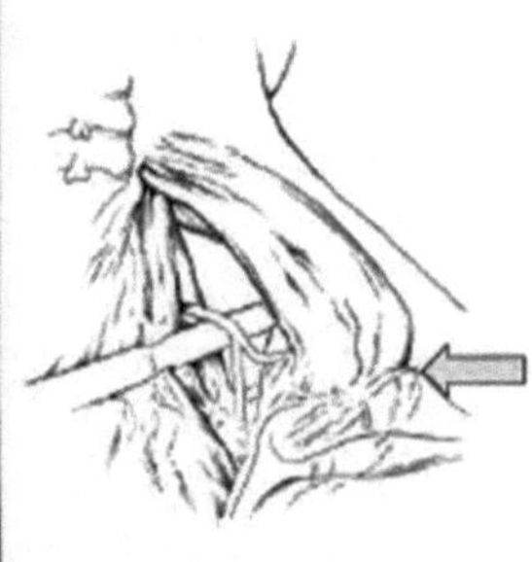

Fig. 7.6 Posterior view of the dorsal scapular nerve piercing the middle scalene muscle (*arrowhead*) and traveling over the probe toward the levator scapulae muscles (*arrow*). From Tubbs et al.[120] Used with permission

Frank et al.[119] found that the nerve innervated the levator scapulae muscles in only 11 of 35 neck specimens. The rhomboid and levator scapulae muscles function collectively to retract and elevate the scapula. Injury to the rhomboid muscles can result in instability of the shoulder.[120] Rare reports suggest that the dorsal scapular nerve may be injured by a traction mechanism during shoulder dislocation. It may also be compressed and entrapped owing to hypertrophy of the middle scalene muscle.[121]

Mechanism of Injury in Sports

There are rare reports of dorsal scapular nerve injury in athletes. One study reported a combined injury to the dorsal scapular nerve and long thoracic nerve as a result of anterior shoulder dislocation during judo.[100] Another report described an isolated injury to the dorsal scapular nerve in a bodybuilder using anabolic steroids. This case was thought to be due to a stretch injury in the hypertrophied middle scalene muscle during exercises of neck flexion and forceful repetitive shoulder shrugging.[122] Presumably, these movements, when made vigorously, can contract the scalene muscles. In addition, rhomboid weakness, mild scapular winging, and electrodiagnostic evidence of dorsal scapular nerve injury with concurrent suprascapular nerve injury has been reported in two sibling volleyball players.[123]

Physical Examination and Diagnostic Tests

The evaluation of an athlete with suspected dorsal scapular nerve injury should include a thorough musculoskeletal and neurovascular examination of the shoulder. Patients may complain of shoulder, neck, or periscapular pain. Pain along the medial border of the scapula may be the sole complaint.[111] In fact, some researchers have determined that dorsal scapular nerve injury can produce underdiagnosed shoulder pain.[124] Entrapment of the dorsal scapular nerve may result in abnormal shoulder motion with mild winging of the scapula that may be subtle and difficult to identify by the physical examination. Rhomboid muscle weakness and scapular winging is best demonstrated by having the patient lower his or her arms from the forward-flexed position.[111] When these muscles are paralyzed, the examiner can more easily place several fingers under the vertebral border of the scapula.[125] The scapula moves laterally and dorsally, especially the lower portion (Table 7.1).[111] If symptoms are of long duration, atrophy of the rhomboids may be present. It may be difficult to differentiate rhomboid muscle atrophy from atrophy of the midportion of the trapezius.

Electrodiagnostic studies are useful for confirming the diagnosis of dorsal scapular nerve injury and ruling out other suspected neuropathies. Needle EMG findings include evidence of acute or chronic denervation of the rhomboid muscles. It is important to conduct a thorough electrodiagnostic study to rule out other causes of scapular winging as well as C5 radiculopathy. It is unclear if imaging studies such as ultrasonography or MRI are useful as diagnostic tools in this nerve injury given the paucity of case reports at this time.

Treatment

Because of the limited number of reported cases of dorsal scapular nerve injury, it is difficult to arrive at conclusions regarding the most effective treatment approach. Given the successful conservative approach to more common peripheral nerve injuries about the shoulder, it is reasonable to manage dorsal scapular neuropathy nonoperatively with pain medication, modalities, and therapeutic exercise. Maximizing the strength of the other shoulder and scapular stabilizers may be adequate to compensate for rhomboid muscle dysfunction.

Thoracodorsal Nerve Injury

Isolated injury to the thoracodorsal nerve is extremely rare, with only a few case reports regarding athletes. The thoracodorsal nerve is a pure motor nerve. It is a branch of the posterior cord of the brachial plexus that derives its fibers from the sixth, seventh, and eighth cervical nerve roots. It follows the course of the subscapular artery along the posterior wall of the axilla to innervate the latissimus dorsi muscle. The latissimus dorsi acts to extend, adduct, and internally rotate the shoulder. It also has a synergistic role in extension and lateral flexion of the lumbar spine.

Isolated injury to the thoracodorsal nerve may be a complication of surgery of the axilla or chest region. It may also be injured by a traction mechanism after vigorous rising of the trunk from a prone or lateral recumbent position. Modelli et al.[122] reported a case of a thoracodorsal nerve injury and postulated a stretch mechanism at the axillary margin of the scapula where it runs with the long thoracic nerve along the posterior wall of the chest, between the subscapular and serratus anterior muscles.

Mechanism of Injury in Sports

Isolated injury to the thoracodorsal nerve was reported by Modelli et al.[122] in a bodybuilder using anabolic steroids. The theorized mechanism of traction is described above. The nerve may be susceptible to entrapment by a hypertrophied subscapularis muscle. An important differential diagnosis is C7 radiculopathy because it is relatively common.

Physical Examination and Diagnostic Tests

The physical examination of suspected thoracodorsal nerve injury should include a thorough musculoskeletal and neurologic evaluation of the shoulder girdle to rule out all other causes of dysfunction in this area. Weakness of the latissimus dorsi muscle may manifest as diminished adduction and internal rotation of the involved shoulder with or without examiner resistance. There may also be ipsilateral weakness in lateral side-bending of the trunk. Atrophy of the posterior wall of the axilla may be observed.

Electrodiagnostic studies may be performed to confirm the clinical diagnosis. Wu et al.[126] described an NCS for the thoracodorsal nerve in which the nerve is stimulated at Erb's point and at the axilla and recorded over the latissimus dorsi. The needle EMG examination is generally more reliable for demonstrating denervation of the latissimus dorsi muscle, although it can be technically challenging as this muscle is not frequently tested. It is sometimes useful to sample the contralateral latissimus dorsi to compare sides.

Treatment

Given the paucity of case reports of isolated thoracodorsal nerve injury in the literature, there is no evidence of the best treatment approach for athletes. A conservative management approach appears to be reasonable, with activity modification and therapeutic stretching and strengthening exercises of the shoulder girdle musculature. If there is adequate return of functional and sport-specific motion and strength, the athlete may return to athletic activity. There are no reports in the literature of surgical procedures to treat thoracodorsal nerve injury. However, the thoracodorsal nerve has been used as a donor nerve in surgical procedures for other peripheral nerve or brachial plexus injuries, including cases of axillary and musculocutaneous nerve damage.[127]

Medial Pectoral Nerve Injury

There are rare reports of medial pectoral nerve injuries in athletes. The medial pectoral nerve is a pure motor nerve that has contributions from the eighth cervical and first thoracic nerve roots. It arises from the medial cord of the brachial plexus. It passes behind the first part of the axillary artery, curves forward between the axillary artery and vein, and unites in front of the axillary artery with a branch from the lateral pectoral nerve. It then enters the deep surface of the pectoralis minor, where it divides into a number of branches that innervate the muscle. The pectoralis minor muscle acts forcefully to rotate the scapula forward. [128] Two or three branches continue on to pierce and terminate in the inferior, sternal portion of the pectoral major muscle. The superior, sternoclavicular portion of the pectoralis major muscle is innervated by the lateral pectoral nerve.

Iatrogenic injury to the medial pectoral nerve during breast and chest wall surgery, specifically as a complication of mastectomy, has been well described.[129–131] In addition, compression of the medial pectoral nerve may occur within a hypertrophied pectoralis minor muscle. The nerve may be susceptible to stretch injury with vigorous chest-expanding strengthening exercise, such as fly exercises with free weights.[132]

Mechanism of Injury in Sports

There are rare case reports of athletes with medial pectoral nerve injury. There is a report of bilateral medial pectoral neuropathy in a weightlifter who was involved in a rigorous, intensive program of bodybuilding over a 3-year period.[132] The athlete denied the use of anabolic steroids. The mechanism of injury in this patient was postulated to be bilateral entrapment of the medial pectoral nerves within hypertrophied pectoralis minor muscles. There is a second report of unilateral medial pectoral neuropathy in a bodybuilder using anabolic steroids. The mononeuropathy manifested a few days after a formebolone injection into the ipsilateral pectoralis major muscle followed by strenuous weight training of the pectoral muscles. In this case, the nerve injury may have occurred because of incorrect self-inoculation of the anabolic steroid, from a stretch injury during vigorous chest-expanding exercises, or from compression within a hypertrophied pectoralis minor muscle.[122]

Physical Examination and Diagnostic Tests

An athlete with an isolated medial pectoral nerve injury may present with painless weakness of the pectoral muscles noted by diminished strength on bench press exercises. Physical examination may reveal atrophy of the inferior sternal portion of the pectoralis major muscle with sparing and maintained bulk of the clavicular portion. There may also be compensatory hypertrophy of the shoulder girdle and arm muscles. Needle EMG may confirm denervation to the inferior portion of the pectoralis major muscle supplied by the medial pectoral nerve while revealing normal motor unit activation and recruitment patterns in the clavicular portion of the pectoralis major muscle, supplied by the lateral pectoral nerve.

Treatment

Generally, resting the affected muscle appears to be appropriate initial management of medial pectoral nerve injury. There was reasonable recovery of strength and muscle mass in the previously described cases that were identified relatively early in their course.[122] A less favorable outcome is seen when the athlete continues to exercise the pectoral muscles, which can contribute to further compression of the nerve and more significant nerve damage.[132] Counseling the athlete regarding the detrimental effects of anabolic steroid use is certainly indicated.

Surgical exploration of sports-related medial pectoral neuropathy has not been described in the literature. As is the case for the thoracodorsal nerve, the medial pectoral nerve may also be used as a donor nerve for other peripheral nerve or brachial plexus injuries.

Musculocutaneous Nerve Injury

Injury to the musculocutaneous nerve occurs rarely in athletes, with only a few case reports describing this injury in sports. Generally, it is seen in athletes who participate in sports requiring vigorous elbow motion. The musculocutaneous nerve originates from the lateral cord of the brachial plexus near the inferior border of the pectoralis minor, receiving contribution from the fifth and sixth cervical nerve roots. It continues between the axillary artery and the median nerve, entering the upper arm by passing obliquely through the coracobrachialis muscle and between the biceps and brachialis muscles (Fig. 7.7).

The musculocutaneous nerve innervates the coracobrachialis muscle and sends branches to the biceps and brachialis muscles before it terminates as the lateral antebrachial cutaneous nerve (LAC). The LAC is purely sensory and exits 2–5 cm proximal to the elbow crease between the brachialis fascia and the thick biceps aponeurosis. It then divides into an anterior and posterior branch and innervates the radial half of the volar forearm and radial third of the dorsal forearm, respectively.

The musculocutaneous nerve is vulnerable to traction injury proximally with shoulder dislocation.[133] It can also be stretched across the humeral head or coracoid with the arm in the throwing position.[77] It can be damaged by blunt trauma to the anterior shoulder, and it is susceptible to direct injury with a clavicular or humeral fracture.[125] The nerve's variable position of penetration through the coracobrachialis muscle can make it susceptible to injury during surgical procedures about the shoulder, including open or arthroscopic procedures.[125,134] Injury can also be due to proximal compression at a hypertrophied coracobrachialis muscle or distal compression at the biceps aponeurosis.

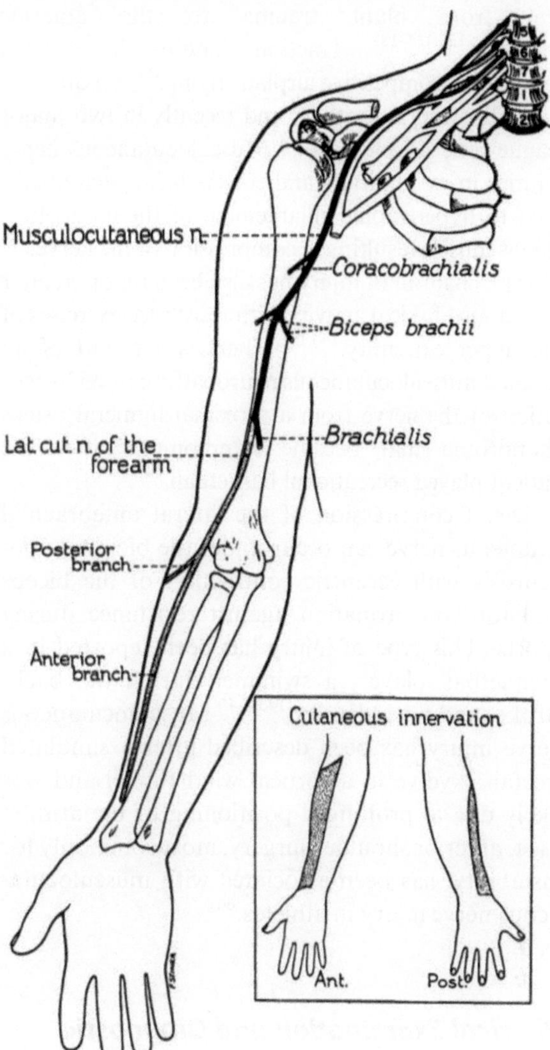

Fig. 7.7 Musculocutaneous nerve course and cutaneous innervation. From Dawson M, Hallett M, Wilbourn A. Entrapment Neuropathies. 3rd ed. Philadelphia: Lippincott-Raven; 1999:335. Used with permission

Mechanism of Injury in Sports

In sports, isolated musculocutaneous nerve injury has been reported in anterior shoulder dislocations and from blunt trauma to the anterior shoulder.[133,135–137] Traction injuries have been reported in competitive airplane flying,[24] in a quarterback throwing a football, and recently in two major league baseball pitchers.[138] Musculocutaneous nerve injuries in weightlifters and rowers have been attributed to hypertrophic enlargement of the coracobrachialis muscle resulting in compression of the nerve.[139] This mechanism of injury has also been reported after strenuous physical activity with resistance exercises of the upper extremity.[140,141] There is a report of an isolated musculocutaneous neuropathy caused by irritation of the nerve from a proximal humeral osteochondroma that became symptomatic after the patient played recreational basketball.[142]

Distal compression of the lateral antebrachial cutaneous nerve can occur under the bicipital aponeurosis with eccentric contraction of the biceps and forearm pronation against resistance during sports. This type of injury has been reported in a racquetball player, a swimmer during the backstroke, and a windsurfer.[143–145] Musculocutaneous nerve injury has been described after a simulated freefall skydive in a vertical wind tunnel and was likely due to prolonged positioning of the arm.[146] Last, anterior shoulder surgery, most commonly for instability, has been associated with musculocutaneous nerve injury in athletes.[66]

Physical Examination and Diagnostic Tests

Athletes with musculocutaneous nerve injury may present with wasting of the biceps and brachialis muscles and weakness of elbow flexion if the nerve is injured proximally. They may report a variable loss of sensation along the lateral aspect of the forearm but generally do not complain of any significant pain. They occasionally have local burning or dysesthetic pain in the forearm. Clinical examination may reveal atrophy of the biceps and brachialis muscles or decreased muscle tone in patients with a partial nerve injury. Elbow flexion is usually weak but may be possible using the brachioradialis muscle, which is innervated by the radial nerve. Elbow flexion strength should be tested with the forearm in supination to minimize activation of the brachioradialis muscle. The biceps reflex may be absent or reduced. There may also be tenderness to palpation of the lateral biceps tendon. Musculocutaneous nerve injury must be differentiated from distal biceps tendon rupture, which is associated with a loss of contour of the muscle belly and superior retraction. If the nerve is injured distally, in the antecubital fossa region, a purely sensory syndrome may result.

Electrodiagnostic evaluation is the best way to differentiate musculocutaneous nerve injury from those injuries associated with more diffuse brachial plexus involvement. Motor NCSs can be performed to the biceps; however, this has the typical technical problems of a proximal NCS. The LAC can also be readily tested. With musculocutaneous nerve lesions, the LAC sensory nerve conduction response is either not elicitable or the amplitude is diminished (when compared to the other side). Needle EMG is the most reliable test, and it helps rule out other lesions such as C5/6 radiculopathy and upper plexus injury. Local injections with steroid and an anesthetic can be used for diagnosis as well as for therapeutic pain relief.[147]

Treatment

Initial treatment consists of conservative management with rest and activity modification. Symptomatic treatment with pain medications and modalities can help mitigate pain. A local injection of steroid and anesthetic to the lateral antebrachial cutaneous nerve at Olson's point (just lateral to the biceps tendon at the elbow crease) may be helpful for reducing painful sensory symptoms in the distribution of the LAC.[147] Full range of motion of the shoulder and the elbow should be maintained; and when strength has reached grade 3/5 on manual muscle testing, progressive resistance exercises may be undertaken. The prognosis for musculocutaneous nerve injury in sports is generally good, with most athletes improving once the offending activity has been stopped.[139] Spontaneous recovery has been reported after both blunt trauma and shoulder dislocations, although higher-energy trauma appears to carry a worse prognosis.[133] The athlete may be allowed to return to the sport once he or she is asymptomatic and has normal strength with appropriate alterations of technique if the nerve injury is secondary to repetitive use or positioning.

Complete lesions of the musculocutaneous nerve that do not demonstrate recovery within 3 months may be considered for surgical exploration.[148] Surgical decompression may be done to release the nerve proximally at the coracobrachialis or distally at the biceps aponeurosis. Decompression of the lateral antebrachial cutaneous nerve at the elbow can be accomplished with triangular wedge resection of the lateral margin of the biceps tendon.[147] Nerve transfer options for musculocutaneous neuropathy include transferring the thoracodorsal nerve to reestablish elbow flexion.[149] Transfer of expendable motor fascicles from the ulnar and median nerves can also reinnervate the biceps and brachialis muscles for strong elbow flexion; in a study by MacKinnon et al., no functional or sensory donor morbidity was seen.[150] Return to the sport is possible after a decompression procedure when the athlete regains full, painless range of motion and reasonable strength. Return to the previous level of athletic activity may be less likely after a nerve transfer procedure.

Parsonage-Turner Syndrome

An idiopathic condition that affects the brachial plexus has been described by a variety of names including Parsonage-Turner syndrome, brachial neuritis, and neuralgic amyotrophy. Many of the proximal neuropathies described above may be confused with brachial neuritis, so this usually self-limiting condition must be kept in mind when examining athletes with proximal upper limb weakness. Many believe that brachial plexitis is due to a viral attack of the upper brachial plexus, akin to Bell's palsy. Pain, often around the medial scapula, is exquisite and occurs before weakness. Pain usually last around 10 days, whereas weakness can persist for a longer period, sometimes months. Brachial plexitis is often bilateral and occurs about one-third of the time. The suprascapular and long thoracic nerves are thought to be the most frequently affected, although the axillary and anterior interosseous nerves have also been implicated.

Case

T.B. is a 35-year-old male recreational volleyball player with no significant past medical history who presented complaining of right shoulder pain of 2 months' duration. He reported no inciting traumatic event or specific injury. He had just finished playing three nights a week in a men's volleyball league during the summer months, which was a clear increase in his activity level from previous months. He reported that he woke up one morning 2 months earlier with a generalized ache in his posterolateral shoulder, and the pain progressively worsened over time. His pain was aggravated by overhead activity, especially while practicing his volleyball serve, and it seemed to get better with rest. He reported progressive weakness in the shoulder as well. He tried ibuprofen and ice with minimum pain relief.

On physical examination, he was a healthy-appearing young man with well developed upper body musculature. He had demonstrable infraspinatus atrophy with concavity of the infraspinatus fossa on the right shoulder. There was no tenderness to palpation in this region. He had full passive range of motion; the active shoulder range of motion was normal and similar to that of the left shoulder. Strength testing revealed weakness in external rotation of the right shoulder compared to the left. Rotator cuff muscle strength was otherwise intact. Provocative maneuvers were negative for supraspinatus impingement. The O'Brien test was negative for labral pathology. The shoulder apprehension test on the right was negative. However, there was mild posterior subluxation of the humeral head on the glenoid rim with a palpable click and mild pain in the posterolateral shoulder region. The neurovascular examination was normal.

Imaging was performed to rule out a labral lesion and to investigate the clinical suspicion of a suprascapular nerve injury with infraspinatus weakness and atrophy noted on examination. MR arthrography of the right shoulder revealed mild posterior subluxation of the humeral head, extensive superior, anterior to posterior labral tearing (SLAP lesion) with a small focus of articular cartilage thinning. In addition, there was a large spinoglenoid notch cyst measuring approximately 2.0 × 2.0 × 1.5 cm. There was evidence of atrophy of the infraspinatus muscle. The muscles and tendons of the rotator cuff were otherwise unremarkable. Thus, the final diagnosis was threefold: (1) SLAP lesion; (2) suprascapular neuropathy at the spinoglenoid notch due to a ganglion cyst; and (3) shoulder instability.

An electrodiagnostic study was not obtained because a spinoglenoid notch cyst is a common cause of suprascapular neuropathy and was presumed to be the etiology of the suprascapular nerve injury in this patient. The findings of atrophy and weakness of the infraspinatus muscle on physical examination along with isolated atrophy of the infraspinatus muscle on imaging were consistent with a lesion at the spinoglenoid notch. It was thought that electrodiagnostic confirmation would not change the treatment options.

One month later his symptoms persisted, and the patient decided to have a surgical intervention. He underwent right shoulder arthroscopy with a superior labral repair and decompression of the spinoglenoid notch cyst as well as a posterior Bankart repair. He participated in a physical therapy program consisting of shoulder stretching, strengthening, and stabilization as well as sport-specific exercises for approximately 4 months. At completion of the physical therapy, T.B. had achieved full range of motion and full strength of his right shoulder. He had no functional limitations and at 6 months returned to playing recreational volleyball at his previous level of competition.

References

1. Vastamaki M, Goransson H. Suprascapular nerve entrapment. Clin Orthop 1993;297:135–44.
2. Zehetgruber H, Noske H, Lang T, et al. Suprascapular nerve entrapment: a meta-analysis. Int Orthop 2002;26:339–43.
3. Rengachary SS, Burr D, Lucas S, et al. Suprascapular entrapment neuropathy: a clinical, anatomical and comparative study. Part 2: Anatomical study. J Neurosurg 1979;5:447–51.
4. Warner J, Krushell R, Masquelet A. Anatomy and relationships of the suprascapular nerve: anatomical constraints to mobilization of the supraspinatus and infraspinatus muscles in the management of massive rotator cuff tears. J Bone Joint Surg Am 1992;74:36–45.
5. Mestdagh H, Drizenko A, Ghestem P. Anatomical basis of suprascapular nerve syndrome. Anat Clin 1981;3:67–71.
6. Alon M, Weiss S, Fischel B, et al. Bilateral suprascapular nerve entrapment due to an anomalous transverse scapular ligament. Clin Orthop 1988;234:31–3.
7. Ozer Y, Grossman J, Gilbert A. Anatomic observations of the suprascapular nerve. Hand Clin 1995;11:539–44.
8. Eversmann W. Entrapment and compression neuropathies. In: Green D, ed. Operative Hand Surgery. 2nd ed. New York: Churchill Livingstone; 1988:1423–78.
9. Weinfeld A, Cheng J, Nath R, et al. Topographic mapping of the superior scapular ligament: a cadaver study to facilitate suprascapular nerve decompression. Plast Reconstr Surg 2002;110:774–9.
10. Hama H, Ueba Y, Morinaga T, et al. A new strategy for treatment of suprascapular entrapment neuropathy in athletes: shaving of the base of the scapular spine. J Shoulder Elbow Surg 1992;1:253–60.
11. Rengachary SS, Neff J, Singer P, et al. Suprascapular entrapment neuropathy: a clinical, anatomical and comparartive study. Part 1: Clinical study. J Neurosurg 1979;5:441–5.
12. Black K, Lombardo J. Suprascapular nerve injuries with isolated paralysis of the infraspinatus. Am J Sport Med 1990;18:225–88.
13. Ringel S, Treihaft M, Carry M, et al. Suprascapular neuropathy in pitchers. Am J Sports Med 1990;18:80–6.
14. Carroll K, Helms C, Otte M, et al. Enlarged spinoglenoid notch veins causing suprascapular nerve compression. Skeletal Radiol. 2003;32:72–7.
15. Fehrman D, Orwin J, Jennings R. Suprascapular nerve entrapment by ganglion cysts: a report of six cases with arthorscopic findings and review of the literature. Arthroscopy 1995;11:727–34.
16. Takagishi K, Saitoh A, Tonegawa M, et al. Isolated paralysis of the infraspinatus muscle. J Bone Joint Surg Br 1994;76:584–7.
17. Sandow M, Ilic J. Suprascapular nerve rotator cuff compression syndrome in volleyball players. J Shoulder Elbow Surg 1998;7:516–21.
18. Osterman A, Babbhulkar S. Unusual compressive neuropathies of the upper limb. Orthop Clin North Am 1996;27:389–408.
19. Weaver HL. Isolated suprascapular nerve lesions. Injury 1983;15:117–26.
20. Bigliani LU, Daisey R, McCann P, et al. An anatomical study of the suprascapular nerve. Arthroscopy 1990;6:262–4.
21. Mallon W, Bronec P, Spinner R, et al. Suprascapular neuropathy after distal clavicle excision. Clin Orthop 1996;29:207–11.
22. Shaffer BS, Conway J, Jobe F, et al. Infraspinatus muscle-splitting incision in posterior shoulder surgery: an anatomic and electromyographic study. Am J Sports Med 1994;22:113–20.
23. Shaffer JW. Suprascapular nerve injury during spine surgery: a case report. Spine 1994;19:70–1.
24. Goodman C. Unusual nerve injuries in recreational activities. Am J Sports Med 1983;11(4):224–7.
25. Jackson D, Farrage J, Hynninen B, et al. Suprascapular neuropathy in athletes: case reports. Clin J Sports Med 1995;5:134–7.

26. Liveson J, Bronson M, Pollack M. Suprascapular nerve lesions at the spinoglenoid notch: report the three cases and review of the literature. J Neurol Neurosurg Psychiatry 1991;54:241–3.
27. Ganzhorn R, Hocker J, Horowitz M, et al. Suprascapular nerve entrapment. J Bone Joint Surg Am 1981;63:492–4.
28. Ferretti A, Cerullo G, Russo G. Suprascapular neuropathy in volleyball players. J Bone Joint Surg Am 1987;69:260–3.
29. Kukowski B. Suprascapular nerve lesion as an occupational neuropathy in a semiprofessional dancer. Arch Phys Med Rehabil 1993;74:768–9.
30. Smith A. Suprascapular neuropathy in a collegiate pitcher. J Athl Train 1995;30:43–6.
31. Bryan W, Wild J. Isolated infraspinatus atrophy: a common cause of posterior shoulder pain and weakness in throwing athletes. Am J Sports Med 1989;17:130–1.
32. Ferretti A, De Carli A, Fontana M. Injury of the suprascapular nerve at the spinoglenoid notch: the natural history of infraspinatus atrophy in volleyball players. Am J Sports Med 1998;26:759–63.
33. Ferretti A, De Carli A, Fontana M. Entrapment of suprascapular nerve at spinoglenoid notch. In: Vastamaki M, Jalovaara P, eds. Surgery of the Shoulder. Amsterdam: Elsevier Science; 1995:385–92.
34. Holzgraefe M, Kukowski B, Eggert S. Prevalence of latent and manifest suprascapular neuropathy in high-performance volleyball players. Br J Sports Med 1994; 28:177–9.
35. Hadley M, Sonntag V, Pittman H. Suprascapular nerve entrapment: a summary of seven cases. J Neurosurg 1986;64:843–8.
36. Agre J, Ash N, Cameron M, et al. Suprascapular neuropathy after intensive progressive resistive exercise: case report. Arch Phys Med Rehabil 1987;68:236–8.
37. Corkill G, Leiberman J, Taylor R. Pack palsy in backpackers. West J Med 1980;132:569–72.
38. Tsur A, Shahin R. Suprascapular nerve entrapment in a basketball player. Harefuah 1997;133:190–2.
39. Krivickas LS, Wilbourn A. Sports and peripheral nerve injuries: report of 190 injuries evaluated in a single electromyography laboratory. Muscle Nerve 1998;21:1092–4.
40. Yoon T, Grabois M, Guillen M. Suprascapular nerve injury following trauma to the shoulder. Trauma 1981;21:652–5.
41. Bencardino J, Rosenberg Z. Entrapment neuropathies of the shoulder and elbow in the athlete. Clin Sports Med 2006;25:465–87.
42. Garcia G, McQueen D. Bilateral suprascapular nerve entrapment syndrome: case report and review of the literature. J Bone Joint Surg Am 1981;63:491–2.
43. Rose D, Kelly C. Shoulder pain: suprascapular nerve block in shoulder pain. J Kans Med Soc 1969;70:135–6.
44. Danguoisse M, Wilson D, Glynn C. MRI and clinical study of an easy and safe technique of suprascapular nerve blockade. Acta Anaesthesiol Belg 1994;45:49–54.
45. Safran M. Nerve injury about the shoulder in athletes. Part 1: Suprascapular nerve and axillary nerve. Am J Sports Med. 2004;32:803–18.
46. Hawkins R, Piatt B, Fritz R, et al. Clinical evaluation and treatment of spinoglenoid notch ganglion cysts. J Shoulder Elbow Surg 1999;8:551.
47. Moore T, Fritts H, Quick D, et al. Suprascapular nerve entrapment caused by supraglenoid cyst compression. J Shoulder Elbow Surg 1997;6:455–62.
48. Tirman P, Feller J, Janzen D, et al. Association of glenoid labral cysts with labral tears and glenohumeral instability: radiographic findings and clinical significance. Radiology 1994;190:653–8.
49. Chochole M, Senker W, Meznik C, et al. Glenoid-labral cyst entrapping the suprascapular nerve: dissolution after arthroscopic debridement of an extended SLAP lesion. Arthroscopy 1997;13:753–5.
50. Iannotti J, Ramsey M. Arthroscopic decompression of a ganglion cyst causing suprascapular nerve compression. Arthroscopy 1996;12:739–45.
51. Bhatia D, de Beer J, van Rooven K, et al. Arthroscopic suprascapular nerve decompression at the suprascapular notch. Arthroscopy 2006;22:1009–13.
52. Barwood S, Burkhart S, Lo I. Arthroscopic suprascapular nerve release at the suprascapular notch in a cadaveric model: an anatomic approach. Arthroscopy 2007;23:221–5.
53. Pollack L, Davis L. Peripheral nerve injuries. Am J Surg 1932;17:462–71.
54. Krivickas LS, Wilbourn A. Peripheral nerve injuries in athletes: a case series of over 200 injuries. Semin Neurol 2000;20:225–32.
55. Duprac F, Boacquet G, Simonet J, et al. Anatomical basis of the variable aspects of injuries of the axillary nerve (excluding the terminal branches in the deltoid muscle). Surg Radiol Anat 1997;19:127–32.
56. Bumbasirevic M, Lesic A, Vidakovic A, et al. Nerve lesions after acute anterior dislocation of the humero-scapular joint: electrodiagnostic study. Med Pregl 1993;46:191–3.
57. De Laat E, Visser C, Coene L, et al. Nerve lesions in primary shoulder dislocations and humeral neck fractures: a prospective clinical and EMG study. J Bone Joint Surg Br 1994;76:381–3.
58. Toolanen G, Hildingsson T, Hedlund T, et al. Early complications after anterior dislocation of the shoulder in patients over 40 years: an ultrasonographic and electromyographic study. Acta Orthop Scand 1993;64:549–52.
59. Visser C, Coene L, Brand R, et al. The incidence of nerve injury in anterior dislocation of the shoulder and its influence on functional recovery: a prospective clinical and EMG study. J Bone Joint Surg Br 1999;81:679–85.
60. Mallon W, Bassett F, Goldner R. Luxatio erecta: inferior glenohumeral dislocation. J Orthop Trauma 1990;4:19–24.
61. Gurmina S, Postacchini F. Anterior dislocation of the shoulder in elderly patients. J Bone Joint Surg Br 1997;79:540–3.
62. Perlmutter G, Apruzzese W. Axillary nerve injury in contact sports: recommendations for treatment and rehabilitation. Sports Med 1998;26:351–61.
63. Visser C, Napoleon L, Coene J, et al. Nerve lesions in proximal humeral fractures. J Shoulder Elbow Surg 2001;10:421–7.
64. Price M, Tillet E, Acland R, et al. Determining the relationship of the axillary nerve to the shoulder joint capsule from an arthroscopic perspective. J Bone Joint Surg Am 2004;86:2135–42.
65. Boardman N, Cofield R. Neurologic complications of shoulder surgery. Clin Orthop 1999;368:44–53.

66. McIlveen S, Duralde X, D'Alessandro D, et al. Isolated nerve injuries about the shoulder. Clin Orthop 1994;306:54–63.
67. Perlmutter G, Leffert R, Zarins B. Direct injury to the axillary nerve in athletes playing contact sports. Am J Sports Med 1997;25:65–8.
68. Petrucci F, Morelli A, Raimondi P. Axillary nerve injuries: 21 cases treated by nerve graft and neurolysis. J Hand Surg [Am] 1982;7:271–8.
69. Neiman E, Swan P. Karate injuries. BMJ 1971;1:233–5.
70. Bateman J. Nerve injuries about the shoulder in sports. J Bone Joint Surg Am 1967;49:785–92.
71. Berry H, Bril V. Axillary nerve palsy following blunt trauma to the shoulder region: a clinical and electrophysiological review. J Neurol Neurosurg Psychiatry 1982;45:1027–32.
72. Paladini D, Dellantonio R, Cinti A. Axillary neuropathy in volleyball players: report of two cases and literature review. J Neuro Neurosurg Psychiatry 1996;60:345–7.
73. Bennett G. Shoulder and elbow lesions of the professional baseball pitcher. JAMA 1941;117:510–4.
74. Goodson J. Brachial plexus injury from the light tight backpack straps. N Engl J Med 1981;305:524–5.
75. Saha A. Surgery of the paralyzed and flail shoulder. Acta Orthop Scand 1967;97(suppl):5–90.
76. Hertel R, Lambert S, Ballmer F. The deltoid extension lag sign for diagnosis and grading of axillary nerve palsy. J Shoulder Elbow Surg 1998;7:97–9.
77. Mendoza F, Main K. Peripheral nerve injuries of the shoulder in the athlete. Clin Sports Med 1990;9:331–42.
78. Filler A, Maravilla K, Tsuruda J. MR neurography and muscle MR imaging for image diagnosis of disorder affecting the peripheral nerves and musculature. Neurol Clin 2004;22:643–82.
79. Duralde XA. Neurologic injuries in the athlete's shoulder. J Athl Train 2000;35:316–28.
80. Alnot J, Valenti PH. Surgical reconstruction of the axillary nerve. In: Post M, Morrey B, Hawkins R, eds. Surgery of the Shoulder. St. Louis: Mosby Year Book; 1990:330–3.
81. Coene LN, Narakas AO. Operative management of lesions of the axillary nerve, isolated or combined with other nerve lesions. Clin Neurol Neurosurg 1992;84(suppl):S64–6.
82. Kline DG, Kim DH. Axillary nerve repair in 99 patients with 101 stretch injuries. J Neurosurg 2003;99:630–6.
83. Kauppila LI. The long thoracic nerve: possible mechanisms of injury based on autopsy study. J Shoulder Elbow Surg 1993;2:244–8.
84. Safran M. Nerve injury about the shoulder in athletes. Part 2: Long thoracic nerve, spinal accessory nerve, burners/stingers, thoracic outlet syndrome. Am J Sports Med 2004;32:1063–76.
85. Foo C, Swann M. Isolated paralysis of the serratus anterior: a report of 20 cases. J Bone Joint Surg Br 1983;65:552–6.
86. Gregg J, Labosky D, Harty M, et al. Serratus anterior paralysis in the young athlete. J Bone Joint Surg Am 1979;61:825–32.
87. Johnson J, Kendall M. Isolated paralysis of the serratus anterior muscle. J Bone Joint Surg Am 1955;37:567–74.
88. Nath R, Lyons A, Bietz A. Microneurolysis and decompression of long thoracic nerve injury are effective in reversing scapular winging: long-term results in 50 cases. BMC Musculoskelet Disord 2007;8:2.
89. Ebraheim N, Lu J, Porshinsky B, et al. Vulnerability of long thoracic nerve: an anatomic study. J Shoulder Elbow Surg 1998;7:458–61.
90. Bora F, Pleasure D, Didzian N. A study of nerve regeneration and neuroma formation after nerve suture by various techniques. J Hand Surg [Am] 1976;1:138–43.
91. Gozna E, Harris W. Traumatic winging of the scapula. J Bone Joint Surg Am 1979;61:1230–3.
92. Disa J, Wang B, Dellon A. Correction of scapular winging by supraclavicular neurolysis of the long thoracic nerve. J Reconstr Microsurg 2001;17:79–84.
93. Horowitz M, Tocantins L. An anatomic study of the role of the long thoracic nerve and the related scapular bursae in the pathogenesis of local paralysis of the serratus anterior. Anat Rec 1938;71:375–85.
94. White A, Witten C. Long thoracic nerve palsy in a professional ballet dancer. Am J Sports Med 1993;21:626–8.
95. Levitz C, Reilly P, Torg J. The pathomechanics of chronic, recurrent cervical nerve root neuropraxia. Am J Sports Med 1997;25:73–6.
96. Overpeck D, Ghormley R. Paralysis of the serratus magnus muscle. JAMA 1940;May:1994–96.
97. Vastamaki M, Kauppila LI. Etiological factors in isolated paralysis of the serratus anterior muscle: a report of 197 cases. J Shoulder Elbow Surg 1993;2:240–3.
98. Woodhead AB. Paralysis of the serratus anterior in a world-class marksman: a case study. Am J Sports Med 1985;13:359–62.
99. Kaplan P. Electrodiagnostic confirmation of long thoracic nerve palsy. J Neurol Neurosurg Psychiatry 1980;43:50–2.
100. Jerosch L, Castro E, Geske B. Damage of the long thoracic and dorsal scapular nerve after traumatic shoulder dislocation: case report and review of the literature. Acta Orthop Belg 1990;56:625–7.
101. Wiater JM, Flatow EL. Long thoracic nerve injury. Clin Orthop 1999;368:17–27.
102. Connor PM, Yamaguchi K, Manifold SG, et al. Split pectoralis major transfer for serratus anterior palsy. Clin Orthop 1997;341:134–42.
103. Post M. Pectoralis major transfer for winging of the scapula. J Shoulder Elbow Surg 1995;4:1–9.
104. Warner JJ, Navarro RA. Serratus anterior dysfunction. Clin Orthop 1998;349:139–48.
105. Basmajian JV. Primary Anatomy. 8th ed. Baltimore: Williams & Wilkins; 1982.
106. Tsairis P. Peripheral nerve injury in athletes. In: Jordan BD, Tsairis P, Warren R, eds. Sports Neurology. Rockville, MD: Aspen; 1989:180.
107. Toth C, McNeil S, Feasby T. Peripheral nervous system injuries in sport and recreation: a systematic review. Sports Med 2005;35:717–38.
108. Cohn BT, Brahms MA, Cohn M. Injury to the eleventh cranial nerve in a high school wrestler. Orthop Rev 1986;15:590–5.
109. Bigliani LU, Compito CA, Duralde XA, et al. Transfer of the levator scapulae, rhomboid major, and rhomboid minor transfer for paralysis of the trapezius. J Bone Joint Surg Am 1996;78:1534–40.

110. Neer CS. Shoulder Reconstruction. Philadelphia: Saunders; 1990:421–85.
111. Saeed MA, Gatens PF. Winging of the scapula. Am Fam Phys 1981;24:139–43.
112. Bigliani LU, Perez-Sanz JR, Wolfe RN. Treatment of trapezius paralysis. J Bone Joint Surg Am 1985;67: 871–7.
113. Olarte M, Adams D. Accessory nerve palsy. J Neurol Neurosurg Psychiatry 1977;40:1113–6.
114. Teboul F, Bizot P, Kakkar R, et al. Surgical management of trapezius palsy. J Bone Joint Surg Am 2004;86(9):1884–90.
115. Wiater JM, Bigliani LU. Spinal accessory nerve injury. Clin Orthop 1999;368:5–16.
116. Aldridge JW, Bruno RJ, Strauch RJ, et al. Nerve entrapment in athletes. Clin Sports Med 2001;20:95–122.
117. Romero J, Gerber C. Levator scapulae and rhomboid transfer for paralysis of trapezius: the Eden-Lange procedure. J Bone Joint Surg Br 2003;85(8):1141–5.
118. Lee HY, Chung IH, Sir W, et al. Variations of the vertral rami of the brachial plexus. J Korean Med Sci 1992;7:19–24.
119. Frank DK, Wenk I, Stern JC, et al. A cadaveric study of the motor nerves to the levator scapulae muscle. Otolaryngol Head Neck Surg 1997;117:671–80.
120. Tubbs RS, Tyler-Kabara EC, Aikens AC, et al. Surgical anatomy of the dorsal scapular nerve. J Neurosurg 2005;102:910–1.
121. Nakano KK. The entrapment neuropathies. Muscle Nerve 1978;1:264–79.
122. Modelli M, Cioni R, Federico A. Rare mononeuropathies of the upper limb in bodybuilders. Muscle Nerve 1998;21:809–12.
123. Ravindran M. Two cases of suprascapular neuropathy in a family. Br J Sports Med 2003;37:539–41.
124. Fisher MA, Gorelick PB. Entrapment neuropathies: differential diagnosis and management. Postgrad Med 1985;77:160–74.
125. Sunderland S. Nerves and Nerve Injuries. 2nd ed. Edinburgh: Churchill Livingstone; 1978:1016.
126. Wu PB, Robinson T, Kingery W, et al. Thoracodorsal nerve conduction study. Am J Phys Med Rehabil 1998;77(4):296–8.
127. Samardzic MM, Grujicic DM, Rasuli LG. The use of thoracodorsal nerve transfer in restoration of irreparable C5 and C6 spinal nerve lesions. Br J Plast Surg 2005;58(4):541–6.
128. Grant JCB, Smith CG. The musculature. In: Schaeffer JP, ed. Morris' Human Anatomy. A Complete Systematic Treatise. Vol 11. New York: McGraw-Hill; 1953:457–8.
129. Giannini F, Cioni R, Paradiso C, et al. Neurophysiological evaluation of pectoralis major muscle after mastectomy. Riv Neurobiol 1992;38:407–12.
130. Scalon EF. The importance of the anterior thoracic nerves in modified radical mastectomy. Surg Gynecol Obstet 1981;152:789–91.
131. Tashiro K, Furukawa M, Nakata T, et al. Electrophysiological study on the atrophied pectoralis major muscle after modified radical mastectomy. Nippon Geka Gakkai Zasshi 1989;90:429–33.
132. Rossi F, Triggs WJ, Gonzalez R, et al. Bilateral medial pectoral neuropathy in a weight lifter. Muscle Nerve 1999;22:1597–9.
133. Jerosch J, Castro WHM, Colemont J. A lesion of the musculocutaneous nerve: a rare complication of anterior shoulder dislocation. Acta Orthop Belg 1989;55: 230–2.
134. Flatow EL, Bigliani LU, April EW. An anatomic study of the musculocutaneous nerve and its relationship to the coracoid process. Clin Orthop 1989;244:166–71.
135. Blom S, Dahlback L. Nerve injuries in dislocations of the shoulder joint and fractures of the neck of the humerus. Acta Chir Scand 1970;136:461–6.
136. Corner NB, Milner SM, Macdonald R, et al. Isolated musculocutaneous nerve lesion after shoulder dislocation. J R Army Med Corps 1990;136(2):107–8.
137. Liveson J. Nerve lesions associated with shoulder dislocation: a electrodiagnostic study of 11 cases. J Neurol Neurosurg Psychiatry 1984;47:742–4.
138. Hsu JC, Paletta GA, Gambardella RA, et al. Musculocutaneous nerve injury in major league baseball pitchers: a report of 2 cases. Am J Sports Med 2007;35(6):1003–6.
139. Kim SM, Goodrich JA. Isolated proximal musculocutaneous nerve palsy: case report. Arch Phys Med Rehabil 1984;65:735–6.
140. Braddom R. Musculocutaneous nerve injury after heavy exercise. Arch Phys Med Rehabil 1978;59:290.
141. Simonetti S. Musculocutaneous nerve lesion after strenuous physical activity. Muscle Nerve 1999;22(5):647–9.
142. Juel VC, Kiely JM, Leone KV, et al. Isolated musculocutaneous neuropathy caused by a proximal humeral exostosis. Neurology 2000;54(2):494–6.
143. Bassett F, Nunley J. Compression of the musculocutaneous nerve at the elbow. J Bone Joint Surg Am 1982; 64:1050–2.
144. Felsenhal G, Mondell D, Reischer M, et al. Forearm pain secondary to compression syndrome of the lateral cutaneous nerve of the forearm. Arch Phys Med Rehabil 1984;65:139–41.
145. Jablecki CK. Lateral antebrachial cutaneous neuropathy in a windsurfer. Muscle Nerve 1999;22:944–5.
146. Mautner K, Keel JC. Musculocutaneous nerve injury after simulated freefall in a vertical wind-tunnel: a case report. Arch Phys Med Rehabil 2007;88(3):391–3.
147. Davidson JJ, Bassett FH, Nunley JA. Musculocutaneous nerve entrapment revisited. J Shoulder Elbow Surg 1998;7:250–5.
148. Kline DG, Hudson AR. Complications of nerve injury and nerve repair. In: Lazar S, Greenfield J, eds. Complications in Surgery and Trauma. Philadelphia: Lippincott; 1983.
149. Novak CB, MacKinnon SE, Tung TH. Patient outcome following a thoracodorsal to musculocutaneous nerve transfer for reconstruction of elbow flexion. Br J Plast Surg 2002;55(5):416–9.
150. MacKinnon SE, Novak CB, Myckatyn TM, et al. Results of reinnervation of the biceps and brachialis muscles with a double fascicular transfer for elbow flexion. J Hand Surg [Am] 2005;30(5):978–85.

Chapter 8
Thoracic Outlet Syndrome

Scott Laker, William J. Sullivan, and Thomas A. Whitehill

Introduction

Thoracic outlet syndrome (TOS) is a neurovascular entrapment syndrome of the upper extremity. It is most broadly separated into vasculogenic (V-TOS) and neurogenic (N-TOS) subtypes. TOS occurs relatively rarely in sports but can be devastating when it does.

Neurogenic TOS has been one of the more controversial diagnoses in medicine. To this day, many clinicians doubt its existence, and its true incidence and prevalence are still widely debated. It lacks a gold standard for diagnosis, presents with a wide variety of symptoms, and poses a significant challenge for timely diagnosis and effective treatment.

Historical Perspective

Sir Astley Cooper identified a connection between a cervical rib and arm ischemia as early as 1818. The first surgery for what could be described as N-TOS was performed in 1861 by Coote; he removed an exostosis of the seventh rib for an ischemic hand. Paget described an axillary vein thrombosis, a form of V-TOS, in 1865 that was hypothesized to be secondary to a cervical rib. Axillary or subclavian vein thrombosis, often from repetitive effort, is often eponymously called *Paget-Schröetter* syndrome, a type of V-TOS. The first cervical rib resection for TOS was performed in 1910 by Murphy. In 1916, Halstead published a collection of 716 cases of cervical ribs with 27 subclavian arterial aneurysms. Later that decade, Stopford and Telford published a report of 10 cases of TOS that were treated with first rib resection and scalenotomy.

Adson and Coffey published what many consider to be the classic article on 31 patients with symptoms of TOS that were treated with first rib resection and 5 others treated with scalenectomy. This same 1927 article described the Adson test, which is still used today for diagnosing TOS. It was not until 1956 that the term *thoracic outlet syndrome* was first used to describe this phenomenon.[1]

Epidemiology

Most of the controversy focuses on N-TOS. Here, patients present with pure neurologic symptoms, typically over time. In contrast, V-TOS is often more acute and divided into arterial and venous injuries. Vascular signs and symptoms include Raynaud's phenomenon, gangrene, claudication, transient ischemia, and loss of pulse. V-TOS tends to present much more acutely and does not create nearly as much of a diagnostic challenge as its neurogenic counterpart.

Vasculogenic TOS is caused by focal vascular trauma from bony abnormalities leading to stenosis of vessels or acute thrombosis due to venous or arterial compression.[2] Paget-Schröetter syndrome may be seen in athletes. Patients with combined

S. Laker (✉)
Department of Rehabilitation, University of Washington, Seattle, WA, USA

V. Akuthota, S.A. Herring (eds.), *Nerve and Vascular Injuries in Sports Medicine*,
DOI 10.1007/978-0-387-76600-3_8, © Springer Science+Business Media, LLC 2009

neurogenic and vascular signs and symptoms tend to have worse outcomes than those with pure vascular symptoms.[3]

Female subjects make up approximately 70% of N-TOS cases.[4,5] This preponderance is hypothesized to be due to the relatively lower location of the brachial plexus in women and the less-developed shoulder girdle musculature. The mean age at injury is around 40 years; and thus far, N-TOS has been exceedingly rare in patients older than 65. Pediatric cases are generally found to be vascular in nature but present in a similar manner.[6]

It is difficult to describe the incidence and prevalence of TOS because of the varying etiology and varying diagnostic criteria used across the field. True N-TOS, where objective neurologic signs of lower plexus motor injury are found, is rare, estimated to be found in just 1 in 1,000,000 cases.[5] Wilbourn coined the term *disputed N-TOS* to describe the more nebulous TOS where pain predominates over any objective neurologic signs.[7] Obviously, the incidence and prevalence of disputed N-TOS is much less clear, although it has been reported to be 0.3%–8.0% in the United States.[7,8]

Neurogenic TOS is thought to be more common than V-TOS, but this may be due to reporting bias and lack of clear diagnostic criteria for the putative disputed N-TOS.[4,8,9] Well described epidemiology does not exist for TOS occurring with sports. However, numerous case reports and case series have described N-TOS and V-TOS singularly and in combination in a variety of sports. Effort thrombosis has drawn particular attention in amateur and professional athletes engaging in overhead repetitive activity.

Anatomy

TOS per se is somewhat of a misnomer as the anatomic region involved is technically the thoracic inlet. It houses a neurovascular bundle comprised of the brachial plexus, subclavian vein, and subclavian artery. There are three distinct compartments with the thoracic outlet.

- Interscalene (or scalene) triangle
- Costoclavicular space
- Retropectoralis minor (or subcoracoid) space

Proximally, the scalene triangle is located supraclavicularly and is bordered by the anterior scalene anteriorly and the middle and posterior scalenes posteriorly (Fig. 8.1). The costoclavicular space is located underneath the clavicle and first rib, with the middle scalene muscle comprising the posterior aspect and the costoclavicular ligament anterior aspect (Fig. 8.2). Distally, the retropectoralis minor (subcoracoid) space is located underneath the pectoralis muscle and the coracoid process. Dynamic imaging studies have shown compression in the abduction external rotation (AER) position in both the costoclavicular and retropectoralis minor spaces but not in the scalene triangle (Fig. 8.3).

Generally, it is thought that the scalene triangle is the most common site of compression as its area is most affected by cervical ribs and scalene muscle

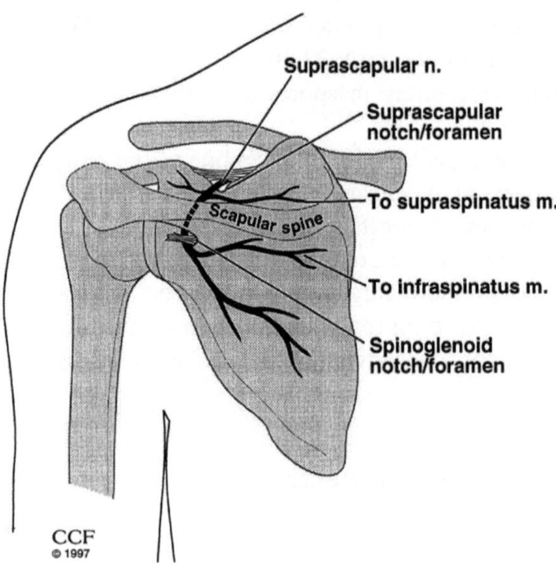

Fig. 8.1 Interscalene triangle (clavicle resected)

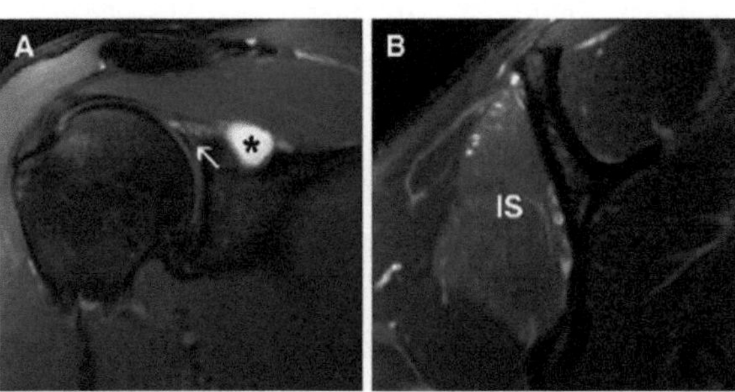

Fig. 8.2 Costoclavicular space

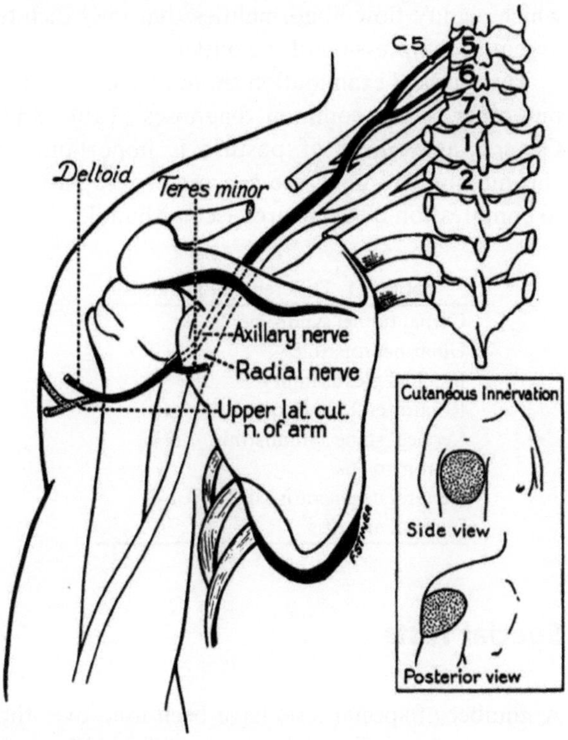

Fig. 8.3 Subcoracoid space

abnormalities. Cadaver studies have shown that cervical ribs are found in approximately 0.5%–1.5% of the population, although 90% are asymptomatic.[10] The lower trunk of the brachial plexus (C8–T1) is six times more commonly involved in N-TOS than upper trunk irritation (C5–7).[4] This is likely due to the fact that the lower truck is in closest proximity to the tendinous portion of the scalene.

Etiology

Trauma is likely the most frequent cause of both V-TOS and N-TOS and is involved in anywhere from 20%–86% of cases.[11–14] It is generally thought that the combination of acute or cumulative trauma and an anatomic predisposition lead to TOS. With trauma, neck hyperextension during a whiplash event appears to be a common mechanism of injury.[11]

Clavicle and first rib fractures can acutely impinge on the components of the neurovascular bundle. Malunion and nonunion of these fractures can also lead to chronic compression of the tissues within the inlet. Clavicle fractures are extremely common in sports and should be kept in mind when evaluating TOS in athletes.

The most common etiology in sports appears to be repetitive overhead motion. In athletes, it has been hypothesized that selective hypertrophy of sport-specific musculature may predispose to TOS. For example, swimmers demonstrate hypertrophy of the pectoralis minor; weightlifters exhibit hypertrophy of the scalenes; figure skaters can have hypertrophy of the subclavius; and overhead athletes (e.g., throwers, tennis players) demonstrate hypertrophy of their throwing arm as well as ipsilateral scapular depression.[15–19]

Anatomic structural variants appear to be common within the thoracic outlet. A study of 250 cadaver dissections showed a 46% incidence of relevant structural abnormalities, anterior more common than posterior, irrespective of age or sex. The same study also found an increased incidence of a scissor-like abnormality, meaning both anterior and posterior findings, in female cadavers. This study also reported the results of 72 surgical cases in which posterior variants were more common than anterior variants.[10] One study demonstrated that only approximately 10% of cadavers had bilaterally normal anatomy.[20]

Roos described nine types of anomalous fibromuscular band based on his own significant surgical and cadaveric experience. Initially, it was thought that 33% of the population had these anatomic variants.[21,22] Currently, 14 types of these bands have been described.[20] Unfortunately, the bands are difficult to visualize on imaging.

Bony abnormalities are also a common indication for surgery. Cervical ribs are estimated to be present in only 0.17%–0.74% of the general population but are much more common in surgical TOS patients.[11] This is partially due to surgical selection of patients with cervical ribs and similar abnormalities. There are also several reports of patients with abnormally elongated transverse processes at C7, as well as combinations of the two.

History and Physical Examination

Patients with TOS are generally seen by an average of 4.7 physicians before appropriate conservative management is prescribed and 6.7 physicians before undergoing surgery.[23] For N-TOS, the length of time from the onset of neurogenic symptoms to surgery has been implicated as a predictive factor for outcome.[24,25] Therefore, a thorough history is essential for moving toward the diagnosis and proper treatment of this syndrome.

A detailed history of the location, duration, quality, and quantity of pain is absolutely necessary. Descriptions of the exacerbating and alleviating factors may help delineate the disorder. Early symptoms often include shoulder (e.g., supraclavicular, scapular) and neck pain and vague achy pain in the medial forearm and hand. Pain can be exacerbated by arm elevation activities. Paresthesias are common in both V-TOS and N-TOS. With N-TOS, paresthesias typically occur in the fourth and fifth digits. Tingling may also occur in the lateral three digits, but carpal tunnel syndrome should be ruled out. It can also be particularly useful to understand any previous litigation or worker compensation issues that may be involved, as this has been shown to affect previous treatment and eventual outcome.[26]

Neurologically, patients can present with a wide variety of complaints, classically paresthesias and numbness in the hand and pain in the arm or neck.[11] Definitive (or true) N-TOS is a primarily motor syndrome, and up to 50% of patients present with weakness, often described early as clumsiness of the hands.[27,28] Intrinsic hand muscle atrophy consistent with lower trunk injuries can be seen in the most severe cases. Because symptoms range from soft findings (pain, paresthesias) to hard deficits (weakness, atrophy), N-TOS is thought to be nebulous and controversial.

With V-TOS involving arterial structures, patients generally present after some type of ischemic event, including ulceration of the digits, gangrene, Raynaud's phenomenon, or pulse deficit. A more detailed history may reveal a more insidious onset of pallor and numbness. These ominous signs require swift surgical treatment to prevent ongoing, permanent tissue loss. Palpation of the supraclavicular fossa can reveal tenderness and occasionally masses that point toward an alternative diagnosis. Sanders' extensive experience with the condition revealed that up to 96% of his surgical patients had unilateral scalene tenderness.[11] Auscultation over the supraclavicular fossa may reveal bruits, which signify flow abnormalities that may dictate urgent decompression of the outlet.

The physical examination should be used to rule out other, more common diagnoses (Table 8.1). General assessment of posture is important, as chronic muscle imbalance can predispose patients to compression of the neurovascular bundle.

Table 8.1 Differential diagnoses

Carpal tunnel syndrome
Ulnar neuropathies
Brachial plexus injury
Rotator cuff tendinosis
Cervical spine sprain/strain
Fibromyositis
Cervical degenerative disc disease
Cervical arthritis

Special Tests

A number of special tests have been used over the years to help confirm a diagnosis of TOS. Many of these tests were originally designed to ascertain the presence of vascular compromise but have more recently been used or adapted to determine N-TOS or nonspecific TOS. As a rule, many of these tests are hampered by a high rate of false positives, with extrapolation of a positive test to reproduction of concordant symptoms rather than diminishment of pulse. In addition to a detailed physical examination, the following items, including the dynamic positioning provocation tests, should be carefully observed in patients with suspected TOS.

- Tenderness over the scalene or supraclavicular region
- Reproducing symptoms by pressure or the Tinel maneuver in the supraclavicular or brachial plexus region
- Upper limb tension testing (ULTT) (e.g., neck side bending to the ipsilateral side causes concordant symptoms)
- Objective neurologic deficits
- Dynamic positioning provocation tests
  - Roos test
  - Wright test
  - Adson maneuver
  - Halstead (costoclavicular) maneuver

A Tinel maneuver or brachial plexus compression test can be performed at the brachial plexus (at Erb's point) and other locations in the upper limb. It is considered positive if it produces tingling in the suspected distribution, although it has a high false-positive rate and poor sensitivity (46%).[27]

The ULTT is performed to elicit irritation of the upper limb neurologic structures. These tests are performed with subtle perturbation in limb position to isolate and stress the various nervous system structures, as described in other chapters. Head tilting toward or away can sometimes irritate nerve structures in TOS.

Four basic dynamic positioning tests are used to provoke symptoms of TOS (Table 8.2), with many modifications having been made to these tests over the years.

Table 8.2 Special tests for thoracic outlet syndrome

Test	Sensitivity (%)	Specificity (%)	PPV (%)	NPV (%)
Roos test	84	30	68	50
Wright's test	90	29	69	63
Adson's maneuver	79	76	85	72
Halstead's maneuver	84	47	74	47

PPV, positive predictive value; NPV, negative predictive value

- The Roos test, or the elevated arm stress test (EAST), is perhaps the most useful component of the physical exam. It is performed by having the patient abduct and externally rotate the shoulders, while repetitively opening and closing the fists for 3 minutes. The test is considered positive if symptoms are reproduced.[21]
- The Wright test, also referred to as the 90° abduction external rotation (AER) position, is performed with the shoulder abducted and externally rotated while palpating the radial pulse; it is classically considered positive if the pulse is obliterated.[27] Over time the test has been modified and is now considered positive if vascular or neurogenic symptoms are reproduced.
- The Adson maneuver is performed by palpating the radial pulse after placing the patient's arms in anatomic position (abducted to approximately 15° while in supination). The patient's neck is then actively rotated toward the affected side. It is considered positive if the radial pulse is obliterated during deep inspiration. In isolation, this is statistically the best of the special tests for TOS.[27]
- The Halstead maneuver, or military position test, is performed with the patient sitting or standing with scapulae retracted and shoulders depressed. This test can be considered positive with either obliteration of the radial pulse or if there is reproduction of symptoms. Historically, this test has been positive in 50%–68% of normal patients and is generally thought not to be reliable.[11]

The sensitivity and specificity of each test is described in Table 8.2.

The scalene muscle block is an office procedure that has been correlated with a successful postsurgical outcome. Sanders found that 94% of patients who had a positive scalene block had a good response to surgery. The block is performed using 4–5 ml of 1% lidocaine into the muscle belly of the anterior scalene. A successful block is defined as decreased tenderness over the anterior scalene compared to that experienced during the preinjection examination. If brachial plexus block is inadvertently achieved, the test is of no diagnostic value. Scalene muscle blocks have not been useful as therapeutic measures.[11]

Imaging

Initial imaging for a patient with TOS is chest radiography including an apical lordotic view, as it can evaluate the presence of cervical ribs, elongated transverse processes, some forms of intrathoracic pathology, and the presence of malunion or nonunion of previous clavicle fractures. Generally, advanced imaging is reserved for the diagnosis of V-TOS and, to a lesser degree, N-TOS. Magnetic resonance imaging (MRI) of the brachial plexus is being used increasingly to assess for a mass effect or soft tissue abnormalities within or around the neurologic structures.

Arterial investigations including MRI, magnetic resonance angiography (MRA), computed tomography (CT), and CT angiography have been used increasingly for diagnosing TOS with varying degrees of diagnostic utility. MRA also is being used increasingly for diagnosing TOS. It appears to be more sensitive with the arms abducted.[2,29] Doppler ultrasonography in the presence of vascular signs and symptoms and a cervical rib is useful to screen for an aneurysm, although angiography is needed when planning surgical intervention.[4,27] Angiography is the gold standard for arterial TOS, even though it is invasive. CT angiography is useful for diagnosing both bony and vascular abnormalities but requires the use of contrast. The benefits of MRA are that is noninvasive and requires neither contrast nor radiation.[2]

Venous investigations typically involve Doppler ultrasonography because of its ease and rapid availability. Compression ultrasonography has a reported sensitivity of 96% and specificity of 93.5% versus color flow Doppler imaging with 100% sensitivity and 93% specificity, which are both better than those of Doppler ultrasonography (81% sensitivity and 77% specificity).[30] Additional modalities are recommended if clinical suspicion is high. MRI is being used increasingly but lacks the sensitivity of other tests for venous thromboses causing V-TOS. However, this may change as higher-power magnets are becoming available. Venography is essentially the gold standard for diagnosis. Although it is an invasive technique used to visualize the vasculature and location of the thrombosis, it is performed often because it provides the opportunity to perform thrombolysis.

Electrodiagnosis

Electrodiagnostic testing is primarily performed to rule out other, more common neurologic entities such as carpal tunnel syndrome. Additionally, many electrodiagnostic techniques have been used to confirm the diagnosis of N-TOS. The classic electrodiagnostic findings are abnormal nerve conduction studies (NCSs) and needle abnormalities in the C8 and especially T1 nerve root pathways (Fig. 8.4). Definitive N-TOS is primarily an axonal motor syndrome but can have subtle sensory findings. However, most patients with TOS undergo normal electrodiagnostic testing.

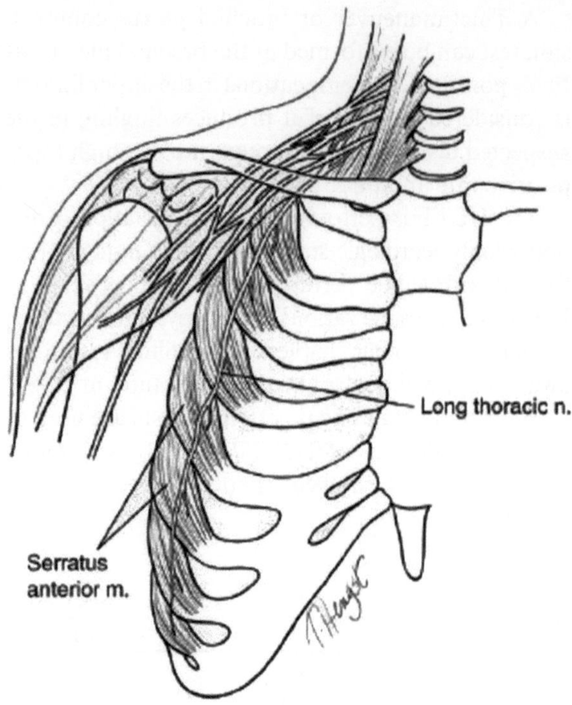

Fig. 8.4 Brachial plexus

Motor NCSs of the median and ulnar nerve may reveal normal- to low-amplitude median compound muscle action potentials (CMAPs). The median motor CMAP has been found to be more significantly affected than the ulnar nerve.[31] This is likely due to the location of the fibers that eventually make up the median nerve being closer to the tendinous portion of the scalene at the level of the lower trunk.[32]

Sensory nerve conduction of the ulnar and medial antebrachial cutaneous (MAC) nerve may show low or relatively low sensory nerve action potential (SNAP) amplitude. The MAC, a sensory nerve derived from the C8 and T1 roots, travels within the lower truck and medial cord of the brachial plexus and gives sensory innervation to the medial aspect of the forearm. In a report of 16 cases, the MAC was significantly affected before abnormalities were noted in any other sensory or motor nerve conduction.[31] Sensory NCS of the median nerve typically remain normal as these nerve fibers stem from the C5–7 nerve root pathways.

Proximal NCSs crossing the brachial plexus are described. However, to assess the lower/medial brachial plexus, recording sites must be placed over median- or ulnar-innervated muscles. Subsequently, a large segment study is generated, thus washing away any subtle injury in the short segment of the brachial plexus within the thoracic outlet. In addition, these studies require large, uncomfortable stimuli that excite other neural tissues, thereby potentially confounding the results. Measurement of distances is also suspect, as they vary considerably when compared to the actual distances these nerves travel, leading to inaccurate calculations of nerve conduction velocities. These studies have not been reproduced consistently over time.

Cervical root stimulation is a relatively controversial, technically challenging technique that seeks to evaluate the trunk levels of the brachial plexus. It involves placing needle electrodes subcutaneous to the level of the nerve root itself. The risks of the procedure include direct nerve injury, pneumothorax, pain, and vasovagal episodes. It requires a high level of electrical stimulation, which can also lead to inaccurate distance measurements.[33,34]

The F-waves of the ulnar or median nerves are nonspecific late responses designed to study the integrity of a nerve over its physiologic course. Case series data showed abnormalities in F-waves only when in provocative positions, although there was no control group in this study.[35] There is work currently being done to quantify F-wave velocity through the axilla; but up to now, the consensus is that more data are needed before relying too heavily on the F-wave in TOS.[34]

Needle electromyography (EMG) is enormously variable depending on the duration and severity of the compression.[31,33,36] Reduced recruitment, positive sharp waves, and fibrillation potentials can be seen, signifying axonal loss. These findings are reported to be most common in the median-innervated abductor pollicis brevis as its motor fibers are located in the lower trunk.[32] Other muscles that have C8 and particularly T1 myotomal involvement may also show changes. Studies of the paraspinal muscles are normal, signifying a lesion distal to the dorsal root ganglion.

Somatosensory evoked potential (SSEP) testing stimulates sensory nerves peripherally at the level of the median or ulnar nerves. The generated far-field potential is then recorded at the level of the wrist, Erb's point, the cervical spine, and the scalp. The amount of time that it takes the stimulation to reach the recording electrode is determined through computer averaging and is used to help localize the lesion. SSEP testing has been used in the diagnosis of TOS but does not add much information to a thorough electrodiagnostic testing regimen. One study found that 86% of patients with abnormal SSEPs had a good response to surgery,[37] but another study showed that 76% of patients with normal SSEPs had a good to excellent response to surgery. Given this conflicting information, some authors prefer ordering the SSEP test only if one has been done previously and then only for comparison.[37] It is thought to be of limited use at this time and depends greatly on the severity of the disease.[38] Cakmur et al. showed that 100% of patients with severe objective signs such as atrophy had SSEP abnormalities. They also found that 67% of patients with less severe signs and symptoms had ulnar SSEP abnormalities; 25% of patients with only subjective symptoms had those same abnormalities.[39]

The literature suggests that a relatively large number of patients with TOS also have evidence of carpal or cubital tunnel syndrome, although the opposite is not necessarily true.[27,36,40] This may be theoretically explained by the double-crush mechanism, where an injury to a nerve proximally predisposes the distal nerve to injury.[41] A reasonable routine electrodiagnostic evaluation of a patient with TOS is described in Table 8.3. One should expect to see positive electrodiagnostic signs in nearly all patients with objective signs such as atrophy or sensory loss in the ulnar distribution or the C8 dermatome. Given the rarity of definitive N-TOS, electrodiagnostic testing is most useful for detecting other, more common disorders.

Conservative Management

The literature surrounding TOS is weighed heavily toward a dedicated trial of appropriate, aggressive, nonsurgical management. In fact, Landry et al. compared operative versus nonoperative cases and found no difference in outcome or progression of symptoms.[22] Treatment is dictated by the type and etiology of the suspected TOS.

Activity modification can be helpful for alleviating symptoms of TOS, so it is reasonable to order a work-site evaluation when clinical suspicion suggests a work-related cause. Avoidance of overhead,

Table 8.3 Routine electrodiagnostic studies for neurogenic thoracic outlet syndrome

Nerve conduction studies
- Median SNAP (C5-T1)
- Ulnar SNAP (C8-T1)
- MABCN SNAP (C8-T1)
- Median CMAP (C8-T1)
- Ulnar CMAP (C8-T1)
- SSEPs (for comparison, if previously performed)

Electromyography
- Sample of muscles comprising C4-T1 myotomes, including median, ulnar, and radial innervated muscles
- Paraspinals

SNAP, sensory nerve action potential; MABCN, medial antebrachial cutaneous nerve; CMAP, compound muscle action potential; SSEPs, somatosensory evoked potentials

exacerbating positions is recommended, including sleep hygiene involving pillows to support the arms.[32] In athletes, changing the biomechanics such that the shoulder does not displace anteriorly and impinge the brachial plexus can also be helpful.

A thorough postural assessment and program of postural reeducation has been shown to be highly effective in many patients. Even patients with significant radiologic findings can benefit from these techniques. Generally, therapists focus on having the patient work on retracting the scapulae and shoulders as well as proper positioning of the head and neck.[40]

Neck exercises have to be performed with caution initially as they can lead to compression of the neurovascular bundle or muscle spasm and pain flares. Therapeutic exercises are aimed at stretching tight anterior structures such as the scalenes and pectoralis minor and strengthen posterior scapular stabilizer muscles such as the serratus anterior. Other exercises for levator scapulae stretching have been described in the literature.[40,42] One study indicated that the most useful technique was scalene muscle activation.[43] Most commonly there is some shortening of the pectoralis minor and scalenes.[40] Peet et al. described an exercise program that has been reviewed and reused in the literature.[1] Functional, multiplanar exercises have also been used to strength muscles dynamically.

Relaxation, deep breathing, and visualization have been used with varying degrees of success, similar in degree to that found in other pain management literature. Other rehabilitation techniques have been utilized but have not been proven to be of use at this time. They include nerve gliding exercises, the Feldenkrais method, scapular manipulation, massage, and biofeedback.[42]

Pharmacologic management runs the gamut from nonsteroidal antiinflammatory drugs (NSAIDs) and muscle relaxants for relief of spasm to opiates.[11] Muscle relaxants generally have little direct effect on muscle tissue, relying on central effects instead. As such, they have significant sedation side effects and a small role in most TOS cases. Neuropathic pain medications, such as tricyclic antidepressants and antiepileptics, can be used for off-label indication of nerve pain in TOS.

Approximately 90%–95% of patients exhibit trigger points during the physical examination; trigger point injections have been used in the management of TOS, but their effectiveness is still in question.[44] Botulinum toxin injections have been increasingly used over the last several years for muscular imbalance and focal spasm control, although little literature exists to date.[45]

Studies generally show that there is an approximately 59%–88% success rate in patients managed conservatively.[43] One study found a nearly 94% success rate, defined by patient satisfaction outcomes, in a group of patients who had previously failed conservative management.[40] Worse outcomes have been associated with concomitant carpal or cubital tunnel syndromes, obesity, and ongoing worker compensation litigation.[22] Obesity has also been correlated with poorer outcomes with conservative management in at least two studies.[22,40]

Conservative management should be attempted for 4–6 months before considering surgery.[46] It is vital to recognize that the therapy should be tailored to the individual and not the disease. Another study reviewed TOS patients managed both conservatively and surgically and found that there were no significant differences in the outcomes when comparing the groups.[22] Given the complexity of this syndrome, it is vital to recognize that a poorly tailored therapy program that is not successful does not mean that therapy has failed. Physicians should carefully review previous therapy programs and consider prescribing a new, more specific therapy course when appropriate before making a surgical referral. Crosby and Wehbe provided a detailed review of nonsurgical treatments.[42]

Effort Thrombosis Syndrome

Paget-Schröetter syndrome, first described during the 1800s by Paget and von Schröetter, is spontaneous thrombosis of the axillary or subclavian vein. Currently, axillary and subclavian vessel deep vein thromboses (DVTs) make up approximately 2%–4% of all DVTs, but they are becoming increasingly more prevalent owing to the use of indwelling venous catheters. The syndrome continues to be rare and is associated with compressive anatomic anomalies.[30] It typically occurs in patients with a recent history of strenuous upper limb activity or trauma and is more typically referred to as effort thrombosis (ET) in many texts. Thus, sports medicine providers must be knowledgeable about this potentially disastrous syndrome.

Clinical presentation in athletes depends on the underlying pathology. Patients with chronic, low-grade compression of axillary or subclavian vasculature can present with vague, dull pain in the upper limb, and varying degrees of arm and hand swelling; occasionally collateral vessels are noted. Acute thrombosis presents with rapid onset of nonpitting edema, cyanosis, and pain. Distal pulses are typically intact unless the thrombosis is massive and acute enough that collateral vascularization has not developed.

Early diagnosis is also important to limit the risk of pulmonary embolism, which has been reported in up to 36% of ET patients.[30] The diagnosis is typically made with the use of Doppler ultrasonography owing to its ease and rapid availability. A hypercoaguability workup is generally indicated, including tests for proteins C and S, factor 5 Leiden, and lupus anticoagulant, although the tests are often negative.

There is no one definitive treatment for Paget-Schröetter syndrome, so the treatment plan must be individualized. Multiple algorithms have been suggested in the literature. In the authors' opinion, however, young athletic patients require prompt, aggressive treatment.

Although no true consensus exists, review of the literature supports an emergent, multifaceted approach to treating acute cases. This approach includes prompt thrombolysis of the clot with confirmation of full lysis by repeat venography. Intravenous anticoagulation with heparin with the goal maintaining the partial thromboplastin time (PTT) at 45–65 seconds is initiated. Conventional venography also defines the amount of fibrous destruction within the vessel, which determines the surgical approach to decompression. If it is < 2 cm, partial venotomy of the stenosed segment is completed along with decompression of the thoracic inlet, including partial first rib resection, removal of the subclavius tendon, division of the anterior scalene tendon, partial division of the middle scalene tendon, venotomy with removal of the fibrotic material, and ultimately patch plasty of the vein.

If the stenotic lesion is ≥ 2 cm, a modified approach with larger exposure is used. Warfarin and an oral antiplatelet agent are initiated after the procedure and continued for 8 weeks. Low-molecular-weight heparin is used as a bridge until the international normalized ratio is therapeutic.

Follow-up duplex ultrasonography is repeated until the patient is symptom-free and fully active and full venous patency is achieved. In that study, 100% of the patients treated within 2 weeks of the onset of symptoms achieved short- and long-term patency.[47] Patients who had residual stenosis on repeat venography were treated with balloon dilatation and stent placement. These vessels remained patent in 100% of patients for follow-up periods of up to 14 years.[47]

Other treatment algorithms recommend initial thrombolysis and venography to evaluate ongoing venous compression and to determine the need for surgery or treatment based on the time since onset of symptoms.[48–50] However, the emergent protocol uses one-time thrombolysis and decompression surgery, which minimizes hospitalization, requires only one 8-week period of anticoagulation, and should have a quicker return to play for the athlete. Because most of these patients are young at the age of onset, the protocol also avoids long-term anticoagulation and its associated risks. Athletes are not allowed to return to contact sports while on anticoagulation. A recent review of competitive athletes treated for ET found an average of 3.5 months before complete return to play was achieved. This study used a 1- to 3-week interval between initial thrombolysis and surgical decompression.[49]

Other treatments of ET in isolation include oral anticoagulation, which does not address underlying compression of the vessels; venolysis and partial decompression, which does not address intrinsic post-thrombotic fibrosis; decompression with angioplasty, which has high recurrence rates; and stenting, which has high rates of stent thrombosis. Multiple studies agree that intravascular stents are not indicated as treatment for Paget-Schröetter syndrome as they have high rates of stent thrombosis.[51] This is thought to be due to both external compression and the underlying low-flow states of the veins compared to that of arteries. The natural history of the syndrome, when treated conservatively, leads to an unacceptable long-term disability in 72% of patients.[52] Athletes should be advised, however, that they have a higher rate of recurrent DVT than the general population.

Surgical Approaches

Surgical referral should be initiated promptly in the appropriate clinical scenario of obvious neurologic signs such as atrophy of the intrinsic hand musculature or when V-TOS is suspected. Once a thorough trial of conservative management has been completed, surgery may be indicated. Surgery for nonspecific or disputed TOS is much more contentious.

There are two generally accepted surgical approaches to TOS: the supraclavicular approach and the transaxillary approach. The supraclavicular approach allows anterior and middle scalenectomy and can include both a cervical and first rib resection. The transaxillary approach allows only resection of the first rib, partial resection of the anterior scalene, and removal of most other anomalous structures.

The transaxillary approach has been used extensively by Roos, Urschel, and Razzuk. It involves safely positioning the patient in the lateral decubitus position. A transverse incision is made in the axilla, the fascia is incised, and blunt dissection is performed toward the chest wall. The intercostobrachial nerve may be visualized during this portion of the operation and should be protected if possible. Injury of the nerve leads to temporary numbness of the axilla and dorsum of the arm. The superior thoracic artery is ligated, and the first rib is palpable at this point. The soft tissue surrounding the first rib is resected, beginning at the anteroinferior surface, then the posterior surface, and finally the superior surface of the rib. A rib cutter is positioned as far posteriorly as is safely possible, and the rib is finally cut. The articulation at the sternum is either removed using clamps and traction or cut anteriorly using the rib cutter. The surgical site is flushed with normal saline to assess for pleural injury. This approach also allows thoracic sympathectomy as well as thromboendarterectomy or aneurysmectomy of the subclavian artery if indicated. The sympathectomy may be part of the reason for initial pain relief as it mitigates sympathetically mediated pain. Because this approach avoids interrupting of the back, shoulder, or chest musculature, it requires little if any physical therapy. Operating time is only 30–45 minutes, and blood loss is minimal. The patient can return home 2–3 days after the surgery and can return to work within 2–3 weeks, depending on his or her occupation.[11,53,55]

The supraclavicular approach begins with a 10-cm incision made parallel and 2 cm above the clavicle. The subcutaneous tissue is dissected, and the sternocleinomastoid and posterior belly of the omohyoid are divided. The fat pad covering the scalenes is dissected, revealing the suprascapular and transverse cervical vessels, which are then ligated. The phrenic nerve is retracted medially, and the anterior scalene is either excised entirely or released at its attachment at the first rib. The scalenectomy should involve as much of the muscle as necessary to free the neurovascular bundle. At this point, the cervical rib can be excised as well.[4,54,55]

Surgical Outcomes

The literature suggests that there is some difference in success rates depending on the surgery performed.[11,23,54] More recent studies with longer periods of follow up have found that these differences are seen purely in the short term.

Compelling arguments have been made for both approaches. The worker compensation studies by Franklin et al. showed that there was no difference in surgeon or surgery type.[25] Sanders reviewed his surgical patients over 23 years and found no differences between the surgical approaches taken.[11] Therefore, it seems that surgeons are well advised to use the approach with which they have the most experience.

Surgical data are difficult to pool given the use of different outcome measures. The lack of clarity as to diagnostic criteria for TOS makes this even more difficult. Nevertheless, there have been several excellent papers published regarding surgical results.

Some report a success rate as high as 99%, whereas others reported rates as low as 23%.[11,54,56] Urschel and Razzuk's extensive review of more than 1700 cases showed that well over 90% of cases had either excellent or good results, regardless of whether the lesion was an upper, lower, or combined trunk lesion.[57] Patients with a repetitive trauma etiology tend to have a lower success rate than those with a singular traumatic cause.[58] The impact that this has on the athlete with TOS is not well understood, especially when comparing the various psychosocial factors involved. When data are compiled, they suggest an 80%–90% success rate.[11]

It has been repeatedly found that patients initially tend to do well after surgery and subsequently have worsening of their symptoms. For example, one study found that 91.5% of patients reported improvement at 6 months, but only 74% reported improvement at 4 years of follow-up.[56] Worse outcomes have generally been associated with longer duration of symptoms (2 years) before surgery.[12]

The worker compensation studies found that the strongest predictors of postoperative disability in their population were the amount of work disability before surgery and the length of time between the injury and its diagnosis. At an average of 4.8 years of follow-up, 72.5% of these patients noted that they were still greatly limited regarding vigorous activities.[25] Even outside the worker compensation system, those with labor jobs tended to have poorer results than nonlaborers after surgery.[59] It has also been noted that patients within the worker compensation system also tend to have a lower success rate compared to other patients.[25,58]

Surgical Complications

The most commonly encountered complication is pneumothorax, which is reported to occur in 33% of patients.[60] There have been reports of injuries involving the long thoracic nerve, intercostobrachial nerve, and thoracic duct as well as apical hematoma, wound infection, and Horner's syndrome. There is an approximately 10% incidence of postoperative phrenic nerve dysfunction.[4,11,12,53,54] Interestingly, there is a report of a patient who suffered rib fractures that were thought to be due to alterations of the mechanical forces around the thoracocervical spine.[56]

Dale's review of the literature in 1982 found no formal reports of true brachial plexus injury. He surveyed members of the International Cardiovascular Society by mail which revealed 273 reports of brachial plexus injury. He also followed a group of 76 patients at 6 months post-operatively and noted one case of complete, though transient, paralysis of the upper limb.[61] Wilbourn followed eight patients with postoperative brachial plexus injury and found that even after 5 years most patients still had significant symptoms and electrodiagnostic evidence of their injuries.[62] Complex regional pain syndrome has also been reported after TOS surgery. In fact, operations on nonspecific or disputed TOS have resulted in significant iatrogenic neurologic sequela.[63]

Recurrent TOS

Patients who have undergone the current combined transcervical scalenectomy and transaxillary first rib resection have a reported recurrence rate of 5%. Patients who underwent earlier procedures, including isolated scalenectomy or first rib resection, have a recurrence of 15%–30%.[64] The recurrences are due to residual scar tissue adhering to any remaining portion of the cervical or first rib or directly to the brachial plexus itself.

One large review of more tha 3900 V-TOS and N-TOS patients showed an overall 31% recurrence rate. These 1221 patients underwent second procedures, and 89% enjoyed initial significant improvement; only 36 patients noted no improvement. Similar to the primary surgery, these success rates drop over time. At 5 years, the number maintaining significant improvement dropped to 75%.[55]

Another reviewer found that 17 of 500 N-TOS patients redeveloped symptoms. These cases were initially managed conservatively with physical therapy but all 17 eventually required surgery. All of these patients experienced excellent or good results and objectively were able to perform all of their activities of daily living; 75% of those who were previously working returned to their professions.[65]

The anatomic findings at the time of surgery generally show fibrocartilaginous scar tissue, although there are reports of retained rib tissue and retention of elongated transverse processes. The surgeries are designed to address the underlying issue and include brachial plexus neurolysis, rib resection, pectoralis minor tenotomy, and subtotal excision of the scalene muscles.

Conclusions

Thoracic outlet syndrome continues to present a difficult clinical scenario 187 years after it was first described. The diagnosis of V-TOS is more objective and has a much clearer treatment plan. N-TOS engenders most of the clinical questions at the heart of the debate. The clinical approach toward the rare, definitive or true N-TOS is not in question. It requires decisive diagnosis and prompt surgery. Unfortunately, disputed TOS is much more common and clinically frustrating.

Great care should be taken to obtain a thorough history and physical examination, complete with proper use and understanding of special tests specific to TOS. Plain films of the cervical spine are the first step in imaging to evaluate for anomalous bony anatomy. MRI, MRA, and CT can be used to determine vascular and soft tissue abnormalities. Thorough and appropriate electrodiagnostic testing should be used to obtain objective proof of neurologic compromise, although an absence of findings on electrodiagnostic tests does not rule out TOS.

An initial trial of appropriate aggressive nonsurgical therapy is advisable in most of these patients once true vascular compromise has been ruled out. Therapy should be performed by therapists familiar with the syndrome, and it should be directed toward the specific etiology of the compression.

Based on the literature, it seems that surgery tends to be highly successful in alleviating the symptoms of TOS. However, proper patient selection is key to successful outcomes as is an appropriate course of conservative management. Each surgeon should choose the operative approach with which they have the most experience and are most confident using. In the end, patients should be well informed of the risks and benefits of the procedure, and expectations should be duly managed.

References

1. Peet RM, Henriksen JD, Anderson TP, Martin GM. Thoracic-outlet syndrome: evaluation of a therapeutic exercise program. Proc Staff Meet Mayo Clin 1956;31(9):281–7.
2. Charon JP, Milne W, Sheppard DG, Houston JG. Evaluation of MR angiographic technique in the assessment of thoracic outlet syndrome. Clin Radiol 2004;59(7):588–95.
3. Divi V, Proctor MC, Axelrod DA, Greenfield LJ. Thoracic outlet decompression for subclavian vein thrombosis: experience in 71 patients. Arch Surg 2005;140(1):54–7.
4. Balci AE, Balci TA, Cakir O, et al. Surgical treatment of thoracic outlet syndrome: effect and results of surgery. Ann Thorac Surg 2003;75(4):1091–6; discussion 6.
5. Gilliatt RW. Thoracic outlet syndrome. BMJ 1983; 287(6394):764.
6. Vercellio G, Baraldini V, Gatti C, et al. Thoracic outlet syndrome in paediatrics: clinical presentation, surgical treatment, and outcome in a series of eight children. J Pediatr Surg 2003;38(1):58–61.
7. Wilbourn AJ. The thoracic outlet syndrome is overdiagnosed. Arch Neurol 1990;47(3):328–30.
8. Roos DB. The thoracic outlet syndrome is underrated. Arch Neurol 1990;47(3):327–8.
9. Brantigan CO, Roos DB. Diagnosing thoracic outlet syndrome. Hand Clin 2004;20(1):27–36.
10. Redenbach DM, Nelems B. A comparative study of structures comprising the thoracic outlet in 250 human cadavers and 72 surgical cases of thoracic outlet syndrome. Eur J Cardiothorac Surg 1998;13(4):353–60.
11. Sanders RJ. Thoracic Outlet Syndrome: A Common Sequelae of Neck Injuries. Philadelphia: Lippincott; 1992.
12. Cheng SW, Reilly LM, Nelken NA, et al. Neurogenic thoracic outlet decompression: rationale for sparing the first rib. Cardiovasc Surg 1995;3(6):617–23; discussion: 24.
13. Sanders RJ, Hammond SL. Etiology and pathology. Hand Clin 2004;20(1):23–6.
14. Strukel RJ, Garrick JG. Thoracic outlet compression in athletes a report of four cases. Am J Sports Med 1978; 6(2):35–9.
15. Karas SE. Thoracic outlet syndrome. Clin Sports Med 1990;9(2):297–310.

16. Esposito MD, Arrington JA, Blackshear MN, et al. Thoracic outlet syndrome in a throwing athlete diagnosed with MRI and MRA. J Magn Reson Imaging 1997;7(3):598–9.
17. Safran MR. Nerve injury about the shoulder in athletes. Part 2: Long thoracic nerve, spinal accessory nerve, burners/stingers, thoracic outlet syndrome. Am J Sports Med 2004;32(4):1063–76.
18. Simovitch RW, Bal GK, Basamania CJ. Thoracic outlet syndrome in a competitive baseball player secondary to the anomalous insertion of an atrophic pectoralis minor muscle: a case report. Am J Sports Med 2006;34(6): 1016–9.
19. Juvonen T, Satta J, Laitala P, et al. Anomalies at the thoracic outlet are frequent in the general population. Am J Surg 1995;170(1):33–7.
20. Roos DB. Congenital anomalies associated with thoracic outlet syndrome: anatomy, symptoms, diagnosis, and treatment. Am J Surg 1976;132(6):771–8.
21. Roos DB. New concepts of thoracic outlet syndrome that explain etiology, symptoms, diagnosis, and treatment. Vasc Surg 1979;13:313–21.
22. Landry GJ, Moneta GL, Taylor LM Jr, et al. Long-term functional outcome of neurogenic thoracic outlet syndrome in surgically and conservatively treated patients. J Vasc Surg 2001;33(2):312–7; discussion 7–9.
23. Donaghy M, Matkovic Z, Morris P. Surgery for suspected neurogenic thoracic outlet syndromes: a follow up study. J Neurol Neurosurg Psychiatry 1999;67(5):602–6.
24. Yavuzer S, Atinkaya C, Tokat O. Clinical predictors of surgical outcome in patients with thoracic outlet syndrome operated on via transaxillary approach. Eur J Cardiothorac Surg 2004;25(2):173–8.
25. Franklin GM, Fulton-Kehoe D, Bradley C, Smith-Weller T. Outcome of surgery for thoracic outlet syndrome in Washington state workers' compensation. Neurology 2000;54(6):1252–7.
26. McGough EC, Pearce MB, Byrne JP. Management of thoracic outlet syndrome. J Thorac Cardiovasc Surg 1979;77(2):169–74.
27. Gillard J, Perez-Cousin M, Hachulla E, et al. Diagnosing thoracic outlet syndrome: contribution of provocative tests, ultrasonography, electrophysiology, and helical computed tomography in 48 patients. Joint Bone Spine 2001;68(5):416–24.
28. Kuschner SH, Fechter JD. Thoracic outlet syndrome: diagnosis and treatment: operative techniques in sports medicine. Orthopedics 1996;4(1):2–7.
29. Demondion X, Bacqueville E, Paul C, et al. Thoracic outlet: assessment with MR imaging in asymptomatic and symptomatic populations. Radiology 2003;227(2):461–8.
30. Prandoni P, Polistena P, Bernardi E, et al. Upper-extremity deep vein thrombosis: risk factors, diagnosis, and complications. Arch Intern Med 1997;157(1): 57–62.
31. Seror P. Medial antebrachial cutaneous nerve conduction study, a new tool to demonstrate mild lower brachial plexus lesions: a report of 16 cases. Clin Neurophysiol 2004;115(10):2316–22.
32. Huang JH, Zager EL. Thoracic outlet syndrome. Neurosurgery 2004;55(4):897–902; discussion 902–3.
33. Dumitru D, Zwarts M. Electrodiagnostic Medicine. 2nd ed. Philadelphia: Hanley & Belfus; 2002.
34. Tolson TD. "EMG" for thoracic outlet syndrome. Hand Clin 2004;20(1):37–42, vi.
35. Cuevas-Trisan RL, Cruz-Jimenez M. Provocative F waves may help in the diagnosis of thoracic outlet syndrome: a report of three cases. Am J Phys Med Rehabil 2003;82(9):712–5.
36. Seror P. Frequency of neurogenic thoracic outlet syndrome in patients with definite carpal tunnel syndrome: an electrophysiological evaluation in 100 women. Clin Neurophysiol 2005;116(2):259–63.
37. Machleder HI, Moll F, Nuwer M, Jordan S. Somatosensory evoked potentials in the assessment of thoracic outlet compression syndrome. J Vasc Surg 1987;6(2):177–84.
38. Aminoff MJ. Use of somatosensory evoked potentials to evaluate the peripheral nervous system. J Clin Neurophysiol 1987;4(2):135–44.
39. Cakmur R, Idiman F, Akalin E, et al. Dermatomal and mixed nerve somatosensory evoked potentials in the diagnosis of neurogenic thoracic outlet syndrome. Electroencephalogr Clin Neurophysiol 1998;108(5):423–34.
40. Novak CB, Collins ED, Mackinnon SE. Outcome following conservative management of thoracic outlet syndrome. J Hand Surg [Am] 1995;20(4):542–8.
41. Upton AR, McComas AJ. The double crush in nerve entrapment syndromes. Lancet 1973;2(7825):359–62.
42. Crosby CA, Wehbe MA. Conservative treatment for thoracic outlet syndrome. Hand Clin 2004;20(1):43–9, vi.
43. Lindgren KA, Oksala I. Long-term outcome of surgery for thoracic outlet syndrome. Am J Surg 1995;169(3):358–60.
44. Atasoy E. Thoracic outlet compression syndrome. Orthop Clin North Am 1996;27(2):265–303.
45. Jordan SE, Ahn SS, Freischlag JA, et al. Selective botulinum chemodenervation of the scalene muscles for treatment of neurogenic thoracic outlet syndrome. Ann Vasc Surg 2000;14(4):365–9.
46. Kenny RA, Traynor GB, Withington D, Keegan DJ. Thoracic outlet syndrome: a useful exercise treatment option. Am J Surg 1993;165(2):282–4.
47. Molina JE, Hunter DW, Dietz CA. Paget-Schroetter syndrome treated with thrombolytics and immediate surgery. J Vasc Surg 2007;45(2):328–34.
48. Shebel ND, Marin A. Effort thrombosis (Paget-Schroetter syndrome) in active young adults: current concepts in diagnosis and treatment. J Vasc Nurs 2006;24(4):116–26.
49. Melby SJ, Vedantham S, Narra VR, et al. Comprehensive surgical management of the competitive athlete with effort thrombosis of the subclavian vein (Paget-Schroetter syndrome). J Vasc Surg 2008;47(4):809–20; discussion 21.
50. Doyle A, Wolford HY, Davies MG, et al. Management of effort thrombosis of the subclavian vein: today's treatment. Ann Vasc Surg 2007;21(6):723–9.
51. Urschel HC Jr, Patel AN. Paget-Schroetter syndrome therapy: failure of intravenous stents. Ann Thorac Surg 2003;75(6):1693–6; discussion 6.
52. Tilney ML, Griffiths HJ, Edwards EA. Natural history of major venous thrombosis of the upper extremity. Arch Surg 1970;101(6):792–6.

53. Roos DB. Transaxillary approach for first rib resection to relieve thoracic outlet syndrome. Ann Surg 1966;163(3): 354–8.
54. Sanders RJ, Hammond SL. Management of cervical ribs and anomalous first ribs causing neurogenic thoracic outlet syndrome. J Vasc Surg 2002;36(1):51–6.
55. Urschel HC Jr, Razzuk MA. Neurovascular compression in the thoracic outlet: changing management over 50 years. Ann Surg 1998;228(4):609–17.
56. Fulford PE, Baguneid MS, Ibrahim MR, et al. Outcome of transaxillary rib resection for thoracic outlet syndrome—a 10 year experience. Cardiovasc Surg 2001; 9(6):620–4.
57. Urschel HC Jr, Razzuk MA. Upper plexus thoracic outlet syndrome: optimal therapy. Ann Thorac Surg 1997;63(4):935–9.
58. Ellison DW, Wood VE. Trauma-related thoracic outlet syndrome. J Hand Surg [Br] 1994;19(4):424–6.
59. Goff CD, Parent FN, Sato DT, et al. A comparison of surgery for neurogenic thoracic outlet syndrome between laborers and nonlaborers. Am J Surg 1998;176(2):215–8.
60. Leffert RD, Perlmutter GS. Thoracic outlet syndrome: results of 282 transaxillary first rib resections. Clin Orthop 1999;(368):66–79.
61. Dale WA. Thoracic outlet compression syndrome: critique in 1982. Arch Surg 1982;117(11):1437–45.
62. Wilbourn AJ. Thoracic outlet syndrome surgery causing severe brachial plexopathy. Muscle Nerve 1988;11(1): 66–74.
63. Leffert RD. Complications of surgery for thoracic outlet syndrome. Hand Clin 2004;20(1):91–8.
64. Atasoy E. Recurrent thoracic outlet syndrome. Hand Clin 2004;20(1):99–105.
65. Ambrad-Chalela E, Thomas GI, Johansen KH. Recurrent neurogenic thoracic outlet syndrome. Am J Surg 2004;187(4):505–10.

Chapter 9
Stingers: Understanding the Mechanism, Diagnosis, Treatment, and Prevention

Stuart M. Weinstein

Introduction

Stingers are the most common source of upper limb peripheral nerve injuries in athletics. They occur frequently in football players, with as many as 50% of college football players reporting at least one stinger in their career. Stingers are localized to injury to either the upper brachial plexus or C5 and C6 nerve roots.

Burners, Stingers, and Burning Hands

The entity known as a *stinger* is synonymous with the term *burner* but not with the neurologic condition characterized by (bilateral) *burning hands*.[1] Therefore, in this chapter the term *stinger* is used to avoid the potential for confusion with burning hands syndrome, which represents the residual neurologic symptoms of a central cord syndrome. Stingers are nerve injuries that occur at a distinct location (although they are not necessarily consistent in any given athlete) within the peripheral neural axis at some point extending from the nerve root to the brachial plexus. Stingers almost always occur in athletes and are sustained during predictable types of athletic competition.

Historically, the incidence of peripheral nerve injuries in athletics is approximately 5%,[2,3] but the true incidence of stingers is not known. Except for certain high profile sports institutions, such as the National Football League (NFL), data are not routinely collected for this type of injury. There are probably two primary reasons why stingers may be underreported in athletic participation. The first reflects the culture of contact and collision sports. Unlike catastrophic head (i.e., major concussion) or spinal trauma (i.e., spinal cord injury), which often receive national media attention, less severe injuries are considered "part of the game." In fact, until the last several years, the same was true for mild concussions, with the expectation that "having your bell rung" or being "dinged" was an accepted part of contact or collision sports; furthermore, the environment surrounding such injuries did not necessitate aggressive medical assessment or management. The second, somewhat parallel, reason may be based on the relative severity of these peripheral nerve injuries. A neurapraxic lesion, such as a typical stinger, is likely to recover sooner than nerve degeneration due to axonotmesis. Prompt spontaneous recovery usually reduces the concern for obtaining medical evaluation. Therefore, for both cultural and neurophysiological reasons, stingers often garner limited attention.

The symptoms associated with first-time stingers generally resolve fairly quickly, although persisting neurologic deficits (especially motor) do occur. The chances of motor deficits are higher with recurrent stinger injuries. Theoretically, the risk of secondary musculoskeletal injury can also occur as a result of significant motor deficit (e.g., rotator cuff tear due to C5 or C6 radiculopathy with weakness). There is also evidence to support significant lost practice and

S.M. Weinstein (✉)
Department of Rehabilitation Medicine, University of Washington, Seattle, WA, USA

V. Akuthota, S.A. Herring (eds.), *Nerve and Vascular Injuries in Sports Medicine*,
DOI 10.1007/978-0-387-76600-3_9,

playing time and increased risk of recurrences following an initial stinger.

The NFL does collect player-injury data through the National Football League Injury Surveillance System and Med Sports Systems (MSS, Iowa City, Iowa) directed by John Powell, PhD, ATC. Injury data have been collected since 1980 for a variety of injury categories, among which are nerve-related injuries. All NFL teams are required to submit injury data to the league from the start of training camp through the Super Bowl. The minimum reportable criterion was 2 days lost playing time from 1980 through 1994 and 1 day lost playing time beginning in 1995. Aggregated NFL injury data for "stingers" were previously reported for the time period 1980–1997.[4] The NFL does not code for a distinct injury category labeled "stinger." Different category basins probably capture this entity, particularly "neck brachial plexus stretch and compression" and secondary categories such as "neck cervical impingement, various levels," "neck cervical plexus stretch and compression," "neck nerve contusion with or without motor and/or sensory loss," "cervical disc herniation, bulge, or rupture, various levels," and "neck neurotrauma." For this data review and to compare to the data presented previously, Table 9.1 shows "neck brachial plexus stretch and compression" injuries alone. Table 9.2 combines those data with "neck cervical impingement, C4–7" and "neck cervical plexus stretch and compression." It must be recognized that this is only an approximate assessment of stingers in the NFL. Not all of these players may have sustained a stinger as defined in this chapter; and, conversely, some NFL players with stingers who might have been coded in a different category would not be included in this data summary. Although not statistically assessed, there appears to be a slight reduction in mean days lost and mean games missed for the most recent 10-year period.

Mechanism of Injury

Undoubtedly, the most important factor when assessing an athlete with a suspected stinger is the distinction between a peripheral nerve injury and an injury to the central nervous system (CNS) (i.e., spinal cord). Quadriplegia/paresis due to a cervical spinal cord injury has vastly different prognostic and rehabilitative consequences than cervical radiculopathy or brachial plexopathy. Nevertheless, much attention has been directed toward the

Table 9.1 Brachial Plexus Stretch and Compression Injuries in the National Football League, 1997–2006 Seasons: Top Five Positions

	Days lost			Games missed	
Position	No. of players	Total	Mean	Total	Mean
Linebacker	80	866	11	79	1
Secondary	59	753	13	65	1
Offensive line	54	977	18	84	1.5
Running back	43	415	10	50	1
Defensive line	38	424	11	25	1

Table 9.2 Combined Injuries in the National Football League: Brachial Plexus Stretch and Compression, Neck Cervical Plexus Stretch and Compression, Neck Cervical Impingement (C4–7), 1997–2006 Seasons: Top Five Positions

	Days lost			Games missed	
Position	No. of players	Total	Mean	Total	Mean
Linebacker	92	978	11	88	1
Secondary	62	828	13	72	1
Offensive line	61	1121	18	104	2
Running back	45	522	12	53	1
Defensive line	43	516	12	33	1

pathomechanics of the stinger itself-specifically whether stingers represent tensile (or stretch) injuries to the brachial plexus or cervical nerve root or compressive injuries to these same neural structures.

A review of the anatomic facts suggests that the cervical nerve root is at greater risk for both tensile and compressive injury than the brachial plexus on the basis that limited perineurial and epineurial tissue courses through the dynamic neuroforamen and it has a relatively linear (in contrast to plexiform) course.[5] Although the literature slightly favors brachial plexus tensile overload[6–12] over nerve root stretch[13–15] or compression injuries[16–18] as the primary mechanism of injury, there is probably a differential mechanism based on the age and experience of the athlete and the sport activity (including position played and specific action). Tensile injuries tend to occur in the less experienced athlete with relatively weaker neck and shoulder girdle musculature, and thus with reduced ability to resist sudden or forceful neck lateral bending to the opposite side of the affected arm. This mechanism occurs more commonly in certain sports, such as during the takedown maneuver in wrestling or in the skeletally immature football player in whom there is widening of the acromiomastoid distance. Conversely, cervical nerve root compression due to narrowing of the neuroforamen from cervical extension and rotation (i.e., a functional Spurling maneuver) is more likely to occur in the older, stronger, more experienced athlete, such as a football defensive back (tackling) or an offensive lineman (pass blocking). A less typical pathomechanism of a stinger is direct brachial plexus compression[19,20] usually resulting from equipment such as padding or a stick.

A closer look at the functional anatomy of the nerve root facilitates an understanding as to why motor deficit appears to be the most common residual neurologic finding after sustaining a stinger. The ventral (or motor) nerve root is more vulnerable than the dorsal (or sensory) nerve root to tensile overload because it lacks the dampening affect of the dorsal root ganglion, has a thinner dural sheath, and directly aligns with the spinal cord. Although the pathomechanics of the stinger is variable, as reported in the literature, the development of myotomal weakness is the one consistent clinical finding.

Clinical Evaluation and Diagnosis

Are the history and physical examination adequate to make the diagnosis of a stinger? Usually, the answer is yes. The sine qua non of diagnosing a stinger is the sudden onset of severe, lancinating, burning pain and dysesthesias in one upper limb following a traumatic event. These symptoms usually follow a single dermatomal distribution, although this level of historical specificity may be lacking. Simultaneous, bilateral stingers almost never occur, so any athlete reporting bilateral upper limb paresthesias or dysesthesias should be carefully evaluated for a spinal cord injury and all necessary precautions observed. (The assessment and treatment of cervical spinal cord injury is beyond the scope of this chapter.) With the first occurrence of a stinger, the symptoms usually resolve quickly, often within seconds to minutes. In fact, the rapid spontaneous reduction or resolution of the burning pain and paresthesias is one of the main reasons these injuries are underreported to coaches, medical personnel, and family. However, recurrent episodes usually lead to more persistent symptoms. Because of potentially unrecognized and untreated initial injuries, more distinct neurologic sequelae result.

In the typical scenario, the athlete exits the playing field unaided, often with the affected limb motionless against the abdomen in a "sling-like" position, complaining of burning pain. Once it is determined to be a neurologic injury, it is imperative to differentiate a peripheral nerve injury from the possibility of a spinal cord injury. The presence of more than one limb's involvement should immediately raise the suspicion of the latter, prompting a full-scale cervical spine rescue protocol. In reality, players with spinal cord injuries rarely leave the field under their own power; thus, an athlete who spontaneously exits the playing field is not likely to have sustained spinal cord trauma.

The sideline evaluation should include the following components: prompt questioning regarding the specific mechanism of injury; a precise distribution and duration of symptoms; active cervical range of motion to assess pain provocation and rigidity (passive cervical range of motion in a symptomatic player is to be avoided on the sideline); palpation for well localized moderate to severe cervical bony tenderness and/or paravertebral muscle guarding; and a detailed neurologic examination with emphasis on motor deficits originating from the C5–7 myotomes (due to the higher prevalence of degenerative changes or hypermobility at these levels). The sideline or locker room motor examination has the potential to be the most informative part of the evaluation, but it is frequently the least well performed aspect of the initial assessment because of the frenetic athletic environment during a game. Because most motor deficits following a stinger affect the C5–7 myotomes, a quick motor examination that assesses only one or two muscle groups, particularly hand intrinsic muscle strength (primarily innervated by C8 and T1), almost always misses identifying any neuropathic muscle weakness. The motor assessment must include testing of at least two muscles in each myotome innervated by different peripheral nerves-e.g., rhomboid (C5, dorsal scapular); infraspinatus (C5/6, suprascapular); deltoid (C5/6, axillary); flexor carpi radialis (C6/7, median); extensor carpi radialis (C6/7, radial); triceps (C7/8, radial); and hand interossei (C8–T1, ulnar). Furthermore, an adequate neurologic examination can assist in ruling out other potential isolated peripheral nerve injuries, including suprascapular and axillary neuropathies.

All athletes with suspected stingers must be carefully monitored for prompt resolution or persistence of symptoms and signs because, at a minimum, it affects return-to-play decisions. As indicated, most first-time episodes resolve quickly, sometimes even before the athlete reaches the sideline. However, the duration of any given episode may vary from seconds to hours, much less commonly lasting for days or longer. In persisting cases, motor deficit is the most common finding, often present without spontaneous pain or sensory symptoms (although symptom provocation with cervical range of motion is still possible and suggestive of heightened nerve irritability). It is important first to assess the athlete serially in the locker room and then the training room or team physician's office. If weakness persists more than 10–14 days or progressively worsens over the first few days after injury, additional ancillary testing and further specialty consultation would be reasonable and necessary to determine the site of injury and degree of axonal damage precisely.

The significance of other altered biomechanical physical findings (i.e., postural faults, muscular flexibility and strength imbalances) that are often present but infrequently emphasized in athletes with recurrent stingers is discussed in the rehabilitation section of this chapter.

Key Diagnostic Tests

There are two primary categories of ancillary testing to consider when evaluating the athlete with a stinger: (1) imaging the cervical spine and shoulder girdle to assess pathoanatomy; and (2) electrodiagnosis of the cervical nerve roots and brachial plexus to assess neural dysfunction. These test results, combined with the clinical assessment, can be used to determine the precise diagnosis, prognosis, treatment, rehabilitation, and return to play.

Imaging

Imaging of the cervical spine can include radiography, magnetic resonance imaging (MRI), and computed tomography (CT). There is probably no absolute indication for cervical radiography following an initial event if the symptoms resolve quickly (e.g., within minutes) and the physical assessment reveals full pain-free cervical range of motion. Even in circumstances of recurrent stingers or persisting symptoms and signs following an initial stinger, the relative value of cervical radiography is limited. A thorough cervical radiographic examination should include an anteroposterior (AP) view, lateral view (including flexion and extension lateral views if instability is suspected), and bilateral oblique views. Some findings that might have clinical relevance include uncovertebral joint degenerative hypertrophy, neuroforaminal encroachment, instability or hypermobility, and loss of normal cervical lordosis.

The utility of the Torg ratio[21] in the assessment of the stinger is controversial. Originally described as a simple radiographic screening tool for the presence of central cervical spinal stenosis but later shown to have a low positive predictive value for true spinal stenosis,[22] abnormalities of the Torg ratio have reportedly been correlated with an increased risk of a "complicated" clinical course following a stinger.[23] However, it is important to emphasize that although more experienced athletes who sustain stingers may have a higher incidence of degenerative disc changes and neuroforaminal stenosis,[24] the Torg ratio was never meant to define relative risk to the peripheral nerves. Therefore, independent of the relative limited utility in predicting central cervical stenosis, the Torg ratio should not be considered a radiographic measure for the presence of cervical neuroforaminal stenosis or the risk of sustaining a stinger in the athletic population.

Advanced imaging studies such as MRI or CT (with sagittal reformatting) more directly demonstrate the presence and extent of neuroforaminal stenosis and disc abnormalities (including disc degeneration and disc herniation). One MRI study of athletes with stingers documented that 87% had evidence for degenerative disc abnormalities at the C4/5, C5/6, and C6/7 levels; and 93% had either disc abnormalities or foraminal narrowing.[24] Although these findings do not indicate an absolute causative association, cervical degenerative changes appear to predispose an athlete structurally to sustaining a stinger.

Electrophysiologic Testing

Electrophysiologic testing is useful in certain clinical circumstances, particularly if persistent or progressive weakness is present beyond 2 weeks after the injury and following recurrent stingers. Needle electromyography (EMG) abnormalities in a resting muscle, if present, represent axonal damage and do not manifest immediately aftert injury, usually requiring a minimum of 7–10 days to show. Furthermore, it has been estimated that injury to a minimum of 30% of the axons is necessary for needle EMG abnormalities to be present.[25] Therefore, milder injury may be difficult to observe with electrodiagnostic testing. Some instances of clinical weakness may represent axonopathy below this 30% threshold, or the weakness may represent a neurapraxic lesion with conduction block. Athletes with the latter condition are more likely to recover spontaneously and quickly. Early evidence (and at times the only evidence) of injury may be seen with abnormal recruitment of motor unit action potentials. Relative healing can include resolution of these recruitment abnormalities and identification of abnormal (often referred to as "chronic or reinnervated") configuration of motor unit action potentials from the affected muscles.

Electrodiagnostic testing should be able to differentiate between a brachial plexus injury and cervical radiculopathy by identifying abnormalities in the cervical paraspinal muscles (with the latter injury) or reduction of distal sensory evoked potential amplitudes (with the former injury). However, early reinnervation of the cervical paraspinals following nerve root trauma may preclude finding needle EMG abnormalities in these muscles. Other conduction techniques have been described including cervical nerve root stimulation, Erb's point timulation, and long latency conductions (e.g., F waves), but the proximal location of these injuries presents technical challenges with any of these nerve conduction studies.

Treatment and Prevention

Can a stinger really be rehabilitated?

Treatment of the athlete with a stinger focuses on three specific areas.

1. Symptoms associated with neuronal injury
2. Specific myotomal weakness secondary to the neurologic injury
3. Postural dysfunction including flexibility and strength imbalances

Ironically, even though a stinger is a primary peripheral nerve injury, there are no specific rehabilitation techniques that clearly accelerate the rate of neural healing. The degree of injury and passage of time generally dictate spontaneous neural regeneration. Left untreated, most athletes recover from a single stinger episode, but the risk of delayed or incomplete recovery increases in proportion to the number of recurrences. Thus, successful rehabilitation implies that the athlete is symptom-free with full range of motion, demonstrates normal strength, *and* has proactively lessened his or her risk for recurrent injury. Beyond the initial stages of healing, rehabilitation of the stinger focuses less directly on the injured nerve and more on the surrounding soft tissue and spinal segmental and postural abnormalities that predisposed the athlete to the injury. For purposes of the following description, the stinger is considered a cervical nerve root injury.

Controlling Symptoms

The first stage of rehabilitation involves controlling pain and inflammation. This includes elimination of the overload forces that caused the initial injury and use of common antiinflammatory and analgesic measures delivered through medications and physical therapy modalities such as thermal agents, gentle stretching, and manual traction techniques. The manual traction technique, more so than mechanical traction, places the athlete at ease, allows graded force application, and provides better control of the neck position maintaining slight cervical flexion. Most athletes experience resolution of painful dysesthesias fairly quickly. Infrequently, and depending on the age of the athlete and level of competition, if symptoms persist despite these measures, consideration should be given to administration of a fluoroscopically guided epidural steroid injection. This can effectively place a localized dose of corticosteroid along the injured nerve root, which may reduce both inflammation and ectopic neural impulses. In most situations, anatomic decompression of neuroforaminal stenosis is not necessary to allow an athlete to recover fully unless the clinical course suggests progressive motor deterioration supported by electrophysiological data. Fortunately, this is a rare occurrence following a stinger. Furthermore, the surgical procedure required to decompress the cervical nerve root adequately might require an anterior discectomy and fusion, leading to a variety of other potential negative consequences, including impact on return to play and longer-term adjacent segment degeneration.

Postural Corrections

Once symptoms are controlled, the second stage of rehabilitation addresses the postural faults that place the athlete at greater risk of sustaining a stinger. In fact, this "forward head" postural attitude is common throughout the general population with a multifactorial basis including sedentary lifestyle, prolonged inactivity following injury, strength and flexibility imbalances about the cervicothoracic spine and shoulder girdle, and a genetic predisposition. In the athletic population, it is the strength and flexibility imbalances that require specific attention. Of note, the radiographic representation of the forward head posture is reduction or absence of the normal cervical lordosis. Although radiographic straightening of the cervical spine can result from acute muscle spasm, more commonly this finding is chronic in duration and is not due to muscle spasm directly. While standard rehabilitation prescriptions include a reference to "correcting lordosis" prior to return to play (which may have more direct bearing on a distinctly unrelated condition known as spear tackler's spine[26]), focused rehabilitation for stingers involves a thorough postural correction.

In general, a chronic forward head posture with loss of normal cervical lordosis results in a relative maldistribution of segmental motion with stiffness in the upper cervical and upper thoracic regions and compensatory increased motion in the mid to lower cervical region. This relative hypermobility may lead to a greater degree of degenerative neuorforaminal stenosis in the mid to lower cervical spine and therefore may explain the increased susceptibility of the nerve root compared to the brachial plexus. As previously shown, a large proportion of athletes who experience a stinger have advanced imaging evidence for these degenerative changes.[24]

Specifically, the segmental and myofascial abnormalities that are typically found with the forward head posture include increased in thoracic kyphosis; excessive scapular protraction and glenohumeral internal rotation; hyperflexion of the lower cervical and upper thoracic segments; hyperextension of the upper cervical segments; segmental hypermobility of the mid to lower cervical segments; and weakening of many muscle groups controlling head and neck motion due to alteration of their normal length–tension relation. Muscles that are shortened (and weakened) include the capital and cervical extensors, sternocleidomastoid, upper trapezius, levator scapula, pectoralis minor and major, anterior deltoid, subscapularis, serratus anterior, and anterior scalene. Those lengthened (and weakened) include the capital and cervical flexors, middle and lower trapezius, rhomboids, thoracic extensors, and latissimus dorsi.

With this understanding of the forward head posture as a basis, a rational approach to the use of manual therapy techniques can be considered. Manual therapy techniques provide analgesic benefit as well as normalization of segmental and myofascial dysfunction with the goal of restoring cervical lordosis. Joint mobilization techniques to improve zygapophysial joint glide must be directed to the hypomobile segments only. Forceful manipulation (the highest grade of mobilization) in the presence of significant neuroforaminal compromise could potentially be aggravating and damaging to the nerve root. Myofascial stretching techniques such as myofascial release and massage should be used to lengthen the shortened and weakened musculature. Improved soft tissue extensibility also improves segmental motion at the hypomobile levels; however, release of tight paraspinal musculature may uncover mid to lower cervical segmental hypermobility. Strengthening exercises are incorporated in the final stage of rehabilitation when the likelihood of nerve root injury is lessened.

Strength Training

The strength training component of rehabilitation following a stinger includes the paraspinal muscles, postural control including the upper thoracic and scapular stabilizer musculature, trunk and core stabilization exercises, and targeted strengthening of the muscles weakened as a result of the inciting neural injury. The rate of progression of exercise is based primarily on persistence of symptoms and secondarily on the results of ancillary electrophysiological and imaging studies. Generally, the less severe the injury and neurologic sequelae, the more rapidly rehabilitation can progress. Theoretically, one does not want to overload muscles that already have been compromised due to a nerve injury. Therefore, electrophysiological data can help guide the aggressiveness of rehabilitation by defining (qualitatively and quantitatively) to what degree residual weakness represents neurapraxia or axonopathy. Conceptually, exercise starts with well protected isometric strengthening of the paraspinal muscles in neutral spine postures, advancing to multiplanar, functional exercises emphasizing strength, agility, balance, and endurance. Finally, sport-specific and position skills training (e.g., blocking and tackling techniques) completes the rehabilitation process.

Protective Equipment

Equipment modifiers such as shoulder pad lifters and cervical rolls are often prescribed and used by athletes (particularly football players) to prevent stingers although there are no research studies that demonstrate a reduction in the incidence of stingers with their use. Furthermore, use of any motion-restricting device must be considered in the context of interfering with an athlete's performance as well as positioning the cervical spine in relative flexion, the latter of which may place the spinal cord at greater risk of traumatic injury. Despite their widespread use, these devices cannot substitute for a complete rehabilitation program.

Guidelines for Safe Return to Play

There are universal return-to-play guidelines that can be applied to most athletic injuries, including resolution of symptoms, regaining range of motion, and recovery of strength and function. In many circumstances, however, athletes return to play before reaching these ideal endpoints, because of some degree of permanence of dysfunction or because they demonstrate an ability to function with a safety margin despite, for example, lack of full range of motion of the affected structure. More specifically, following a noncatastrophic cervical spine injury, the goal of normal cervical lordosis may not be achievable and would not represent an absolute contraindication to return to play. Following a stinger, return-to-play decisions are based on a combination of clinical, electrophysiological, and imaging findings. Furthermore, weight is given to whether this was an initial or a recurrent injury. Finally, the player should have completed the key aspects of a comprehensive rehabilitation program as described above.

Electrodiagnostic testing is generally not required to determine return to play if the clinical assessment demonstrates normal motor testing. However, if weakness persists beyond 2–4 weeks following the injury, electrodiagnostics can play a role in determining return to play. The presence of moderate fibrillation potentials or positive waves is indicative of significant axonopathy and suggests the possibility of a more prolonged clinical course. Repeat studies should be considered especially if some degree of weakness persists despite adequate rehabilitation. A follow-up study may be a guide to returning an athlete to competition, particularly if the study does not reveal these spontaneous potentials and motor unit recruitment reveals evidence for motor unit reinnervation (i.e., increased numbers of polyphasic, arger-amplitude action potentials). Also, the athlete should achieve other rehabilitation goals, and the degree of residual weakness should not place him at risk for secondary injury (e.g., weak infraspinatus increasing the risk for a rotator cuff tear). Reestablishment of a "normal" electrodiagnostic test is not a criterion for return to play if the remaining or residual abnormalities are indicative of reinnervation and not acute axonal dysfunction. If a recurrent stinger occurs, then new electrophysiologic testing may be useful.

The primary abnormality on an advanced imaging study such as MRI that would potentially delay return to play is a cervical disc herniation resulting in nerve root compression that correlates with the clinical scenario. As described above, there is a high prevalence of neuroforaminal stenosis in athletes with stingers. Because there is no nonsurgical treatment to correct this condition absolutely, the presence of neuroforaminal stenosis should not be an absolute contraindication to return to play. If the athlete has participated in the comprehensive rehabilitation program, measures to correct soft tissue restrictions, segmental stiffness, and postural faults should effectively increase the dynamic diameter of the foramen and reduce the potential for mechanical stress on the nerve root. Unfortunately, other unexpected anatomic abnormalities may be identified on cervical MRI in athletes including central spinal canal stenosis. Although central stenosis has no direct clinical relevance to the stinger and may in fact be asymptomatic, this finding prompts additional concerns about return to play unrelated to the stinger injury.

Finally, the timing of return to play following a stinger depends not only on the factors already discussed but also on the number of previous stingers the athlete has sustained; generally, more severe and persistent motor deficits occur in athletes who have experienced recurrent stingers. The following is a general guide to assist with deciding return to play. It is based on a combination of clinical experience, neurophysiological principles, and extrapolation of information from other athletic and nonathletic peripheral nerve injuries. Following a first-time stinger, the athlete may return to same game competition if full recovery occurs within 15 minutes of the injury, and the athlete may return to competition in 1 week if full clinical recovery occurs within 48–72 hours. In any other scenario, further assessment is pursued. There are no distinct rules on how to approach an athlete whose symptoms resolve between days 4 and 10. Even if symptoms resolve relatively quickly after a first episode, any postural dysfunction and relative weaknesses should be addressed. An athlete's strength and fitness program should be revisited more comprehensively in the off-season. More caution is taken if an athlete sustains more than one stinger during the same season. In part, this is because there is a greater likelihood of residual neuropathic weakness, and there are likely significant underlying biomechanical issues as well as technique issues that must be addressed. The athlete should be held from practice and competition at a minimum for the number of weeks that corresponds to the number of that stinger (e.g., 2 weeks for the second stinger, 3 weeks for the third stinger). After the third stinger in the same season, consideration should be given to ending that season, particularly in the presence of significant weakness, electrodiagnostic findings suggesting acute moderate axonopathy, or MRI revealing focal disc herniation resulting in nerve root compression. Again, these should be considered guidelines only. As with any athletic injury, other medical and nonmedical factors contribute to the decision-making process regarding when an athlete can return to play.

References

1. Maroon JC. "Burning hands" in football spinal cord injuries. JAMA 1977;238:2049–51.
2. Hirasawa Y, Sakakida K. Sports and peripheral nerve injury. Am J Sports Med 1983;11:420–6.
3. Takazawa H, Sudo N. Statistical observation of nerve injuries in athletes. Brain Nerve Injuries 1971;3:11–7.
4. Weinstein SM, Herring SA. Assessment and rehabilitation of the athlete with a stinger. In: Cantu RC, ed. Neurologic Athletic Neck and Spine Injuries, Philadelphia: Saunders; 2000:81–191.
5. Sunderland S. The brachial plexus normal anatomy. In: Nerves and Nerve Injuries. New York: Churchill Livingstone; 1978:856.
6. Archmbault JL. Brachial plexus stretch injury. J Am Coll Health 1983;31:256–60.
7. Clancy WG, Brand RL, Bergfeld JA. Upper trunk brachial plexus injuries in contact sports. Am J Sports Med 1977;5:209–15.
8. Funk FJ, Wells RE. Injuries of the cervical spine in football. Clin Orthop 1975;109:50–8.
9. Hunter C. Injuries to the brachial plexus: experience of a private sports medicine clinic. J Osteopath Assoc 1982; 91:757–60.
10. Jackson DW, Lohr FT. Cervical spine injuries. Clin Sports Med 1986;5:373–86.
11. Robertson WC, Eichman PL, Clancy WG. Upper trunk brachial plexopathy in football players. JAMA 1979; 241:1480–2.
12. Wroble RR, Albright JP. Neck and low back injuries in wrestling. Clin Sports Med 1986;5:295–325.
13. Chrisman OD, Snook GA, Stanitis JM, et al. Lateral flexion injuries in contact sports. JAMA 1965;192:613–5.
14. Marshall TM. Nerve pinch injuries in football. J Ky Med Assoc 1970;October:68:648–9.
15. Speer KP, Bassett FJ III. The prolonged burner syndrome. Am J Sports Med 1990;18:591–4.
16. Poindexter DP, Johnson EW. Football shoulder and neck injury: a study of the "stinger." Arch Phys Med Rehabil 1984;65:601–2.
17. Rockett FX. Observations on the "burner:" traumatic cervical radiculopathy. Clin Orthop 1982;164:18–9.
18. Watkins RG. Neck injuries in football players. Clin Sports Med 1986;5:215–46.
19. DiBennedetto M, Markey F. Electrodiagnostic localization of traumatic upper trunk brachial plexopathy. Arch Phys Med Rehabil 1984;65:15–7.
20. Markey KL, DiBennedetto M, Curl WW. Upper trunk brachial plexopathy: the stinger syndrome. Am J Sports Med 1993;21:650–5.
21. Pavlov HJ, Torg JS, Robie B, et al. Cervical spinal stenosis: determination with vertebral body ratio method. Radiology 1987;164:771–5.
22. Herzog RJ, Wiens JJ, Dillingham MF, et al. Normal cervical spine morphometry and cervical spinal stenosis in asymptomatic professional football players: plain radiography, multiplanar computed tomography, and magnetic resonance imaging. Spine 1991;16:S178–86.
23. Meyer SA, Schulte KR, Callaghan JJ, et al. Cervical spinal stenosis and stingers in collegiate football players. Am J Sports Med. 1994;22:158–66.
24. Levitz CL, Reilly PJ, Torg JS. The pathomechanics of chronic, recurrent cervical nerve root neurapraxia: the chronic burner syndrome. Am J Sports Med 1997;25: 73–6.
25. Wilbourn A, Bergfeld J. Value of EMG examination with sports related nerve injury. Electroencephalogr Clin Neurophysiol 1983;55:42P–54P.
26. Torg JS, Sennet B, Pavlov HJ, et al. Spear tackler's spine: an entity precluding participation in tackle football and collision activities that expose the cervical spine to axial energy inputs. Am J Sports Med 1993;21:640–9.

Part III
Lower Limb Syndromes

Chapter 10
Peripheral Nerve Entrapment and Compartment Syndromes of the Lower Leg

Andrea J. Boon and Mansour Y. Dib

Introduction

Peripheral nerve injuries are quite rare in the athlete, accounting for less than 1% of sporting injuries.[1–4] Nevertheless, they can be a career-ending event for the athlete and have ramifications for many functional activities outside of sports. Therefore, it is imperative that nerve involvement be diagnosed promptly, allowing early intervention prior to irreversible loss of nerve function. Sports medicine physicians must have an in-depth knowledge of peripheral nerve anatomy and physiology to diagnose the level of injury accurately and provide appropriate treatment and prognostic information to the athlete. The diagnosis is primarily based on the history, physical examination, and electrodiagnostic testing. Treatment is usually conservative and can include relative rest, technique modification, physical therapy, antiinflammatory medication, splinting, and steroid injection. Occasionally, surgical decompression or reconstruction is necessary. Similarly, compartment syndromes in the athlete can have a major impact on performance, often limiting participation in the case of exertional compartment syndrome or causing irreparable loss of function in the case of acute compartment syndrome. Exertional compartment syndromes can be difficult to diagnose and may masquerade as a peripheral nerve injury because of the associated neural compression that occurs with increased compartment pressures. One must maintain a high index of suspicion and pursue a definitive diagnosis, including measurement of compartment pressures, to diagnose this condition in a timely manner. This chapter discusses nerve entrapment and compartment syndromes in the leg, reviewing the anatomy, mechanisms of injury, clinical presentation, evaluation, treatment, and prevention.

Mechanism of Nerve Injury

Nerves can be injured through a variety of mechanisms. Acutely, a nerve can be crushed or transected because of a direct blow or laceration. Typically, this carries the worst prognosis owing to partial or complete axonal loss. Compression of the nerve can occur acutely (e.g., from ill-fitting equipment) or chronically. Chronic tension or compression of the nerve can result in repetitive microtrauma, usually related to a prominent or abnormal band of muscle, tendon, fascia, or a bony prominence. Traction or stretch injury is the most common mechanism of injury in athletes but is most often seen in the upper limb, with involvement of the brachial plexus.[1,2] A severe traction injury can completely disrupt the nerve fibers, which portends a grave prognosis. Iatrogenic injury in athletes is most often related to the treatment of other sporting injuries, such as after cast application or as a complication of arthroscopic surgery.

In addition, athletes are as prone to non-sports-related causes of nerve dysfunction as the general population. When evaluating a nerve injury in an athlete, particularly in the absence of an obvious

A.J. Boon (✉)
Department of Physical Medicine and Rehabilitation, Mayo Clinic, Rochester, MN, USA

V. Akuthota, S.A. Herring (eds.), *Nerve and Vascular Injuries in Sports Medicine*,
DOI 10.1007/978-0-387-76600-3_10, © Springer Science+Business Media, LLC 2009

inciting event, it is important to consider the possibility of nontraumatic peripheral nerve injury, which may be related to inflammatory, infectious, metabolic, neoplastic, paraneoplastic, toxic, inherited, or degenerative causes. The history should include a personal and family history of neurologic conditions, including an inherited tendency to pressure palsies or brachial plexitis. The physical examination should include a full motor and sensory examination, as well as testing of the deep tendon reflexes to evaluate for more diffuse involvement as might be seen with a peripheral neuropathy, polyradiculoneuropathy, mononeuritis multiplex, or motor neuron disease. Appropriate laboratory studies may include screening for connective tissue disorders, diabetes, thyroid dysfunction, amyloidosis, sarcoidosis, renal dysfunction, heavy metal intoxication (particularly lead and copper), and alcohol or nutritional supplement misuse. In addition to electrodiagnostic testing, high-resolution ultrasonography or magnetic resonance imaging (MRI) of the nerve may provide additional helpful information.

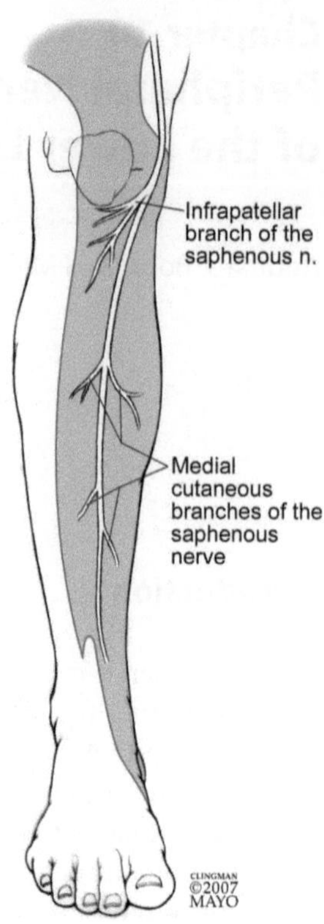

Fig. 10.1 Cutaneous sensory distribution of the saphenous nerve. Used with permission of Mayo Foundation for Medical Education and Research

Saphenous Nerve

Anatomy

The saphenous nerve is a terminal cutaneous branch of the femoral nerve, derived from the L3/4 nerve roots, providing sensory innervation to the medial calf and proximal medial side of the foot (Fig. 10.1). It branches off the femoral nerve just distal to the inguinal ligament and enters Hunter's canal (the roof of which is formed by dense connective tissue bridging the adductor magnus and longus muscles medially and the vastus medialis muscle laterally). The nerve exits the canal in the distal third of the thigh by piercing the subsartorial fascia, then travels deep to, or occasionally pierces, the sartorius muscle before emerging between the tendons of the sartorius and gracilis muscles. The nerve gives off the infrapatellar plexus and then descends along the medial border of the tibia, in close proximity to the saphenous vein, to end in two terminal branches, one supplying the skin of the medial ankle and the other supplying the skin of the medial foot.[5]

Etiology

The saphenous nerve can be entrapped anywhere along its course but is most vulnerable at the level where it pierces the roof of Hunter's canal in the distal thigh because of sharp angulation as it exits the tough connective tissue in conjunction with repetitive shear forces associated with local muscle contraction. Saphenous neuropathy is rare in athletes but has been reported after patellar dislocation,[6] in surfers,[7] in a bodybuilder (the saphenous neuropathy was thought to be due to hypertrophied muscles),[5] and in a runner in association with a swollen pes anserine bursa.[8] The saphenous nerve can also be injured iatrogenically as a complication of both knee and ankle arthroscopy[9–11] and after injection around the knee.[12]

Clinical Presentation

Saphenous neuropathy typically presents with deep, aching pain and occasionally paresthesias in the distribution of the nerve. Pain can be localized anywhere along the course of the nerve, from the thigh to the proximal medial foot, but is most often felt in the region of the medial knee or calf. Consequently, saphenous neuropathy can mimic various musculoskeletal complaints, such as a medial meniscal tear in the knee, pes anserine bursitis, medial tibial stress syndrome, or stress fracture.[8] The infrapatellar branch can be injured as it pierces the sartorius tendon or courses subcutaneously across the medial femoral epicondyle, where it is prone to damage from arthroscopic procedures or direct blows to the knee. Patients may note paresthesias in the region of the knee that get worse with knee flexion or with compression from tight equipment or braces.

The differential diagnosis should include L4 radiculopathy, lumbar plexopathy, or a more proximal femoral neuropathy. Physical examination may show a well demarcated area of altered sensation within the distribution of the saphenous nerve, symptom provocation with passive thigh hyperextension, and pain or paresthesias with deep palpation proximal to the medial femoral condyle. Because the saphenous nerve is purely sensory, there should be no associated weakness. Any weakness, atrophy, or loss of the quadriceps deep tendon reflex should prompt further evaluation for a more proximal nerve lesion.

Evaluation

Electrodiagnostic studies can be helpful for diagnosing saphenous neuropathy but are more helpful for excluding other causes of neuropathic medial leg pain. Saphenous nerve conduction studies (NCSs) are technically challenging, and the response can be absent even in normal subjects. For these reasons, it is imperative that NCSs are performed bilaterally to allow side-to-side comparison, with more than 50% loss of amplitude in the affected limb considered diagnostic of saphenous nerve injury. Although femoral NCS can be performed if a more proximal femoral neuropathy is suspected, the needle examination is usually more helpful. With a true saphenous neuropathy, the needle examination is completely normal; however, given the differential diagnosis, it is important to check both femoral and obturator innervated muscles. The quadriceps muscle is involved in femoral neuropathy, whereas in the case of a plexopathy or L4 radiculopathy the adductor longus and tibialis anterior may also show changes, in which case lumbar paraspinal muscles should be examined as well.

Management

Once the diagnosis has been established, treatment is symptomatic. If symptoms are merely numbness or hypesthesia, simple reassurance often suffices. If pain is the main complaint, a local anesthetic and steroid injection may be both diagnostic and therapeutic.[5] In athletes, elimination of any provocative factors such as tight clothing or equipment along the course of the saphenous nerve is important. Surgical release is rarely indicated, but occasionally excision of a neuroma is necessary.[11]

Sural Nerve

Anatomy

The sural nerve, a purely cutaneous nerve, is derived from the S1 nerve root, which is formed just distal to the popliteal fossa by the medial sural branch of the tibial nerve and the lateral sural branch of the common peroneal nerve. The nerve travels deep between the two heads of the gastrocnemius muscle before becoming subcutaneous in the distal third of the leg. It passes superficially and laterally behind the lateral malleolus to provide sensation to the lateral aspect of the ankle and foot (Fig. 10.2).

Etiology

The sural nerve is most frequently injured at the level of the ankle, usually because of a severe sprain or fracture and typically (1) as it exits through the fascia just above the ankle or (2) behind the lateral malleolus. It can also be injured during ankle arthroscopy and with an avulsion fracture of the base of the fifth metatarsal.[13] The nerve can be injured anywhere along its course because of ill-fitting shoes, boots, or other athletic equipment.

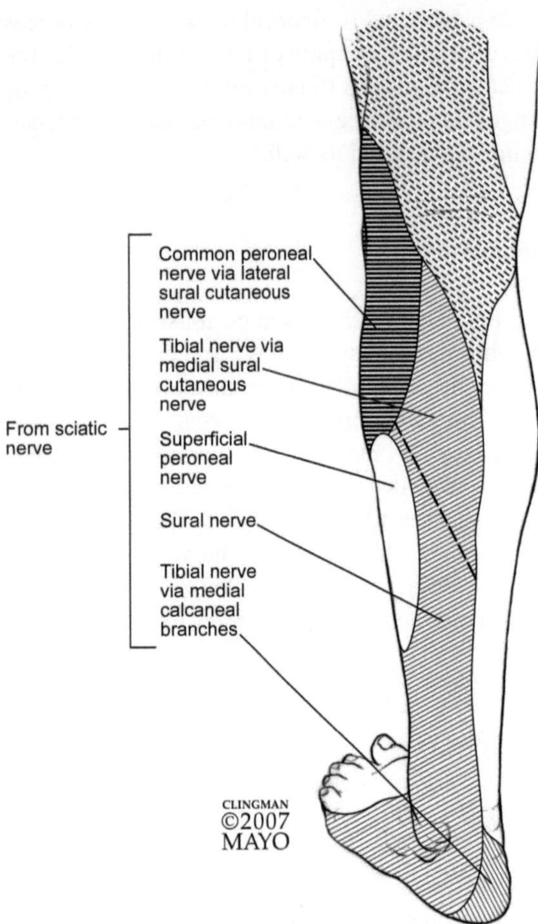

Fig. 10.2 Cutaneous sensory distribution of the sural nerve. Used with permission of Mayo Foundation for Medical Education and Research

Proximally, it may be injured during knee arthroscopy or because of pressure from a Baker's cyst.[14]

Clinical Presentation and Evaluation

Clinically, sural neuropathy usually presents as numbness or pain in the lateral ankle or foot, with or without objective sensory loss on examination. A Tinel sign may be present at the site of compression. Sural NCSs are easy to perform and technically reliable in patients under the age of 60 years, but they only detect neuropathies involving the nerve proximal to the site of recording at the ankle. Side-to-side comparison is helpful when low amplitudes are suspected on the symptomatic side. Other possible causes for lateral foot pain or numbness include S1 radiculopathy, tibial neuropathy, and length-dependent peripheral neuropathy. These causes can be ruled out by careful physical examination and further electrodiagnostic studies including peroneal and tibial motor NCSs and needle examination of L5 and S1 innervated muscles.

Management

Treatment is typically conservative and is directed at removing the source of compression. Symptomatic management of pain is also emphasized. Occasionally, surgery is necessary to relieve entrapment caused by displaced bone fragments or dense scar tissue. Complex regional pain syndrome (or reflex sympathetic dystrophy) can be seen following severe trauma to any peripheral nerve, including sural neuropathy[5]; and in such cases a multifaceted treatment approach is necessary.

Peroneal Nerve

Anatomy

The peroneal nerve is a division of the sciatic nerve, arising from the posterior divisions of the sacral plexus (L4–S2). The sciatic nerve splits at or slightly above the popliteal fossa to form the tibial and common peroneal nerves. The common peroneal nerve then passes laterally and anteriorly over the posterior aspect of the fibular head before winding around the lateral aspect of the fibular neck. At this level, it is superficial and vulnerable to direct external compression. It then runs deep to the proximal part of the peroneus longus muscle (a potential site of entrapment) and divides into its two terminal branches: the superficial and deep peroneal nerves.

The superficial peroneal nerve travels in the lateral compartment of the leg between the peroneus longus and brevis muscles, which it innervates. About 10 cm proximal to the tip of the lateral malleolus it pierces the fascia to become subcutaneous, dividing shortly thereafter into intermediate and medial dorsal cutaneous nerves, which supply sensation to the dorsum of the foot with the exception of the first web space (Fig. 10.3).

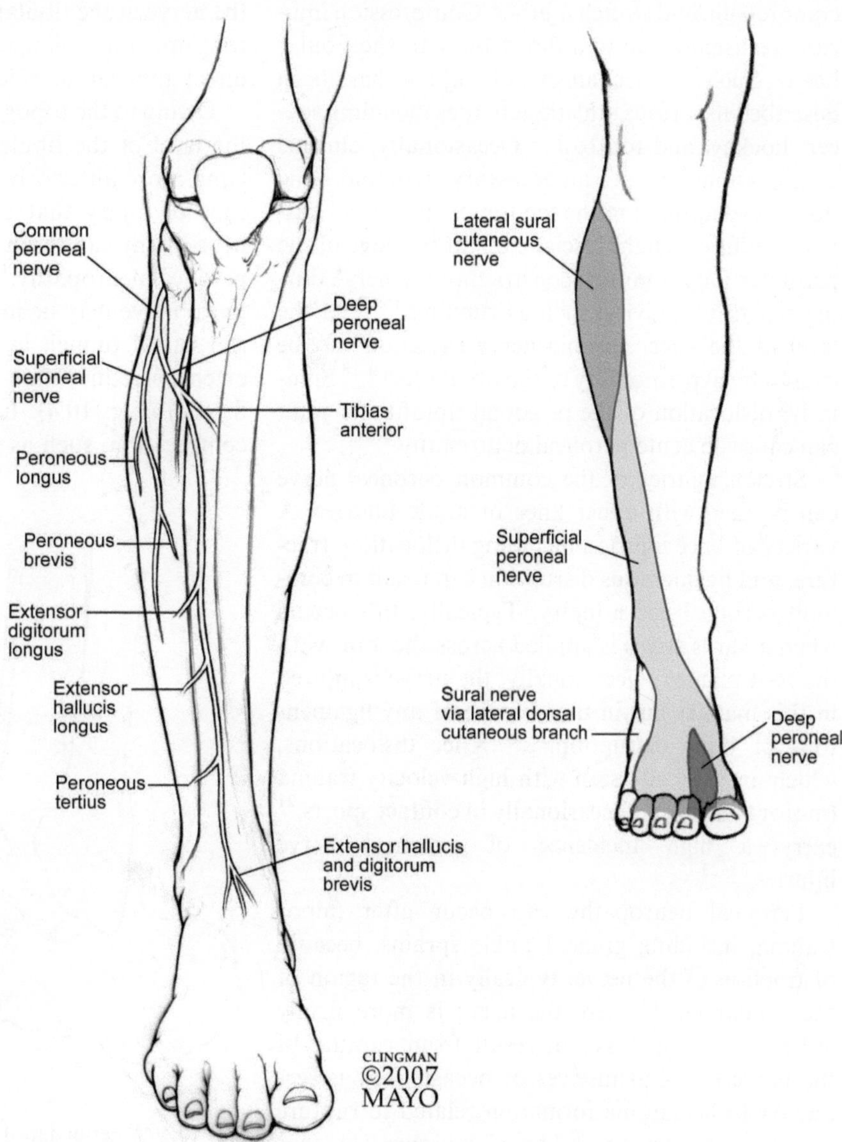

Fig. 10.3 Motor and sensory territory of the peroneal nerve. Used with permission of Mayo Foundation for Medical Education and Research

After leaving the common peroneal nerve, the deep peroneal nerve penetrates the intermuscular septum (between the lateral and anterior compartments). This is a potential site of entrapment. The nerve then enters the anterior compartment, traveling with the anterior tibial artery between the tibialis anterior and extensor hallucis longus (EHL) muscles. It provides innervation to the muscles of the anterior compartment (EHL, tibialis anterior, extensor digitorum longus, and peroneus tertius). Distally, it passes underneath the extensor retinaculum (sometimes referred to as the anterior tarsal tunnel) and innervates the EDB before sending a small cutaneous branch to the first web space (Fig. 10.3).

Etiology

The common peroneal nerve is the most frequently involved nerve in lower limb sport-related injuries.[1] Because of its close proximity to the bone and its superficial course while wrapping around the fibular neck, this nerve is susceptible to both compression and stretch injuries. Compression injuries are usually due to a direct blow to the fibular head. Such a mechanism of injury has been described in various athletic activities including soccer, hockey, and football.[15] Occasionally, chronic compression is due to an accessory sesamoid bone (fabella syndrome) in the tendon of the lateral gastrocnemius or a tight fascial band at the edge of the peroneus longus muscle constricting the nerve during repetitive activity, such as running.[16,17] At the level of the knee, chronic nerve irritation can be caused by hypermobility of the fibular head.[18] Similarly, dislocation of the proximal tibiofibular joint can cause an acute peroneal neuropathy.[16]

Stretch injuries of the common peroneal nerve can be seen with either knee or ankle injuries. A variety of knee injuries, including dislocation, fracture, and ligamentous disruption can result in common peroneal nerve injury. Typically, this occurs when a varus stress is applied across the joint with the foot planted. Occasionally, the nerve is injured in this manner but in the absence of any ligamentous or bony disruption.[19,20] Knee dislocations, which are typically seen with high-velocity trauma (motor sports) and occasionally in contact sports,[21] carry a high incidence of peroneal nerve injuries.[21–23]

Peroneal neuropathy can occur after minor trauma, including grade 1 ankle sprains, because of traction of the nerve, typically in the region of the fibular head where the nerve is more firmly tethered.[24] Axon loss can result from rupture of the nerve fibers themselves or occasionally is secondary to hematoma formation related to rupture of the nutrient arteries.[20] There is a higher incidence of peroneal nerve involvement in high-grade ankle sprains, with one study documenting fibrillation potentials in peroneal innervated muscles in 86% of grade III sprains.[25] Peroneal neuropathy with footdrop has been reported in association with bungee jumping; however, this was in a professional jumper who made more than 2000 jumps over a period of 6 months and was presumably due to repetitive traction from the harness tied around the ankles.[26]

Iatrogenic common peroneal nerve injuries can arise as complications of surgical procedures around the knee, both arthroscopic and open.[27,28] Because of the shallow, subcutaneous location of the nerve at the fibular head, it is highly susceptible to temperature changes, and injury can be caused by direct application of ice in that area.[29]

Owing to the topography of the nerve fascicles at the level of the fibular neck, with the deep fibers lying more anteriorly, many of the same mechanisms of injury that produce a common peroneal neuropathy can result in an isolated proximal deep peroneal neuropathy.[16] More distally, the deep peroneal nerve may be injured at the level of the anterior tarsal tunnel, as it passes under the inferior extensor retinaculum (anterior tarsal tunnel syndrome) (Fig. 10.4). Injury can be due to external compression, such as from tight ski or snowboard

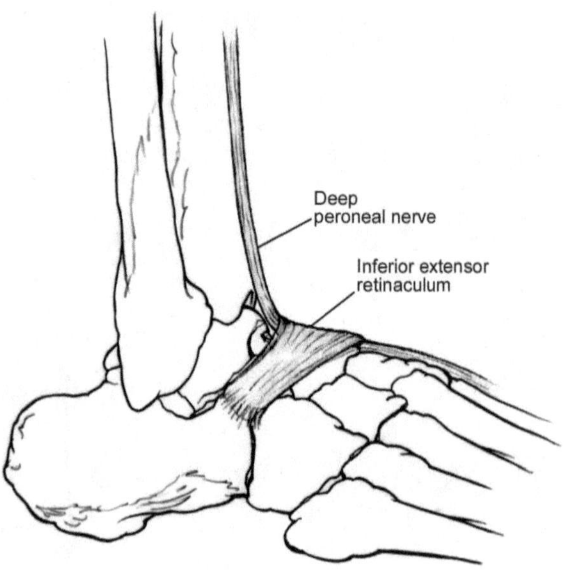

Fig. 10.4 Anterior tarsal tunnel. The deep peroneal nerve passes deep to the inferior extensor retinaculum. Used with permission of Mayo Foundation for Medical Education and Research

boots or shoes,[30,31] repetitive contact with the ball while playing soccer,[5] or repetitive traction of the nerve over the anterior ankle as with ballet dancing that involves excessive plantarflexion.[5] In the foot, intrinsic compression of the deep peroneal nerve can occur as it passes over the talonavicular or metatarsophalangeal (MTP) joints due to osteophytes arising from the tarsal bones or as the nerve passes underneath the extensor hallucis brevis muscle.[5]

The superficial peroneal nerve is rarely injured in isolation proximally but is prone to injury in the distal leg and ankle as it exits the fascia and divides into the medial and intermediate dorsal cutaneous nerves. It is at risk during surgical fixation of ankle fractures[32] as well as during ankle arthroscopy. According to Ferkel et al., more than half the nerve injuries related to ankle arthroscopy involve the superficial peroneal nerve.[9,33] Both the deep and superficial peroneal nerves can be involved in compartment syndromes, which are discussed in more detail later in the chapter.

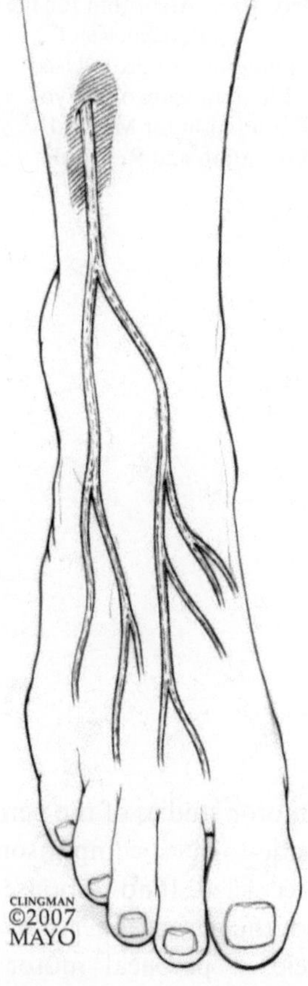

Fig. 10.5 Site of entrapment of the superficial peroneal nerve as it emerges through the fascia proximal to the ankle. Used with permission of Mayo Foundation for Medical Education and Research

Clinical Presentation

With proximal involvement of the deep peroneal nerve, the athlete complains of foot slap or catching of the toes, which tends to be worse when walking barefoot. On physical examination, there is weakness of the ankle dorsiflexors with normal strength of the ankle plantarflexors, hamstrings, and hip abductors. There may be sensory changes in the first web space. When the nerve is entrapped more distally, at the level of the anterior tarsal tunnel or in the foot, there may be atrophy of the EDB muscle (except when that muscle is supplied by an accessory deep peroneal nerve, which passes behind the lateral malleolus), vague pain in the ankle and dorsum of the foot, and burning pain or numbness involving the first web space.[31]

Athletes with proximal superficial peroneal nerve involvement may present with recurrent ankle sprains or ankle instability because of weakness of the ankle evertors and altered sensation/proprioception in the lateral leg or dorsum of the foot. If the superficial peroneal nerve is entrapped where it exits the fascia proximal to the ankle (Fig.10.5), there is numbness over the dorsal ankle and foot (not including the first web space), and there may be a palpable area of fullness or swelling with the Tinel sign at potential muscle herniation sites in the area of the fascial defect.

The differential diagnosis in a patient with peroneal neuropathy should include more proximal nerve involvement (sciatic neuropathy, lumbosacral plexopathy, L5 radiculopathy) as well as acute or exertional compartment syndromes. With an isolated peroneal neuropathy in the absence of inciting trauma or obvious compression, nonathletic causes should be kept in mind, such as inherited neuropathy with a tendency to pressure palsies or painful mononeuritis multiplex.[34] If there is no pain or numbness associated with footdrop, motor neuron disease should also be considered, particularly if the painless weakness progresses to involve other nerves or limbs. A juvenile-inherited form of motor neuron disease is occasionally present in teenagers or young adults. Figure 10.6 gives an algorithmic approach to the differential diagnosis of footdrop.

Evaluation

Electrodiagnostic evaluation of the peroneal nerve can be helpful, for both excluding other potential diagnoses (e.g., sciatic neuropathy, lumbar plexopathy, L5 radiculopathy) and providing prognostic information for the athlete. NCSs should include

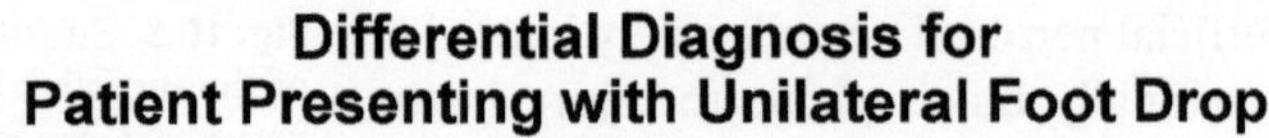

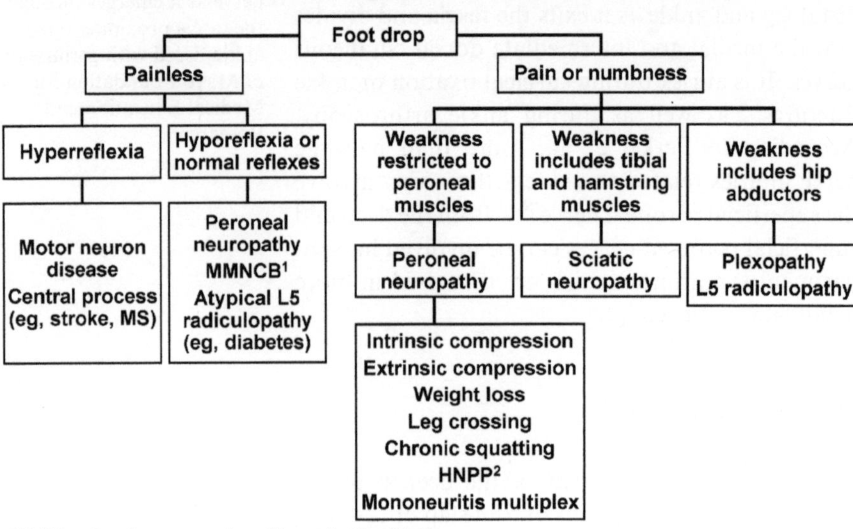

Fig. 10.6 Algorithm for the differential diagnosis of unilateral foot drop. Used with permission of Mayo Foundation for Medical Education and Research

motor studies of the peroneal and tibial nerve, with side-to-side comparison if low amplitudes are recorded. If no response is elicited with stimulation of the peroneal nerve recording over the EDB muscle, a peroneal motor NCS can be performed recording over the tibialis anterior muscle, as this is a more robust response and may be relatively preserved even in the case of severe peroneal neuropathy. It is important to stimulate the peroneal nerve both above and below the fibular head to evaluate for conduction block or focal conduction slowing indicative of focal demyelination. If present, this typically carries a better prognosis, assuming that the cause of compression can be relieved. A superficial peroneal sensory NCS should be performed, as this sense is usually preserved in the setting of L5 radiculopathy but diminished in peroneal neuropathy. The amplitude of the sensory nerve action potential should be compared with the contralateral response because the superficial peroneal sensory response can be low or absent even in young, normal subjects.

Needle examination is essential for evaluating the severity of axonal loss in muscles innervated by the superficial and deep peroneal nerves and excluding a more proximal neuropathic process. L5, non-peroneal-innervated muscles, such as the tibialis posterior or flexor digitorum longus (FDL) muscle, should be examined; if changes are present, it implies that the nerve injury is outside the peroneal distribution. The short head of the biceps femoris can be examined to exclude more proximal peroneal or sciatic neuropathy. Proximal L5 muscles, such as the gluteus medius or tensor fascia lata, are involved in the setting of lumbar plexopathy or radiculopathy; in such cases, the lumbar paraspinals are then examined to differentiate between plexopathy and radiculopathy.

Management

Treatment of peroneal nerve injuries depends on the etiology and severity of the injury. If compression is present, it must be removed. In the case of intrinsic compression related to a tight fascial band, abnormal bony prominence, or perineural cyst, surgical release may be indicated if there is evidence of a conduction block on NCSs, axonal loss on needle electromyography (EMG), or functional impairment related to the neuropathy. In the case of a stretch injury, usually observation is prudent, with surgical intervention typically indicated only in the case of a severe traction injury in which there has been complete or nearly complete disruption of the axons. While awaiting recovery, it is important to protect the nerve-splinting or bracing may be helpful to prevent recurrent ankle sprain with associated traction to the nerve-and to strengthen the involved muscles gradually. Proprioceptive retraining of the ankle muscle groups can be helpful for avoiding repetitive nerve injury related to weak ankle evertors and recurrent ankle sprain.

Tibial Nerve

Anatomy

The tibial nerve is derived from nerve roots L5–S2. It branches off the sciatic nerve at or just above the popliteal fossa. Within the popliteal space, the tibial nerve gives off branches that supply the popliteus, the soleus, both heads of the gastrocnemius, and the plantaris muscles. It then passes under the soleus arch on its way to the deep posterior compartment of the leg. Here it travels in close proximity to the tibia and the posterior tibial artery and innervates the tibialis posterior (PT), FDL, and flexor hallucis longus (FHL) muscles. At the ankle, it enters the tarsal tunnel and divides into the medial calcaneal, medial plantar, and lateral plantar nerves, supplying sensation to the plantar aspect of the foot and innervating the intrinsic foot muscles.

Etiology

The tibial nerve, lying deep in the posterior compartment of the leg, is less vulnerable to injury than the peroneal nerve. At the level of the knee, the tibial nerve may be compressed by space-occupying lesions in the popliteal fossa (e.g., a Baker's cyst), but it is most often injured in association with knee dislocations or severe injuries to the posterior knee capsule. Typically, these injuries are also associated with peroneal nerve and popliteal vascular bundle injury.[35] A complete tibial neuropathy has been reported in an equestrian, secondary to rupture of the popliteus muscle with associated swelling in the popliteal fossa. The equestrian was able to return to sport gradually with conservative management.[36] In the leg, the tibial nerve can be entrapped underneath the fibromuscular arch of the soleus,[5,37] injured in association with fractures of the tibial shaft, or involved in a posterior compartment syndrome. Distal tibial neuropathies are reviewed later in the chapter.

Clinical Presentation

Symptoms related to tibial nerve injury vary depending on the level of the injury. If the nerve is injured at the knee, the athlete develops weakness of the ankle plantarflexors, invertors, toe flexors, and intrinsic foot musculature. Long-standing weakness of the intrinsic foot muscles can lead to clawing of the toes and foot deformity. Burning pain, numbness, or altered sensation may involve the posterior calf (medial sural cutaneous nerve) or lateral aspect of the foot (sural nerve) if the injury occurs above the level at which these nerves branch from the tibial nerve and/or the plantar aspect of the foot (medial and lateral plantar and medial calcaneal nerves). A Tinel sign may be present in the area of nerve injury.

In athletes presenting with weakness of the ankle plantarflexors or sensory disturbance in the sole of the foot, the differential diagnosis includes S1 radiculopathy, sciatic neuropathy, and lumbosacral plexopathy. A more generalized length-dependent peripheral neuropathy, either inherited or acquired, may start with unilateral symptoms; and it can usually be differentiated from a tibial neuropathy based on the NCSs. In the case of an isolated tibial neuropathy, it is important to consider nonathletic causes of nerve injury such as an inflammatory process causing mononeuritis multiplex.[34]

Evaluation

Electrodiagnostic evaluation of the tibial nerve can be used for localization and grading the severity. The NCSs should include tibial and personal motor studies with side-to-side comparison if an abnormality is found. Sensory studies should include the sural response-which comes off the tibial nerve just below the popliteal fossa and is typically the most robust sensory response in the lower limb-in addition to a medial plantar sensory study. The latter is more sensitive for early length-dependent peripheral neuropathy but may be absent in normal adults over the age of 55 years.

The needle examination should include tibial innervated muscles, such as the gastrocnemius, soleus, PT, FDL, and intrinsic foot muscles. If abnormalities are found within a tibial nerve distribution, peroneal innervated muscles should be examined to evaluate for a more generalized peripheral neuropathy, and proximal sciatic innervated muscles (e.g., hamstrings) should be examined to exclude a sciatic neuropathy. The gluteus maximus and sacral paraspinal muscles should be examined to exclude a sacral plexopathy and an S1 radiculopathy, respectively.

Treatment

Treatment of tibial neuropathy depends on the cause of the injury. In the case of nerve laceration, immediate exploration and repair may be indicated. With entrapment, relief of the compression should be achieved, which may require surgical intervention in the case of intrinsic compression. Traction injuries are usually best managed conservatively-with observation, protection of the ankle joint, maintenance of flexibility (heel cord stretching is important to avoid biomechanical overuse problems as the athlete recovers and returns to activity), ankle proprioceptive retraining, and calf and intrinsic foot muscle strengthening.

If there is significant weakness of the gastrosoleus muscle group, an ankle foot orthosis may be helpful to assist with the pushoff phase of gait and to help stabilize the ankle. Clawing of the toes can lead to skin breakdown, particularly if the foot is insensate from the nerve injury. Prescription footwear or a custom foot orthosis may be necessary.

If pain is a significant problem, it can be treated with neuropathic pain medication, such as tricyclic antidepressants or membrane-stabilizing agents such as gabapentin. Topical neuropathic pain medications can be helpful but must be applied several times per day, and they have to be custom-made by a pharmacist; for example, a compound containing amitriptyline, gabapentin, and ketamine can be used.

Neuropathies in the Region of the Foot and Ankle

Anatomy

Sensory symptoms in the ankle or foot can be related to entrapment of multiple nerves: the tibial nerve or one of its three major branches (medial calcaneal, medial plantar, lateral plantar); the interdigital nerves; or the dorsal cutaneous branches of the peroneal and sural nerves.

At the ankle, the tibial nerve passes behind the medial malleolus underneath the flexor retinaculum, accompanied by the posterior tibial vascular axis and the tendons of the deep compartment muscles (PT, FDL, FHL), to form the contents of the tarsal tunnel. The tarsal tunnel components are arranged in the following order from medial to lateral: PT tendon, FDL tendon, PT artery, PT vein, PT nerve, and FHL tendon (the latter being the most laterally situated structure (Fig. 10.7).

Within the tarsal tunnel at the level of the medial malleolus, the tibial nerve divides into three branches: medial calcaneal, medial plantar, and lateral plantar nerves. These nerves provide sensory innervation to the sole of the foot (Fig. 10.8) and motor innervation to the intrinsic foot muscles. Sensation to the dorsum of the foot is provided by medial, intermediate, and lateral dorsal cutaneous nerves; the latter is the terminal branch of the sural nerve and the former are terminal branches of the superficial peroneal nerve.

The medial calcaneal nerve passes between the deep fascia of the abductor hallucis muscle and the medial aspect of the anterior calcaneus to supply sensory innervation to the skin of the medial heel. The medial plantar nerve supplies sensation to the medial aspect of the sole of the foot and the plantar surface of the first 3 ½ toes. It supplies motor innervation to the abductor hallucis, flexor hallucis brevis, flexor digitorum brevis, and the most medial lumbrical muscle. The lateral plantar nerve gives off the first branch of the lateral plantar nerve (FBLPN) behind the medial malleolus before passing under the abductor hallucis muscle and between the flexor digitorum brevis and quadratus plantae muscles, which provides sensation to the lateral sole of the foot, the plantar aspect of the fifth toe, and the lateral half of the fourth toe. The lateral plantar nerve innervates the flexor digiti minimi, adductor hallucis, quadratus plantae, remaining three lumbrical, and all of the interosseous muscles.

The FBLPN (also known as the inferior calcaneal nerve, Baxter's nerve, or the nerve to the abductor digiti quinti) penetrates the abductor hallucis fascia and then passes inferiorly between the

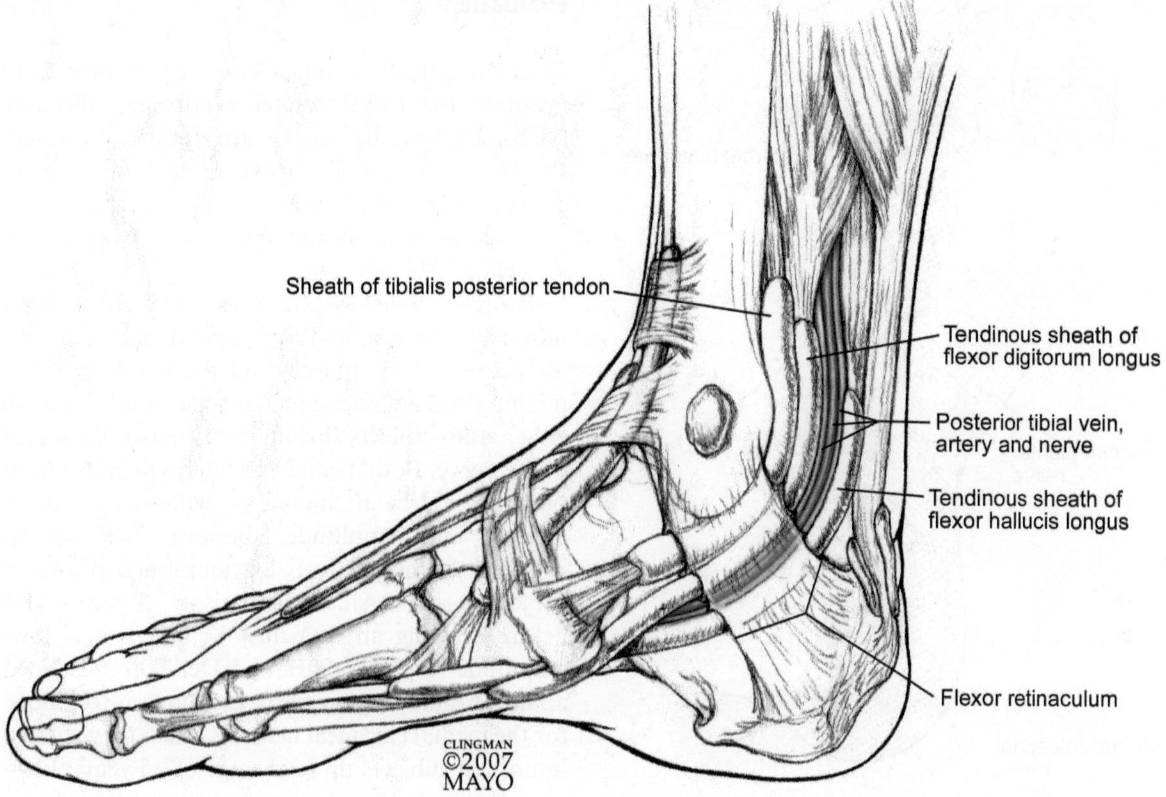

Fig. 10.7 Contents of the tarsal tunnel. Used with permission of Mayo Foundation for Medical Education and Research

abductor hallucis medially and the quadratus plantae muscle laterally. The nerve turns abruptly, passing toward the lateral foot between the flexor digitorum brevis inferiorly and quadratus plantae superiorly to divide into terminal branches supplying the abductor digiti minimi, the flexor digitorum brevis, and the medial calcaneal periosteum.[38] It does not provide any cutaneous sensory innervation.

Tarsal Tunnel Syndrome

Etiology

A number of etiologic factors have been implicated in tarsal tunnel syndrome, most often space-occupying lesions such as accessory calf muscles,[39,40] ganglion cysts,[41,42] tumors, or bone fragments.[43] The nerve can also be irritated by tenosynovitis of any of the tendons traversing the tunnel or by external compression from tight equipment or footwear (e.g., ski boots).[41,44] Fibrosis within the tarsal tunnel secondary to recurrent ankle sprains has also been described as an etiology.[15] Abnormal foot or ankle biomechanics, such as overpronation with running, are thought to result in repetitive stretching of the tibial nerve, making it more susceptible to injury in the region of the tarsal tunnel.[6,45]

Clinical Presentation

If compression occurs at the level of the tarsal tunnel, there can be involvement of the main tibial nerve or any of its three terminal branches. Patients often present with pain or aching in the region of the medial malleolus or more distally in the arch or the sole of the foot. The pain may be burning, stabbing, or throbbing and is usually

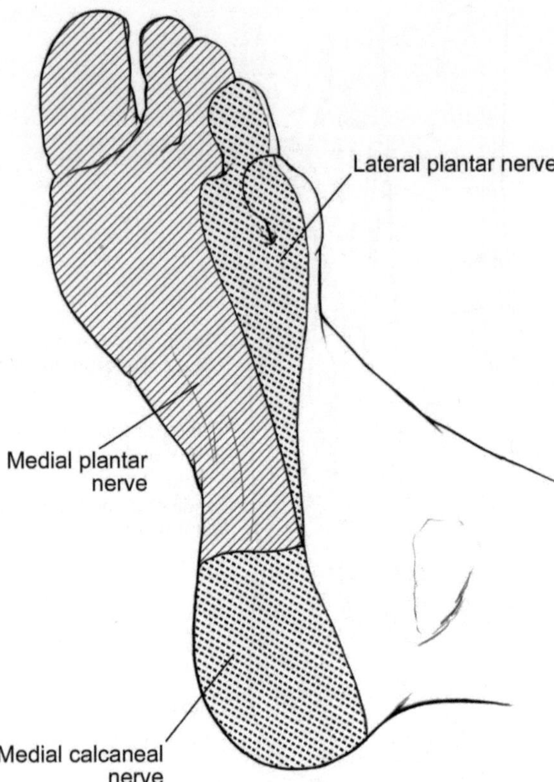

Fig. 10.8 Cutaneous innervation of the plantar foot. Used with permission of Mayo Foundation for Medical Education and Research

worse at night, particularly after excessive weight bearing or repetitive activity involving the ankle. Tarsal tunnel syndrome pain tends to be better first thing in the morning (helping to differentiate it from plantar fasciitis).[41] There may be numbness or burning paresthesias as well as decreased sensation at the sole of the foot and a Tinel sign over the tarsal tunnel. Typically, tarsal tunnel syndrome does not cause muscle atrophy or weakness of the intrinsic foot muscles, although with severe or prolonged nerve compression it is possible.

Tarsal tunnel syndrome causing neuropathy is rare; thus, other musculoskeletal causes of foot and ankle pain should be investigated. Plantar fasciitis, calcaneal fat pad atrophy, calcaneal or navicular stress fracture, osteochondritis of the talus, sinus tarsi syndrome, synovial impingement, and tenosynovitis are some of the conditions that may present with foot or ankle pain.

Evaluation

Electrodiagnostic studies can be performed to evaluate for tarsal tunnel syndrome, although NCSs and needle EMG are rarely abnormal. Electrophysiologically proven tarsal tunnel syndrome is most often seen when the symptoms are due to a space-occupying lesion within the tunnel.[35]

If tarsal tunnel syndrome is suspected, a tibial motor response should be recorded from both the abductor hallucis muscle and the abductor digiti minimi pedis muscle; a prolonged distal latency on either study reflects slowing in the most distal part of the nerve. Both medial and lateral plantar mixed NCSs should be attempted to evaluate both distal latency and amplitude. Because the normal response can be relatively low amplitude in normal subjects, side-to-side comparison is important before drawing any conclusions based on a low-amplitude response. Park and Del Toro described an antidromic sensory nerve conduction technique for the medial calcaneal nerve,[42] which they studied in normal subjects up to the age of 45 years; however, this technique does not appear to be in common clinical use at this time.

Needle examination should include intrinsic foot muscles (e.g., abductor hallucis, abductor digiti minimi pedis, first dorsal interosseous muscles). If abnormalities are found, more extensive proximal needle examination should be performed, as outlined earlier for the evaluation of tibial neuropathies. Evaluation of the contralateral intrinsic foot muscles can also be helpful, because it may be difficult for the patient to activate motor unit potentials voluntarily, and some increase in spontaneous activity can be seen in these muscles in normal subjects, presumably due to direct muscle or nerve terminal trauma from daily activities.[46]

Treatment

Conservative management of tarsal tunnel syndrome involves relative rest (which may include use of a short leg cast or ankle foot orthosis), nonsteroidal antiinflammatory drugs (NSAIDs), improved arch support/correction of overpronation, and local anesthetic/steroid injection. Often therapeutic exercise to improve hip abductor strengthening and mitigate overpronation can be a helpful treatment of tarsal tunnel syndrome in runners. However, surgical release of the entrapment may be necessary to allow athletes to return to their former level of function, particularly in the setting of a space-occupying lesion.

Medial Plantar Nerve

A number of entrapment neuropathies in the foot have been described, particularly in runners. Entrapment of the medial plantar nerve has been termed *jogger's foot*, with compression of the nerve occurring between the abductor hallucis muscle and the overlying navicular bone, likely related to overpronation.[45] Patients may present with achy pain in the arch or burning pain in the medial heel and are often misdiagnosed as having plantar fasciitis. On examination, there is tenderness and possibly a Tinel sign just posterior to the navicular tuberosity, and there may be numbness in the medial plantar aspect of the foot. Flexion of the toes against resistance should not induce pain and can be helpful for differentiating entrapment from tenosynovitis. Injection with local anesthetic can confirm the diagnosis, and treatment consists of antiinflammatory medication, avoidance of rigid high-arched orthotics, modification of running technique to correct overpronation, and occasionally surgical release.[5]

Medial Calcaneal Nerve

Compression of the anterior branch of the medial calcaneal nerve has been reported in runners and soccer players, with entrapment typically occurring between the abductor hallucis muscle and the medial aspect of the calcaneus, resulting in chronic heel pain.[47] These symptoms are often attributed to plantar fasciitis, but careful clinical examination demonstrates maximum tenderness over the medial anterior heel pad and the abductor hallucis muscle, rather than the plantar fascia. Pressure over the nerve can often reproduce pain.[47] Numbness, if present, is noted in the plantar aspect of the heel. Conservative therapy is similar to that for medial plantar neuropathy. Failing that, surgical decompression, with release of the abductor hallucis fascia, may allow the athlete to return to sports.[47]

Lateral Plantar Nerve

Isolated entrapment of the lateral plantar nerve is rare; however, entrapment of the FBLPN is more common, particularly in runners.[38] There are several potential sites of entrapment, but the most common is probably as the nerve changes direction deep to the abductor hallucis muscle (Fig. 10.9), particularly if this muscle is hypertrophied, which may occur in runners.[16,38] The nerve can also be impinged by calcaneal spurs as it courses laterally, immediately anterior to the calcaneus.[48] Entrapment of the FBLPN is thought to occur in 10%–15% of cases of chronic plantar fasciitis[5,38] owing to proximal edema of the flexor digitorum brevis muscle and edema of the plantar fascia. Entrapment of the FBLPN by scar tissue has also been reported in a gymnast after sustaining a minor injury followed by repetitive trauma to the heel.[49]

Patients usually complain of vague burning pain in the medial heel with occasional radiation into the lateral aspect of the foot.[49,50] Tenderness to palpation is most pronounced at the medial heel, superior to the plantar fascia origin, although there may be mild tenderness over the plantar fascia origin. There should be no sensory deficit present. Treatment involves relative rest, footwear modification with additional cushioning of the heel, stretching of the Achilles tendon and plantar fascia, NSAIDs, and corticosteroid injection. If surgical intervention is necessary, removal of a calcaneal spur or release of the plantar fascia may be required, in addition to release of the abductor hallucis fascia to decompress the nerve adequately.[6,41]

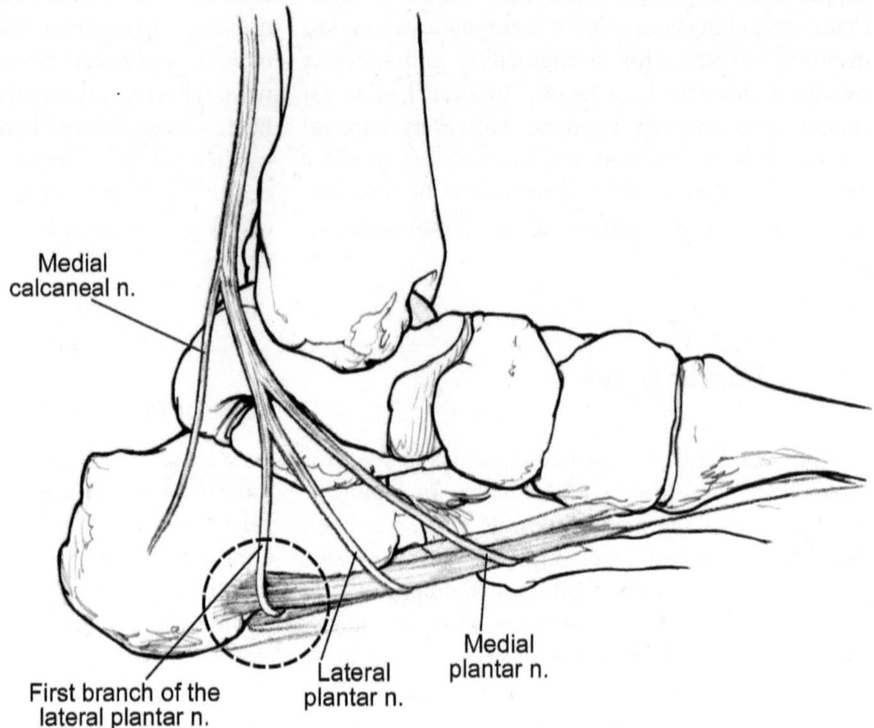

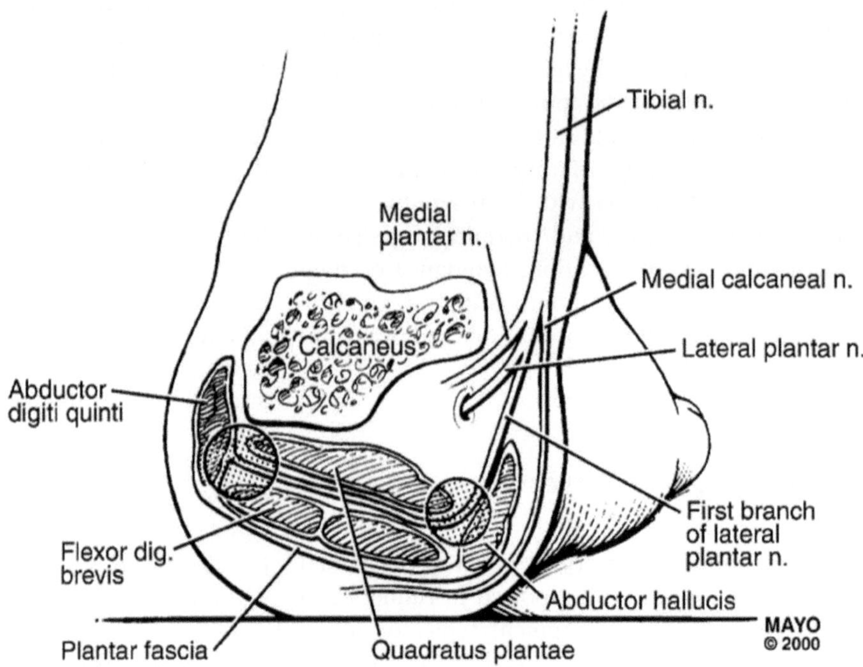

Fig. 10.9 Site of entrapment of the first branch of the lateral plantar nerve as it changes abruptly from an inferior to lateral direction between the abductor hallucis and quadratus plantae muscles. Used with permission of Mayo Foundation for Medical Education and Research

Interdigital Neuroma

Anatomy

The interdigital nerves are implicated in the most common entrapment neuropathy in the foot, commonly referred to as *Morton's neuroma.*[51] The interdigital nerves are terminal branches of the medial and lateral plantar nerves. Most often it is the interdigital nerve within the second or third web space that is involved with these neuromas (Fig. 10.10).

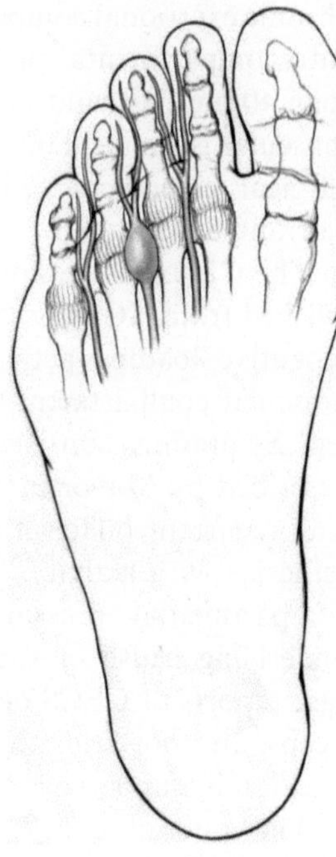

Fig. 10.10 The most common site of an interdigital neuroma is shown at the third web space between the third and fourth metatarsal heads. Used with permission of Mayo Foundation for Medical Education and Research

Etiology

The underlying pathophysiology is thought to be recurrent impingement of the interdigital nerve underneath the intermetatarsal ligament, resulting in a compressive neuropathy. Overpronation or hypermobility of the fourth metatarsal and the wearing of nonphysiologic shoes with pointy toes or high heels are potential predisposing factors.[52,53] Occasionally, the symptoms start after an acute dorsiflexion injury to the MTP joints. In runners, second MTP joint synovitis can develop related to localized capsular swelling and subsequently crowds the interdigital nerve. Over time, characteristic pathologic changes develop within the nerve, including demyelination, juxtaneural and intraneural fibrosis, and fibrinoid degeneration.[5,52]

Transient paresthesia due to repetitive compression of the interdigital nerves has been reported in military recruits and with the use of exercise equipment, such as stair-stepper machines. Symptoms typically resolve after discontinuing the provocative activity.[5] Because it has not yet been determined whether such transient symptoms predispose to the development of a neuroma, it seems prudent to counsel the athlete to use appropriate footwear, with adequate width of the toe box and good cushioning, and to cross-train to avoid prolonged symptoms during provocative activities.

Clinical Presentation

Athletes with an interdigital neuroma usually present with pain in the plantar aspect of the foot either in the metatarsal area or radiating into the involved toes. Typically, they can point to the site of the pain with one finger. Symptoms may be worse first thing in the morning and are provoked during the pushoff phase of gait or with activities that involve pressure on the ball of the foot (e.g, ballet) as the nerve is stretched over the distal edge of the intermetatarsal ligament. Shearing or torsional stress to the metatarsals (e.g., when walking on uneven terrain) can be quite provocative. Symptoms are usually relieved by rest and sometimes just by removing the offending shoe.[50]

On examination, there may be a Tinel sign and tenderness to palpation on the plantar aspect of the foot between the metatarsals. With compression of the metatarsal heads with one hand and simultaneous compression of the web space using the thumb and forefinger of the other hand, the patient's pain is reproduced, and the examiner often feels a *Mulder's click* as the neuroma is squeezed between the two metatarsals (squeeze test).[52] There may be decreased sensation to pinprick in the two involved toes. For example, with a neuroma in the third web space, there would be hypesthesia along the lateral aspect of the third toe and the medial aspect of the fourth toe.

The differential diagnosis for interdigital neuroma includes more proximal nerve entrapment, including tarsal tunnel syndrome, peripheral neuropathy, lumbosacral radiculopathy, metatarsalgia, subluxation or synovitis of the MTP joint, metatarsal stress fracture, Freiberg's infarction, and soft tissue or bony tumor of the forefoot.

Evaluation

The value of electrodiagnostic studies in the diagnosis of interdigital neuroma lies solely in ruling out more proximal causes of nerve entrapment, as a reliable NCS for the interdigital nerves is not currently available. High-resolution ultrasonography or MRI can demonstrate the neuroma, although typically clinical evaluation and response to diagnostic local anesthetic injection are sufficient to make a confident diagnosis.

Treatment

Conservative treatment of an interdigital neuroma includes eliminating provocative footwear and using a shoe with good cushioning, a wide toe box, and a low heel. Use of a metatarsal pad and infiltration of local anesthetic and steroid (usually performed from a dorsal approach into the involved web space) can help manage symptoms. Repeat injection is not recommended.[50] In the case of failed conservative treatment, surgical success rates of 80% or greater have been reported.[54] The recommended surgical approach is a dorsal incision (to avoid painful scar formation on the sole of the foot) with partial resection of the intermetatarsal ligament and resection of the nerve, allowing the proximal portion to retract up into the soft tissues of the mid-foot.

Compartment Syndromes

Compartment syndromes can be acute or chronic exertional varieties. An increase in the intracompartmental pressure is the common theme between these two entities; however, the pathophysiology, symptoms, and management differ. A separate discussion of compartment syndromes is provided in a subsequent chapter.

Although acute compartment syndrome (ACS) has been reported in athletes in the absence of trauma,[55] it typically occurs after severe trauma to the involved extremity, with or without bone fracture. A space-occupying lesion (e.g., muscle edema, hematoma) develops within a confined space, creating an acute rise in the compartment pressure and impeding the vascular supply. The resulting neuromuscular ischemia causes more edema and hence more ischemia. The pain starts out dull but rapidly becomes excruciating, increasing with passive stretch of the involved muscles. The symptoms do not respond to rest or elevation as is the case with chronic exertional compartment syndrome (CECS). Intracompartmental pressures are typically higher than 40 mm Hg, and the risk of permanent neuromuscular ischemic damage is such that this is a true surgical emergency, with immediate fasciotomy warranted.[56]

The CECS is a condition that should be distinguished from ACS and occurs in athletes following repetitive loading activities. It can occur in any muscular compartment but is most common in the leg. Symptoms consistent with CECS were first described by Mavor in 1956 in a patient experiencing recurrent bilateral anterior leg pain and paresthesias with activity.[57] In 1975, increased intracompartmental pressure was identified as the underlying cause of such symptoms.[58] There are case reports of CECS occurring in the arms, quadriceps, and posterior thigh; but the most common location by far is the leg compartments.

The anterior compartment is most commonly affected[59,60]; this compartment contains the tibialis anterior, EHL, extensor digitorum longus, and peroneus tertius muscles, all of which receive innervation from the deep peroneal nerve. The deep posterior compartment is also frequently involved in CECS; it contains the PT, FDL, and FHL muscles, which are innervated by the tibial nerve.[61] The lateral and superficial posterior compartments are less commonly involved in CECS.[62,63]

This syndrome (CECS) is more common than many people think. One study reported a prevalence of 14% in athletes complaining of leg pain.[64] Symptoms are often bilateral in young athletes and are equally prevalent in males and females. A sudden increase in training intensity increases the risk of developing CECS. With exercise, muscle volume can increase by 20%,[56] and when this occurs in a compartment with tight, unyielding fascial boundaries the pressure inside would be expected to rise. Another possible explanation for the rise in pressure is the mechanical damage theory. Exercise is well known to cause myofibrillar damage and release of protein-bound ions. According to that theory, excessive release of ions during periods of exercise can result in high osmotic pressure, drawing water into the muscle and increasing intracompartmental pressure. It is generally agreed that the elevated pressure impedes the vascular supply to the muscle, creating neuromuscular ischemia and pain.[65] However, a study using a radioisotope to measure muscular blood flow did not find any difference between symptomatic and normal athletes[66]; thus, the etiology of CECS has yet to be definitively identified.

Athletes with CECS usually complain of tightness, cramping, or burning in the affected compartment. The discomfort is usually bilateral, typically begins at a predictable time during exercise, and is relieved by rest.[58,60,67] The pain may be accompanied by paresthesias or weakness in the distribution of the affected nerve. Physical examination when the patient is at rest is often normal but reveals a muscle hernia in the affected compartment in 20%–60% of patients.[68] Physical examination performed immediately after exercise reveals compartment fullness and tenderness to palpation over the affected muscles (in contrast to the periosteal tenderness seen with stress reactions). The neurovascular examination is typically normal; in fact, any abnormal physical findings warrant a workup to rule out vascular or neurologic causes.

The differential diagnosis of CECS is wide and includes vascular, neurologic, and musculoskeletal causes of leg pain.[67] Problems to be ruled out before assigning a diagnosis of CECS include medial tibial stress syndrome, stress fractures, tenosynovitis, radiculopathy, neurogenic claudication, peripheral nerve entrapment, arterial insufficiency from various etiologies, deep venous thrombosis, infection, and tumors. Diagnostic tests such as plain radiography, bone scans, lower extremity or spine MRI, and Doppler ultrasonography should be considered to help exclude other diagnoses.

The gold standard test for diagnosing CECS is intracompartmental pressure testing. The measurement is obtained by placing a large-bore needle or a wick catheter in the compartment and connecting it to a pressure monitor; such pressure measuring kits are commercially available. During testing, the needle positioning, depth of penetration, and the knee and ankle positions should be controlled. Measurement of the deep posterior compartment is technically more difficult because of the anatomic location of the compartment.

Multiple authors have suggested various diagnostic criteria.[59,69,70] The most widely accepted method is to measure the compartment pressure at rest, exercise the patient until the symptoms appear, and repeat the measurements at 1 and 5 minutes after exercise.[68] The normal resting pressure in asymptomatic subjects is 5–10 mm Hg. Diagnostic criteria for CECS are (1) resting pressure $\geq$15 mm Hg; (2) a 1-minute post-exercise pressure >30 mm Hg; and (3) a 5-minute post-exercise pressure $\geq$ 20 mm Hg. Not all of these criteria are necessary to make the diagnosis of CECS, but the diagnostic confidence increases as more of these criteria are fulfilled.

Other methods for diagnosing CECS have been proposed recently. In a study by Hayes et al., single-photon emission computed thallium chloride scintigraphy was able to identify increased pressure and reversible areas of ischemia in a compartment.[71] Although this could potentially be a sensitive diagnostic tool, more studies on a larger scale are needed. Another study, using pre- and post-exercise NCSs, showed loss of the normal post-exercise amplitude potentiation effect in patients with CECS.[72] Such methods, although innovative, have yet to replace the pressure monitoring technique.

Once CECS is diagnosed, conservative treatment should be attempted initially. Relative rest, with cross-training to maintain fitness (e.g., cycling, swimming, water-jogging) should initially be prescribed followed by a gradual return to the provocative activity, with initiation of intensive stretching of the involved muscles prior to exercise. Changes in footwear and running surface may be of benefit.[59] Unfortunately, such conservative measures often fail to alleviate the symptoms once normal activity is resumed[59,70]; so if the athlete wishes to continue the provocative activity, surgical intervention is necessary. Therefore, it is imperative that the diagnosis be carefully confirmed before proceeding to fasciotomy or fasciectomy.

Decompressive fasciotomy is the surgery of choice, and success with such a procedure has been reported in the range of 75%–90% of cases.[59,70,73] Multiple techniques have been described to perform the fasciotomies; newer techniques focus on small skin incisions providing adequate fascial release.[74,75] Special care should be taken to ensure full release of the fascia and avoid injuries to the superficial peroneal nerve as it pierces the anterior muscular septum.[51] Posterior compartment fasciotomies have a lower success rate for reasons that are not totally clear.[61] If fasciotomy fails to relieve the symptoms, the differential diagnosis should be revisited and non-CECS-related causes again excluded. Failure to decompress the affected compartment fully or to identify the appropriate compartment for decompression are other potential causes for surgical failure.[51]

Following surgery, partial weight bearing is initiated within the first week; early mobilization to minimize scarring is advocated by many surgeons.[76,77] Activity is then gradually progressed over the next 2–3 weeks and may include isokinetic muscle strengthening, stationary cycling, and swimming. Running is usually introduced around 6 weeks. The goal is a return to full activity at about 12 weeks.

Conclusion

Although nerve injury in the leg is relatively rare in athletes, it can have a major impact on the athlete's ability to participate, particularly if not recognized early before significant axon loss has occurred. Nerve injury can be related to a wide variety of causes, but in athletes the most common mechanisms of injury are compression or traction. Both acute and exertional compartment syndrome can be associated with nerve injury. It is important to rule out more proximal causes of nerve entrapment and to exclude more common musculoskeletal conditions that may present similarly. In conjunction with a detailed history and careful neurologic examination, electrodiagnostic evaluation is often helpful for localizing the level of nerve involvement and providing prognostic information on the degree and temporal profile of recovery. Treatment is generally conservative, but surgical intervention to relieve compression or salvage the nerve is occasionally necessary.

Case Study

History

A 25 year-old elite female soccer player presented with a 2-month history of deep aching pain in the anterolateral right leg that would occur at about 20 minutes into an intense training session or when running. She complained of a sense of tightness in the anterior leg when the symptoms were present. If she stopped and walked, the symptoms would be relieved, only to recur fairly quickly if she tried to run again. If she attempted to run through the pain, she was unable to continue the activity, as she would develop numbness of the foot, catch her toes, and trip. Past medical history was notable for prior fracture of the right tibia and fibula, which was treated operatively with intramedullary rodding of the tibia when the woman was age 21 years.

Physical Examination

Physical examination revealed a fit, muscular, healthy-appearing woman. Lumbar spine motion was full and pain-free, including with quadrant loading. Neurologic examination was normal at baseline, but after she ran for 20 minutes repeat evaluation showed weakness of the ankle dorsiflexors, evertors, and toe extensors, with decreased sensation to pinprick over the dorsum of the foot. There was mild tenderness to palpation over the lateral compartment of the leg; percussion and palpation over the tibia and anterior compartment was not provocative. Percussion over the proximal fibula was painful, with tingling reproduced in the dorsum of the foot, and this finding was much more pronounced after running for 20 minutes.

Differential Diagnosis

Differential diagnosis included exertional compartment syndrome, peroneal neuropathy, L5 radiculopathy, fibular stress fracture, and tibial stress syndrome.

Diagnostic Studies

Her bone scan was negative for tibial stress syndrome or stress fracture. MRI of the lumbar spine showed mild spondylotic changes, without significant neural foraminal narrowing. Compartment pressure measurements before and after 20 minutes of running were normal. NCSs (peroneal and tibial motor studies, superficial peroneal and sural sensory studies) were normal at baseline. Needle examination (tibialis anterior, peroneus longus, medial gastrocnemius, tibialis posterior, tensor fascia lata muscles) showed some long-duration motor unit potentials in the tibialis anterior and peroneus longus muscles, without fibrillation potentials. After the patient had run for 20 minutes and was markedly symptomatic, the peroneal motor NCS was rechecked, and a conduction block of 50% with slowing of conduction velocity across the fibular head was noted.

Diagnosis

Common peroneal neuropathy with conduction block across the fibular head was the diagnosis.

Management and Outcome

Because of an inability to participate at an elite level and lack of an obvious cause of extrinsic compression, the athlete underwent exploratory surgery. The peroneal nerve was seen to be compressed as it wound around the fibular neck and passed underneath the musculotendinous attachments of the peroneus longus (Fig. 10.11). Successful neurolysis was achieved by releasing the fascial attachments. A gradual rehabilitation program was initiated 2 weeks postoperatively, emphasizing ankle proprioception; and she was able to return to full participation 4 weeks after surgery.

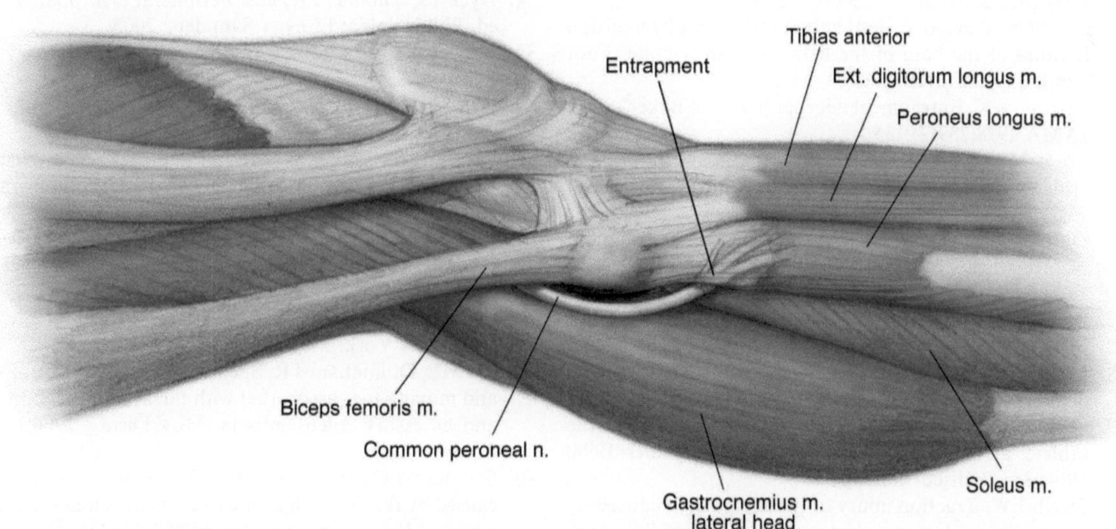

Fig. 10.11 Entrapment of the common peroneal nerve as it winds around the fibular neck and passes underneath the tendinous edge of the peroneus longus muscle. Used with permission of Mayo Foundation for Medical Education and Research

References

1. Krivickas LS, Wilbourn AJ. Peripheral nerve injuries in athletes: a case series of over 200 injuries. Semin Neurol 2000;20(2):225–32.
2. Hirasawa Y, Sakakida K. Sports and peripheral nerve injury. Am J Sports Med 1983;11(6):420–6.
3. Kimura J. Electrodiagnosis in Diseases of Nerve and Muscle: Principles and Practice. 2nd ed. Philadelphia: Davis; 1989.
4. Daube JR. Clinical Neurophysiology. 2nd ed. New York: Oxford University Press; 2002.

5. Schon LC. Nerve entrapment, neuropathy, and nerve dysfunction in athletes. Orthop Clin North Am 1994;25(1):47–59.
6. Gleeson AP, Kerr JG. Patella dislocation neurapraxia: a report of two cases. Injury 1996;27(7):519–20.
7. Fabian RH, Norcross KA, Hancock MB. Surfer's neuropathy. N Engl J Med 1987;316(9):555.
8. Hemler DE, Ward WK, Karstetter KW, et al. Saphenous nerve entrapment caused by pes anserine bursitis mimicking stress fracture of the tibia. Arch Phys Med Rehabil 1991;72(5):336–7.
9. Ferkel RD, Heath DD, Guhl JF. Neurological complications of ankle arthroscopy. Arthroscopy 1996;12(2):200–8.
10. Logue EJ 3rd, Drez D Jr. Dermatitis complicating saphenous nerve injury after arthroscopic debridement of a medial meniscal cyst. Arthroscopy 1996;12(2):228–31.
11. Worth RM, Kettelkamp DB, Defalque RJ, et al. Saphenous nerve entrapment: a cause of medial knee pain. Am J Sports Med 1984;12(1):80–1.
12. Iizuka M, Yao R, Wainapel S. Saphenous nerve injury following medial knee joint injection: a case report. Arch Phys Med Rehabil 2005;86(10):2062–5.
13. Gould N, Trevino S. Sural nerve entrapment by avulsion fracture of the base of the fifth metatarsal bone. Foot Ankle 1981;2(3):153–5.
14. Nakano KK. Entrapment neuropathy from Baker's cyst. JAMA 1978;239(2):135.
15. Lorei MP, Hershman EB. Peripheral nerve injuries in athletes: treatment and prevention. Sports Med 1993; 16(2):130–47.
16. Dawson DM, Hallett M, Wilbourn AJ, eds. Entrapment Neuropathies. 3rd ed. Philadelphia: Lippincott-Raven; 1999.
17. Leach RE, Purnell MB, Saito A. Peroneal nerve entrapment in runners. Am J Sports Med 1989;17(2):287–91.
18. Moller BN, Kadin S. Entrapment of the common peroneal nerve. Am J Sports Med 1987;15(1):90–1.
19. Seckler MM, DiStefano V. Peroneal nerve palsy in the athlete: a result of indirect trauma. Orthopedics 1996; 19(4):345–7; discussion 7–8.
20. Streib EW. Traction injury of peroneal nerve caused by minor athletic trauma: electromyographic studies. Arch Neurol 1983;40(1):62–3.
21. Wascher DC, Dvirnak PC, DeCoster TA. Knee dislocation: initial assessment and implications for treatment. J Orthop Trauma 1997;11(7):525–9.
22. Malizos KN, Xenakis T, Mavrodontidis AN, et al. Knee dislocations and their management: a report of 16 cases. Acta Orthop Scand Suppl 1997;275:80–3.
23. Montgomery TJ, Savoie FH, White JL, et al. Orthopedic management of knee dislocations: comparison of surgical reconstruction and immobilization. Am J Knee Surg 1995;8(3):97–103.
24. Meals RA. Peroneal-nerve palsy complicating ankle sprain: report of two cases and review of the literature. J Bone Joint Surg Am 1977;59(7):966–8.
25. Nitz AJ, Dobner JJ, Kersey D. Nerve injury and grades II and III ankle sprains. Am J Sports Med 1985;13(3):177–82.
26. Torre PR, Williams GG, Blackwell T, et al. Bungee jumper's foot drop peroneal nerve palsy caused by bungee cord jumping. Ann Emerg Med 1993;22(11):1766–7.
27. Putukian M, McKeag DB, Nogle S. Noncontact knee dislocation in a female basketball player: a case report. Clin J Sport Med 1995;5(4):258–61.
28. Peicha G, Pascher A, Schwarzl F, et al. Transection of the peroneal nerve complicating knee arthroscopy: case report and cadaver study. Arthroscopy 1998;14(2): 221–3.
29. Moeller JL, Monroe J, McKeag DB. Cryotherapy-induced common peroneal nerve palsy. Clin J Sport Med 1997;7(3):212–6.
30. Lindenbaum BL. Ski boot compression syndrome. Clin Orthop 1979(140):109–10.
31. Gessini L, Jandolo B, Pietrangeli A. The anterior tarsal syndrome: report of four cases. J Bone Joint Surg Am 1984;66(5):786–7.
32. Redfern DJ, Sauve PS, Sakellariou A. Investigation of incidence of superficial peroneal nerve injury following ankle fracture. Foot Ankle Int 2003;24(10):771–4.
33. Takao M, Ochi M, Shu N, et al. A case of superficial peroneal nerve injury during ankle arthroscopy. Arthroscopy 2001;17(4):403–4.
34. Dyck PJ, Thomas PK, eds. Peripheral Neuropathy. 4th ed. Philadelphia: Elsevier Saunders; 2005.
35. Krivickas LS. Lower-extremity nerve injuries. In: Feinberg JH, Spielholz NI, eds. Peripheral Nerve Injuries in the Athlete. Champaign, IL: Human Kinetics; 2003: 106–41.
36. De Ruiter GC, Torchia ME, Amrami KK, et al. Neurovascular compression following isolated popliteus muscle rupture: a case report. J Surg Orthop Adv 2005; 14(3):129–32.
37. Peri G. The "critical zones" of entrapment of the nerves of the lower limb. Surg Radiol Anat 1991;13(2):139–43.
38. O'Connor FG, Wilder RP. Textbook of Running Medicine. New York: McGraw-Hill; 2001.
39. Pla ME, Dillingham TR, Spellman NT, et al. Painful legs and moving toes associated with tarsal tunnel syndrome and accessory soleus muscle. Mov Disord 1996;11(1): 82–6.
40. Sammarco GJ, Stephens MM. Tarsal tunnel syndrome caused by the flexor digitorum accessorius longus: a case report. J Bone Joint Surg Am 1990;72(3):453–4.
41. Jackson DL, Haglund B. Tarsal tunnel syndrome in athletes: case reports and literature review. Am J Sports Med 1991;19(1):61–5.
42. Park TA, Del Toro DR. The medial calcaneal nerve: anatomy and nerve conduction technique. Muscle Nerve 1995;18(1):32–8.
43. Stefko RM, Lauerman WC, Heckman JD. Tarsal tunnel syndrome caused by an unrecognized fracture of the posterior process of the talus (Cedell fracture): a case report. J Bone Joint Surg Am 1994;76(1):116–8.
44. Yamamoto S, Tominaga Y, Yura S, et al. Tarsal tunnel syndrome with double causes (ganglion, tarsal coalition) evoked by ski boots: case report. J Sports Med Phys Fitness 1995;35(2):143–5.
45. Rask MR. Medial plantar neurapraxia (jogger's foot): report of 3 cases. Clin Orthop 1978(134):193–5.
46. Boon AJ, Harper CM. Needle EMG of abductor hallucis and peroneus tertius in normal subjects. Muscle Nerve 2003;27(6):752–6.

47. Henricson AS, Westlin NE. Chronic calcaneal pain in athletes: entrapment of the calcaneal nerve? Am J Sports Med 1984;12(2):152–4.
48. Park TA, Del Toro DR. Isolated inferior calcaneal neuropathy. Muscle Nerve 1996;19(1):106–8.
49. Fredericson M, Standage S, Chou L, et al. Lateral plantar nerve entrapment in a competitive gymnast. Clin J Sport Med 2001;11(2):111–4.
50. Mann R. Entrapment neuropathies of the foot. In: DeLee J, Drez D, eds. Orthopaedic Sports Medicine. Philadelphia: Saunders; 1995:1831–41.
51. Spindler KP, Pappas J. Neurovascular problems. In: Nicholas JA, Hershman EB, eds. The Lower Extremity and Spine in Sports Medicine. St. Louis: Mosby; 1995: 1345–58.
52. Wu KK. Morton's interdigital neuroma: a clinical review of its etiology, treatment, and results. J Foot Ankle Surg 1996;35(2):112–9; discussion 87–8.
53. Jones DC, Singer KM. Soft-tissue conditions of the ankle and foot. In: Nicholas JA, Hershman EB, eds. The Lower Extremity and Spine in Sports Medicine. 2nd ed. St. Louis: Mosby; 1995.
54. Mann RA, Reynolds JC. Interdigital neuroma: a critical clinical analysis. Foot Ankle 1983;3(4):238–43.
55. Lipscomb AB, Ibrahim AA. Acute peroneal compartment syndrome in a well conditioned athlete: report of a case. Am J Sports Med 1977;5(4):154–7.
56. Bourne RB, Rorabeck CH. Compartment syndromes of the lower leg. Clin Orthop 1989;(240):97–104.
57. Mavor GE. The anterior tibial syndrome. J Bone Joint Surg Br 1956;38(2):513–7.
58. Reneman RS. The anterior and the lateral compartmental syndrome of the leg due to intensive use of muscles. Clin Orthop 1975;(113):69–80.
59. Fronek J, Mubarak SJ, Hargens AR, et al. Management of chronic exertional anterior compartment syndrome of the lower extremity. Clin Orthop 1987;(220):217–27.
60. Martens MA, Moeyersoons JP. Acute and recurrent effort-related compartment syndrome in sports. Sports Med 1990;9(1):62–8.
61. Rorabeck CH. Exertional tibialis posterior compartment syndrome. Clin Orthop 1986(208):61–4.
62. Kirby NG. Exercise ischaemia in the fascial compartment of soleus: report of a case. J Bone Joint Surg Br 1970;52(4):738–40.
63. Mubarak SJ, Owen CA, Garfin S, et al. Acute exertional superficial posterior compartment syndrome. Am J Sports Med 1978;6(5):287–90.
64. Qvarfordt P, Christenson JT, Eklof B, et al. Intramuscular pressure, muscle blood flow, and skeletal muscle metabolism in chronic anterior tibial compartment syndrome. Clin Orthop 1983;(179):284–90.
65. Styf JR, Korner LM. Diagnosis of chronic anterior compartment syndrome in the lower leg. Acta Orthop Scand 1987;58(2):139–44.
66. Amendola A, Rorabeck CH, Vellett D, et al. The use of magnetic resonance imaging in exertional compartment syndromes. Am J Sports Med 1990;18(1):29–34.
67. Edwards PH Jr, Wright ML, Hartman JF. A practical approach for the differential diagnosis of chronic leg pain in the athlete. Am J Sports Med 2005;33(8):1241–9.
68. Pedowitz RA, Hargens AR, Mubarak SJ, et al. Modified criteria for the objective diagnosis of chronic compartment syndrome of the leg. Am J Sports Med 1990; 18(1):35–40.
69. Puranen J, Alavaikko A. Intracompartmental pressure increase on exertion in patients with chronic compartment syndrome in the leg. J Bone Joint Surg Am 1981;63(8):1304–9.
70. Rorabeck CH, Bourne RB, Fowler PJ. The surgical treatment of exertional compartment syndrome in athletes. J Bone Joint Surg Am 1983;65(9):1245–51.
71. Hayes AA, Bower GD, Pitstock KL. Chronic (exertional) compartment syndrome of the legs diagnosed with thallous chloride scintigraphy. J Nucl Med 1995;36(9):1618–24.
72. Rowdon GA, Richardson JK, Hoffmann P, et al. Chronic anterior compartment syndrome and deep peroneal nerve function. Clin J Sport Med 2001;11(4): 229–33.
73. Almdahl SM, Samdal F. Fasciotomy for chronic compartment syndrome. Acta Orthop Scand 1989;60(2):210–1.
74. Mouhsine E, Garofalo R, Moretti B, et al. Two minimal incision fasciotomy for chronic exertional compartment syndrome of the lower leg. Knee Surg Sports Traumatol Arthrosc 2006;14(2):193–7.
75. Raikin SM, Rapuri VR, Vitanzo P. Bilateral simultaneous fasciotomy for chronic exertional compartment syndrome. Foot Ankle Int 2005;26(12):1007–11.
76. Schepsis AA, Martini D, Corbett M. Surgical management of exertional compartment syndrome of the lower leg: long-term followup. Am J Sports Med 1993; 21(6):811–7; discussion 7.
77. Styf JR, Korner LM. Chronic anterior-compartment syndrome of the leg: results of treatment by fasciotomy. J Bone Joint Surg Am 1986;68(9):1338–47.

Chapter 11
Peripheral Nerve Injuries of the Proximal Lower Limb in Athletes

Marla S. Kaufman and Mark E. Domroese

Introduction

Sports injuries that affect the peripheral nerves of the proximal lower limb (above the knee) are relatively uncommon. Injuries involving the lumbosacral plexus occur more often than peripheral nerve injuries. Of peripheral nerve injuries in athletes, sciatic neuropathy is the most common.[1] In this chapter we cover injuries to the following nerves.

- Iliohypogastric nerve
- Lateral femoral cutaneous nerve
- Obturator nerve
- Femoral and saphenous nerves
- Superior gluteal nerve
- Inferior gluteal nerve
- Sciatic nerve (including piriformis syndrome)
- Cluneal nerves
- Posterior cutaneous nerve of the thigh
- Pudendal nerve

In addition, we discuss nerve injuries involved with the *sportsman's hernia*. Peripheral nerve injuries involving the distal lower limb (knee and distal) are discussed in a separate chapter.

M.S. Kaufman (✉)
Department of Rehabilitation Medicine and Department of Orthopaedics and Sports Medicine, University of Washington Medical Center, UW Medicine Sports and Spine Physicians, Seattle, WA, USA

Anatomy

All of the peripheral nerves of the lower limb originate from the lumbar and sacral plexuses. These plexuses lack the distinct subcomponent structures that the brachial plexus has (e.g., trunks and cords), but do have branches and divisions that terminate in the peripheral nerves that supply the entire lower leg. Because the plexuses are interconnected and both supply the lower limb, they are often referred to jointly as the lumbosacral plexus (Fig. 11.1). The two plexuses are in close proximity but innervate different regions of the lower limb. Lumbar plexus innervation is limited to the musculature of the anterior and medial thigh as well as the skin of the medial side of the leg and foot. The sacral plexus innervates the muscles of the buttock, muscles and skin of the posterior thigh, and muscles inferior to the knee.

The lumbar plexus arises deep within the abdomen and is formed from the ventral rami of L1–4, with a variable contribution from T12 and L5. When L3 is the lowest nerve to enter the lumbar plexus, the plexus is said to be *prefixed* or *high*. When L5 is the lowest nerve, the plexus is termed *postfixed* or *low*. The lumbar plexus lies on the inner surface of the posterior abdominal wall and at its origin is embedded in the psoas major muscle. The terminal peripheral nerves exit from the psoas muscle and pass into the lower part of the abdominal wall or into the thigh.

Although the lumbar plexus lacks the consistent subcomponent structure of the brachial plexus, it does divide into anterior and posterior divisions. L1 divides into two branches (upper and

V. Akuthota, S.A. Herring (eds.), *Nerve and Vascular Injuries in Sports Medicine*,
DOI 10.1007/978-0-387-76600-3_11, © Springer Science+Business Media, LLC 2009

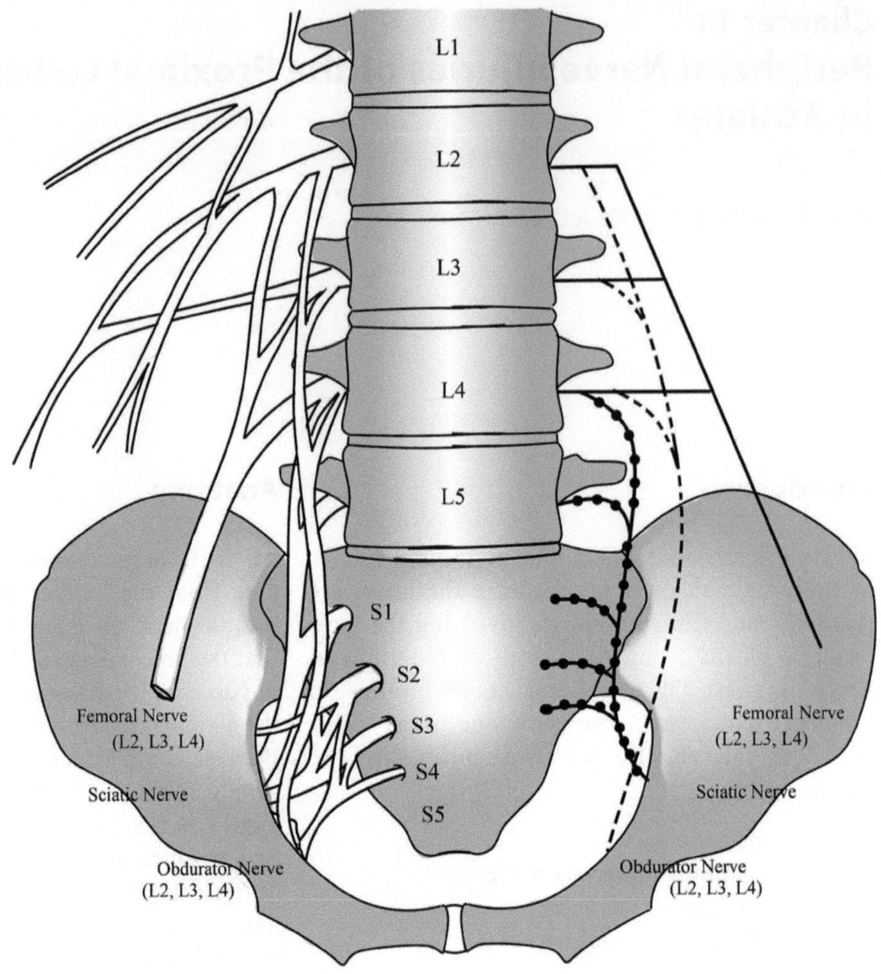

Fig. 11.1 Lumbosacral plexus

lower). The upper branch is the larger of the two and, with contribution from T12, divides into the iliohypogastric and ilioinguinal nerves. The lower, smaller branch joins a branch of L2 to form the genitofemoral nerve. L2–4 divide into anterior and posterior divisions. The anterior divisions of L2–4 form the obturator nerve. A small branch of the posterior divisions of L2 and L3 join to form the lateral femoral cutaneous nerve, whereas large branches from L2 and L3 unite with the posterior division of L4 to form the femoral nerve (Table 11.1).

The sacral plexus is formed by the ventral rami of L4–S3 or S4. The ventral ramus of part of L4 and that of L5 form the lumbosacral trunk. This trunk then joins with the ventral rami of S1 through S3 or S4 to form the sacral plexus. The sacral plexus is located partly inside and partly outside the posterior pelvis. It traverses between the piriformis muscle and the fascia of the pelvis and also through the greater sciatic foramen.

As does the lumbar plexus, the sacral plexus divides into anterior and posterior divisions. The

Table 11. 1 Branches of the lumbar plexus

Nerve	Roots	Division (if applicable)
Iliohypogastric	T12, L1	N/A
Ilioinguinal	T12, L1	N/A
Genitofemoral	L1, L2	N/A
Lateral femoral cutaneous	L2, L3	Posterior
Femoral	L2, L3, L4	Posterior
Obturator	L2, L3, L4	Anterior

anterior divisions of L4–S3 usually form the tibial nerve, which is the anterior and medial portion of the sciatic nerve. Posterior branches of L4–S2 form the common peroneal nerve, which is the posterior and lateral portion of the sciatic nerve. The tibial and common peroneal fibers form a single, large sciatic nerve until they separate just proximal to the knee. The superior gluteal nerve is formed by the posterior divisions of the lumbosacral trunk and S1, and the inferior gluteal nerve is derived from the posterior division of the lumbosacral trunk joining with S1 and S2. The posterior femoral cutaneous nerve is formed by portions of both anterior and posterior divisions of the plexus (S1–3). Anterior portions of S2 and S3 join a portion of S4 to form the pudendal nerve, which is the lowest branch of the sacral plexus. In addition, the anterior division of the sacral plexus gives off the nerve to the piriformis muscle, the nerve to the quadratus femoris, nerves to the gemellus inferior and superior, and the nerve to the obturator internus (Table 11.2).

Table 11. 2 Select branches of the sacral plexus

Nerve	Roots	Division
Tibial	L4–S3	Anterior
Common peroneal	L4–S2	Posterior
Superior gluteal	L4–S1	Posterior
Inferior gluteal	L4–S2	Posterior
To piriformis muscle	S2	Posterior
Posterior femoral cutaneous	S1–3	Anterior and posterior
To quadratus femoris	L4–S2	Anterior
To inferior gemellus	L4–S2	Anterior
To superior gemellus	L5–S2	Anterior
To obturator internus	L5–S2	Anterior
Pudendal	S2–4	Anterior

Iliohypogastric Nerve

The iliohypogastric nerve is formed from the upper branch of fibers from the primary ventral rami of T12 and L1. It courses through the psoas muscle, behind the lower pole of the kidney, and crosses obliquely in front of the quadratus lumborum. Near the iliac crest, the nerve perforates the posterior portion of the transversus abdominis, giving off its muscular branches, and then divides into anterior and lateral cutaneous branches near the anterosuperior iliac spine. Branches of the iliohypogastric nerve innervate the abdominal wall muscles and the skin of the upper buttock and a small area over the pubis.

Iliohypogastric neuropathy, or injury to either of its two branches, is rare.[2] The main trunk of the nerve may be injured by retroperitoneal tumors or large surgical incisions (e.g., for nephrectomy) resulting in sensory abnormalities and weakness of the lower abdominal muscles. Surgical incision of the lower quadrant of the abdomen may result in injury to the anterior portion, causing a suprapubic sensory deficit.[3] Compression of the lateral branch where it crosses the iliac crest results in a sensory deficit over the upper buttock.[4]

In athletes, these rarely occurring injuries generally result from direct trauma to the lateral pelvis during collision sports.[5] The most common symptom caused by this injury is pain, but sensory loss may also be noted. It remains unclear whether iliohypogastric nerve injury can occur with a *footballer's hernia,* which is lower abdominal bulging, but should always be excluded prior to surgical herniorrhaphy.[5,6]

Ziprin et al. described 25 male athletes who presented with groin pain. Their principal sport, according to the original article, was rugby or football in 19 individuals and cycling, hockey, marathon running, and cricket in 4 of the other 6 athletes. Interestingly, 23 of the 25 athletes were noted to have single or multiple tears in the external oblique aponeurosis, in which the neurovascular bundles containing the terminal branches of the iliohypogastric nerve are housed. It was assumed that the tear(s) resulted in nerve entrapment, and treatment was focused on surgical repair of the tears and division of the neurovascular bundles.[7]

Sportsman's Hernia

The term *sportsman's hernia* has been used in the literature to refer to the condition of chronic groin pain. The terms *Gilmore's groin,*[8] *groin disruption,*[9] and *pubalgia*[10] have been used somewhat synonymously with sportsman's hernia. When describing this condition, Gilmore noted a combination of a torn external oblique aponeurosis, a torn conjoined tendon, and dehiscence between the inguinal ligament and torn conjoined tendon. In contrast, Williams and Foster described chronic groin pain due to a tear in only the external oblique aponeurosis at the site of emergence of the terminal branches of the iliohypogastric neurovascular bundle.[11] Although there does not appear to be an overall consensus regarding the specifics of the underlying pathophysiology, it is generally accepted that a tear occurs at the external oblique muscle, which may result in an occult hernia.[12]

The clinical findings include chronic groin pain that is aggravated by sudden and twisting movements, especially the action of kicking a ball, coughing, sneezing, or even rolling over in bed. The literature available warns that sportsman's hernia is a diagnosis of exclusion and that the more common causes of groin pain (e.g., musculotendinous injuries and osteitis pubis) must be ruled out first. Also, signs and symptoms have been described as being diffuse and nonspecific. Williams and Foster did point out, however, that groin strain is a common complaint, particularly in soccer players, and that early surgical groin exploration should be considered, as it often results in good outcomes with repair to only the external oblique aponeurosis.[11]

Lateral Femoral Cutaneous Nerve

The lateral femoral cutaneous nerve (also known as the lateral cutaneous nerve of the thigh) is formed from the posterior divisions of the ventral primary rami of L2 and L3. The nerve remains retroperitoneal along the inner wall of the pelvis, passing through the psoas muscle and over the iliacus muscle. It emerges through an orifice formed by the lateral attachment of the inguinal ligament to the anterosuperior iliac spine.[13] In the proximal anterior thigh, it crosses the proximal edge of the sartorius muscle and then splits into anterior and posterior branches, piercing the fascia lata and becoming superficial. The lateral femoral cutaneous nerve is a pure sensory nerve, supplying the skin of the anterolateral aspect of the thigh. Pain and sensory impairment overlying this area occur as a result of injury to this nerve, a condition termed *meralgia paresthetica*.

Generally the etiology of meralgia paresthetica is not clearly identified, but it is assumed to be secondary to compression of the nerve at the inguinal ligament. Autopsy studies demonstrated lesions of the nerve at this location in about 50% of cases.[14] In athletics, compression or entrapment of the nerve in this area could occur in contact sports as a result of direct trauma, as in football (soccer) and rugby.[15] Female gymnasts have reported this injury with repeated soft tissue trauma to this area secondary to work on the uneven bars.[16] Scuba divers wearing weight belts can also have direct trauma to the nerve and experience symptoms of anterolateral thigh tingling.[5] Meralgia paresthetica resulting from upper thigh trauma has also been reported in a soccer player.[17] In addition, symptoms of lateral femoral cutaneous nerve entrapment have been reported in long-distance backpackers.[18]

Conservative treatment has reportedly been successful in more than 90% of cases,[13] and it has been reported that many cases of meralgia paresthetica resolve spontaneously.[19] Boulware noted that paresthesias in long-distance hikers were quite bothersome during the activity but resolved after the hike was finished.[18] Surgical exploration of the nerve should be reserved for resistant, painful cases.

Obturator Nerve

The obturator nerve originates from the anterior divisions of the ventral rami of L2–4, descending through the psoas muscle, and passing into the lesser pelvis. As it traverses the obturator tunnel, a fibroosseus passageway located under the pubic ramus, toward its exit into the anteromedial thigh at the obturator foramen, it divides into three branches.

- Branch innervating the obturator externus
- Main anterior branch innervating the adductor longus, adductor brevis, gracilis, and occasionally the pectineus as well as providing sensation to the skin and fascia of the distal two-thirds of the medial thigh
- Main posterior branch innervating the adductor magnus and obturator externus as well as providing sensation to the articular capsule, cruciate ligaments, and synovial membrane of the knee

Although injury to the obturator nerve has been reported rarely, injury to the nerve can lead to adductor group muscle weakness and sensory impairment with associated pain localized to a region of the medial thigh. The course of the obturator nerve in the pelvis and the obturator canal protect it from direct trauma but also place it at risk of compression from space-occupying pelvic masses or hematomas. The obturator nerve can also be injured in association with pelvic fractures.[5]

Sport-related injury to the obturator nerve is rare. Entrapment due to compression by a fascial band at the outlet of the obturator canal has been described in rugby and Australian-rules football players.[20] The injury was reported to be quite responsive to surgical neurolysis. Obturator hernia, although rare and difficult to diagnose, should be included in the differential diagnosis of obturator neuropathy, as it may respond to surgical intervention.[21,22]

Femoral and Saphenous Nerves

The femoral nerve is formed by the posterior divisions of the ventral rami of the L2–4 nerve roots (Fig. 11.2). The nerve roots come together to form the femoral nerve within the psoas muscle, which then emerges from the lateral border of the psoas, passing along the surface of the iliacus muscle below the iliacus fascia. It passes under the inguinal ligament lateral to the femoral artery and vein and into the upper thigh, where it divides into motor branches to the quadriceps group, sartorius, and pectineus muscles, as well as sensory branches to the skin of the anterior thigh.

The clinical presentation of femoral neuropathy includes pain localized at or below the inguinal region, quadriceps weakness, and reduced or absent patellar reflex. Sensory impairment is less common than motor symptoms. The most common injury to the femoral nerve reported in the sports medicine literature is secondary to psoas bursitis or muscular strain of the iliopsoas with associated hematoma and nerve compression.[5,23,24] Hyperextension of the hip as a cause of acute femoral injury has been reported in gymnasts, football players, basketball players, and long jumpers.[25]

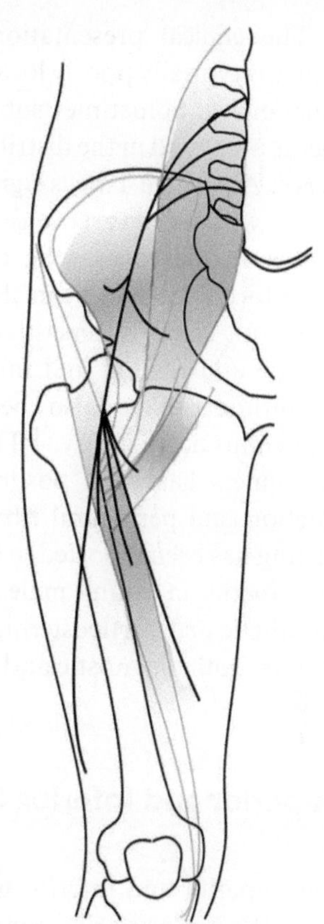

Fig. 11.2 Femoral nerve

Femoral mononeuropathies have also been reported in cross-country skiers.[26,27] Dancers who perform maneuvers requiring simultaneous hip extension and knee flexion are at risk for femoral neuropathy.[15,28] It has also been reported that gymnasts carry out maneuvers and attain body postures that place them at risk for femoral neuropathy, especially with the involvement of trampolines.[29] In addition, localized injury to a motor branch of the femoral nerve supplying the vastus lateralis has been described in a bodybuilder. The injury was thought to be due to repetitive stretch and compression, leading to selective atrophy of the distal portion of the vastus lateralis muscle.[30]

The exclusively sensory saphenous nerve is the continuation of the femoral nerve. It runs along the medial border of the sartorius muscle, entering the subsartorial canal (also known as the adductor canal) of Hunter with the femoral artery and vein. It emerges from the canal by piercing the anteromedial intermuscular septum about 10 cm above the knee.

The clinical presentation of saphenous nerve injury is typically poorly localized pain in the medial knee or leg. Sometimes subjective sensory impairments are found in the distribution of the saphenous nerve. A positive Tinel's sign can sometimes help in cases without overt sensory impairment.[6] The saphenous nerve may be compressed by bursitis close to the knee joint in the distal portion of the adductor canal.[6] Repetitive knee flexion during cycling and rowing and muscular hypertrophy in weightlifters have also been reported to cause saphenous nerve injury.[31] The mechanism of injury in runners has been posited to be secondary to traction and perineural fibrosis. Prolonged wave-surfing has been reported to be a cause of saphenous neuropathy in young males.[32] A local block with anesthetic and corticosteroid in the adductor canal may be both diagnostic and therapeutic.[33,34]

Superior and Inferior Gluteal Nerves

The superior and inferior gluteal nerves originate from the posterior divisions of L4–S1 and L4–S2, respectively. Along with the sciatic nerve, pudendal nerve, and posterior cutaneous nerve of the thigh, they pass through the sciatic notch into the deep gluteal region. The superior gluteal nerve passes above the piriformis muscle and enters the deep gluteal region to innervate the gluteus medius, gluteus minimus, and tensor fascia lata muscles. The inferior gluteal nerve passes below the piriformis muscle and supplies the gluteus maximus muscle. These nerves do not have cutaneous innervation.

The superior gluteal nerve is not commonly injured, but superior gluteal neuropathies have been noted to result from local buttock trauma, pelvic fractures, hip surgery, and buttock injections.[35,36] As it courses above the piriformis muscle, unlike other deep gluteal nerves, it may be injured in isolation. The inferior gluteal nerve, however, is generally injured in association with the sciatic nerve, pudendal nerve, and/or the posterior cutaneous nerve of the thigh, as they all pass below the piriformis muscle. Local trauma secondary to space-occupying lesions has been reported as the etiology of inferior gluteal neuropathy.[37] Although controversial, it has been hypothesized that hypertrophy of the piriformis muscle can result in a compression neuropathy of either of these two nerves.[38] Treatment includes surgical exploration of the nerves, and spontaneous resolution has been reported for postsurgical or traumatic lesions.[39]

Sciatic Nerve

The sciatic nerve is the largest nerve that arises from the lumbosacral plexus. It is made up of anterior and posterior division fibers from the ventral rami of L4–S3. The anterior division fibers of L4–S2 form the common peroneal portion of the sciatic, and the posterior division fibers of L4–S3 form the tibial portion of the sciatic nerve. The sciatic nerve exits through the greater sciatic foramen, passing between the piriformis superiorly and the superior gemellus inferiorly. Occasionally, the sciatic nerve may pass through, or over, the piriformis muscle.[40] The nerve runs through the deep gluteal region, covered by the gluteus maximus, passing between the ischial tuberosity medially and the greater trochanter of the femur laterally. It lies close to the posterior capsule of the hip joint in this location. From there the nerve continues distally toward the popliteal fossa where it splits into its tibial and peroneal nerve components. Within the posterior thigh, the tibial portion of the sciatic nerve gives off muscle branches to the hamstring muscles, with the exception of the short head of the biceps femoris, which is innervated by a branch from the peroneal portion of the sciatic nerve above the level of the knee. No cutaneous branches arise from the sciatic nerve as it passes through the posterior thigh.

Sciatic nerve trauma in sports commonly occurs in contact sports as a result of local trauma, such as a fall onto the buttocks that compresses the nerve against the posterior portion of the hip capsule.[15] Clinical symptoms of sciatic nerve injury include buttock pain radiating down the lower extremity into the leg with associated paresthesias. Muscle weakness is sometimes detected in the hamstrings or in muscles below the knee. Complete, rapid recovery is reported as the general rule, with conservative management comprised of rest and antiinflammatory drugs.

Hip fractures and dislocations may also compress the sciatic nerve.[2] Spencer suggested that if a dense sciatic nerve injury is present after an injury, a dislocated hip should be suspected as the etiology.[41] Focal nerve entrapment of the sciatic nerve has been described at the level of the ischial tuberosity at the attachment of the biceps femoris, due to either a fibrous edge of the muscle or a fibrous aponeurotic band. Puranen and Orava called this the *hamstring syndrome* and reported that surgical division of the fibrous bands cured the symptoms present in a series of cases.[42]

Piriformis syndrome as a clinical entity has been widely debated, and its existence remains controversial. Even among those who tout the clinical relevance of the syndrome, there is no consensus regarding its definition. For purposes of this discussion, we assume that piriformis syndrome exists as first described by Robinson in 1947.[43] He reported that sciatica was a symptom-not a disease entity-and that piriformis syndrome was sciatica caused by an abnormal condition of the piriformis muscle, which was usually traumatic. He described five cardinal features: a history of local trauma to the gluteal region; pain localized to the sacroiliac joint, greater sciatic notch, and piriformis muscle and extending distally along the course of the sciatic nerve, causing difficulty with ambulation; pain worsened by lifting or bending over but alleviated with traction; a palpable and tender piriformis muscle; and a positive Lasègue sign. In addition, he reported that patients may have gluteal atrophy.

In 1938, Beaton and Anson[44] examined 240 cadavers in order to describe six variations of sciatic nerve exit. They implicated piriformis spasm in sciatica, especially when the piriformis muscle is pierced by the sciatic nerve. McCrory and Bell[5] coined the term *deep gluteal syndrome,* doubting that all pain elements could be attributed exclusively to the piriformis muscle/sciatic nerve combination. Similarly, Papadopoulos and Khan[45] used the term *pelvic outlet syndrome* to encompass all extraspinal nerve compression of structures in proximity to the sciatic notch, with resultant lower extremity pain.

In any athlete presenting with aching or cramping buttock pain, ± radiation to the ipsilateral thigh, ± extension below the knee (*sciatica*), ± weakness/numbness, the piriformis syndrome should be present on the differential diagnosis, although more common etiologies such as hip pathology, radiculopathy, and sacroiliac joint pathology need to be ruled out first. Symptoms associated with piriformis syndrome are generally thought to be exacerbated by the FADIR position (hip *f*lexion, *ad*duction, *i*nternal *r*otation) and tenderness to palpation with a rectal or pelvic examination. Magnetic resonance imaging (MRI) and computed tomography (CT) may be used as part of the workup,[46] although they are generally more helpful for ruling out other etiologies rather than ruling in piriformis syndrome. Although needle electromyography (EMG) is generally normal, Fishman and Zybert[47] and Fishman et al.[48] used the delayed H-reflex test with hip flexion, adduction, internal rotation (FAIR = FADIR) to help with the diagnosis. Measurement error may confound interpretation using the Fishman method.

There have been several case reports of piriformis syndrome diagnosed in athletes. As a history of buttock trauma, even remote, is a key feature in this syndrome, it would be reasonable to consider this diagnosis in any athlete participating in contact sports or with a history of local gluteal trauma. One report[49] related the case of a 19-year-old football player who had been hit by another player and fell to the ground, landing on his buttock. He had reported shooting pain from his buttock down the back of his thigh and calf to his lateral foot. After examination and workup, he was diagnosed with piriformis syndrome and was treated with a program consisting of stretching, manipulation, and chiropractic palpation. Another author reported a case of a female runner with buttock pain aggravated by exercise. Again, stretching was effective as a treatment modality.[50] Treatment options include physical therapy, oral medications, and emerging but experimental treatment such as local injections of corticosteroids and botulinum toxin as well as surgical release.

Cluneal Nerves

The cluneal nerves, derived from both lumbar and sacral roots, provide cutaneous innervation to the gluteal region. The superior cluneal nerve, formed by the lateral branches of the dorsal rami of L1–3 (and possibly T12), innervates the superior two-thirds of the skin overlying the buttock. It emerges from the deep fascia just superior to the iliac crest. The middle cluneal nerve is formed by the lateral branches of the dorsal rami of S1–3 through a sacral anastomosis and becomes superficial along a line drawn connecting the posterosuperior iliac spine (PSIS) to the tip of the coccyx, supplying the skin overlying the coccyx and the adjacent buttock. The inferior cluneal nerve is derived from the gluteal branch of the posterior femoral cutaneous nerve (ventral rami of S1–3) and courses around the inferior border of the gluteus maximus muscle.[51]

Maigne and Doursounian's cadaveric study described the most medial of the cluneal nerves (mediosuperior cluneal nerve) as originating from the L1 root 60% of the time and the L2 root 40% of the time. Despite variations in derivation, the mediosuperior cluneal nerve crosses the posterior iliac crest approximately 7 cm from the midline, where it becomes shallower and passes through a space formed by the thoracolumbar fascia and the iliac crest. These authors hypothesized that entrapment of the nerve could occur at this point.[52]

Mediosuperior cluneal nerve entrapment has been reported in two young athletes, a 17-year-old tennis player and a 16-year-old volleyball player.[53] Both girls had a difficult time sitting for long periods of time because of pain, and both had palpable trigger points para-midline over the iliac crest. The authors of these cases proposed simultaneous full flexion of the ipsilateral hip and knee joints as a provocative test that reproduced their symptoms. It was hypothesized that during sports activities such as tennis and volleyball, where the player positions the hip throughout the range of flexion, the nerve is subjected to stretching forces that lead to irritation and edema; if left untreated, it can progress to scarring and inflammatory cell infiltration with consequential entrapment. The athletes reportedly were both successfully treated with injection of a combination of anesthetic and corticosteroid.[53]

Posterior Cutaneous Nerve of the Thigh

The posterior cutaneous nerve of the thigh (PCNT) originates from the ventral rami of S1–3. Along with the sciatic nerve, pudendal nerve, and gluteal nerves, it passes through the sciatic notch. The PCNT courses below the piriformis muscle and medial to the sciatic nerve and then superficially down the posterior thigh to the knee, providing cutaneous innervation to the skin of the lower buttock and posterior thigh. Additionally, the perineal branches (also referred to as the inferior cluneal nerve) partially innervate the skin of the perineum and genitals, along with branches from the pudendal nerve.

Lesions of the PCNT relating to sports are rare. Falls onto the buttock and bicycle riding for a prolonged period of time may compress the nerve while it is in the pelvis.[2] In addition, prolonged sitting may put pressure on the distal edge of the gluteus maximus, resulting in nerve entrapment. Numbness and tingling along the sensory distribution are the most common symptoms.[5,6] It has been hypothesized that PCNT entrapment may be the actual etiology in symptoms incorrectly diagnosed as piriformis syndrome.[5] Treatment may consist of surgical exploration.

Pudendal Nerve

The pudendal nerve contains nerve fibers from the ventral rami of the S2–4 nerve roots. It courses through the greater sciatic foramen, over the sacrospinous ligament, and then back into the lesser sciatic foramen, passing anterior to the sacrotuberous ligament. The inferior rectal branch innervates the external anal sphincter and provides sensation to the lower anal canal and perianal skin. After giving off the inferior rectal branch, the pudendal nerve enters the pudendal canal along the medial aspect of the ischial tuberosity up toward the inferior pubic ramus. Within the pudendal canal, the pudendal nerve gives off the perineal nerve branch that innervates the muscles of the perineum, urethral sphincter, and erectile tissue of the penis; and it provides sensation to the perianal and scrotal or labial areas. The final continuation of the pudendal nerve is the dorsal nerve of the penis or clitoris.

Direct injuries to the pudendal nerve are rare owing to its relatively protected course. Surgical manipulation of pelvic fractures has been reported as a potential cause of pudendal nerve damage.[54] There are several reports of injury to the pudendal nerve in cyclists as a result of prolonged compression by narrow bicycle seats.[55–60] Symptoms reported include recurrent numbness of the penis and scrotum after prolonged cycling. Transient impotence lasting up to several weeks has been reported.[61] Female cyclists have reported similar perineal numbness with prolonged cycling.[62]

Conclusion

Despite their relative rarity, one must be aware of peripheral nerve injuries of the proximal lower limb in athletes, especially among certain populations and sports. If not properly diagnosed in a timely manner, these nerve injuries can lead to long-lasting, sometimes permanent deficits, affecting not only athletic performance but also the ability to perform day-to-day activities. Hence, an early, correct diagnosis is imperative.

Peripheral nerve injuries in the proximal lower limb may be divided into two categories: acute (generally resulting from direct trauma) and chronic (secondary to repetitive microtrauma or entrapment). It is important for the physician treating athletes to have an intimate knowledge of the anatomy, as well as the typical patterns of nerve injury, to diagnose peripheral nerve injuries of the proximal lower extremity. Some sports involve highly specific maneuvers that may lead to injury, and providers need to understand the intricacies of the sports of their patients so they can properly diagnose nerve injuries.

Diagnosis may be one of exclusion, after ruling out more common musculoskeletal sport-related injury. Electrodiagnostics are often an integral component to the workup for potential peripheral nerve injury, as they can rule in or out specific nerve injuries.

In most cases, peripheral nerve injuries in the proximal lower limbs of athletes can be managed with conservative treatment, such as rest, antiinflammatory agents, and physical therapy. Some neuropathies may even resolve spontaneously. Surgical consultation and exploration of the nerve, however, may be required for resistant cases.

References

1. Krivickas LS, Wilbourn AJ. Peripheral nerve injury in athletes: a case series of over 200 injuries. Semin Neurol 2000;20(2):225–32.
2. Stewart J. Focal Peripheral Neuropathies. 2nd ed. New York: Raven Press; 1993.
3. Stulz P, Pfeiffer KM. Peripheral nerve injuries resulting from common surgical procedures in the lower portion of the abdomen. Arch Surg 1982;117: 324–7.
4. Mumenthaler M, Schliack H. Peripheral Nerve Lesions: Diagnosis and Therapy. New York: Thieme; 1991.
5. McCrory P, Bell S. Nerve entrapment syndromes as a cause of pain in hip, groin and buttock. Sports Med 1999;27:261–74.
6. Cavaletti G, Marmiroli P, Alberti G, et al. Sport-related peripheral nerve injuries: part 2. Sport Sci Health 2005;1:61–7.
7. Ziprin P, Williams P, Foster ME. External oblique aponeurosis nerve entrapment as a cause of groin pain in the athlete. Br J Surg 1999;86(4):566–8.
8. Gilmore OJA. Gilmore's groin. Sports Med Soft Tissue Trauma 1992;3:12–4.
9. Per AFH, Renstrom PA. Tendon and muscle injuries in the groin area. Clin Sports Med 1992;11(4):815–31.
10. Taylor DC, Meyers WC, Moylan JA, et al. Abdominal musculature abnormalities as a cause of groin pain in athletes: inguinal hernias and pubalgia. Ann J Sports Med 1991;3:239–42.
11. Williams P, Foster ME. 'Gilmore's groin'—or is it? Br J Sports Med 1995;29:2068.
12. Fon LJ, Spence RAJ. Sportsman's hernia. Br J Surg 2000;87:545–52.
13. Williams P, Trzil K. Management of meralgia paraesthetica. J Neurosurg 1991;74:76–80.
14. Jefferson D, Eames R. Subclinical entrapment of the lateral femoral cutaneous nerve: an autopsy study. Muscle Nerve 1979;2:145–54.
15. Lorei MP, Hershman EB. Peripheral nerve injuries in athletes. Sports Med 1993;16:130–47.
16. MacGregor J, Moncur J. Meralgia paraesthetica: a sport lesion in girl gymnasts. Br J Sports Med 1977;11:16–7.
17. Ulkar B, Yildiz Y, Kunduracioglu B. Meralgia paresthetica: a long-standing performance-limiting cause of anterior thigh pain in a soccer player. Am J Sports Med 2003;31:787–9.
18. Boulware DR. Backpacking-induced paresthesias. Wilderness Environ Med 2003;14(3):161–6.
19. Ecker A, Woltman H. Meralgia paraesthetica: a report of 150 cases. JAMA 1938;110:1650–2.
20. Bradshaw C, McCrory P, Bell S. Obturator nerve entrapment: a cause of groin pain in athletes. Am J Sports Med 1997;25:402–8.
21. Sowell A, Ljungdahl I, Spanger L. Thigh neuralgia as a symptom of obturator hernia. Acta Chir Scand 1976;142:457–9.
22. Kozlowski JM, Beck JM. Obturator hernia: an elusive diagnosis. Arch Surg 1977;112:1001–2.

23. Guillani G, Poppi M, Acciarn N., et al. CT scan and surgical treatment of traumatic iliacus hematoma with femoral neuropathy: case report. J Trauma 1990;30: 229–31.
24. Brozin IH, Martlet J, Goldberg I, et al. Traumatic closed femoral nerve neuropathy. J Trauma 1982;22:158–60.
25. McCrory P, Bell S, Bradshaw C. Nerve entrapments of the lower leg, ankle and foot in sports. Sports Med 2002;32:371–91.
26. Boyle H, Johnson RJ, Pope MN, et al. Cross country skiing injuries. In: Johnson RJ, Mote CJ, eds. Skiing Trauma and Safety: Fifth International Symposium ASTM STP 1104. Philadelphia: American Society for Testing and Materials; 1985:411–2.
27. Muellner T, Ganko A, Bugge W, et al. Isolated femoral mononeuropathy in the athlete: anatomic considerations and report of two cases. Am J Sports Med 2001;29: 814–7.
28. Sammarco GJ, Stephens MM. Neurapraxia of the femoral nerve in a modern dancer. Am J Sports Med 1991;19:413–4.
29. Toth C, McNeil S, Feasby T. Peripheral nervous system injuries in sport and recreation. Sports Med 2005;35(8): 717–38.
30. Padua L, D'Aloya E, LoMonaco M, et al. Mononeuropathy of a distal branch of the femoral nerve in a body building champion. J Neurol Neurosurg Psychiatry 1997;63:669–71.
31. Schon LC, Baxter DE. Neuropathies of the foot and ankle in athletes. Clin Sports Med 1990;9:489–508.
32. Fabian RH, Noreross KA, Hancock MB. Surfer's neuropathy. N Engl J Med 1987;316:555.
33. Mozes MM, Ouaknine G, Nathan H. Saphenous nervous entrapment simulating vascular disorder. Surgery 1975;77:299–303.
34. Romanoff ME, Cory PC, Kalenak A, et al. Saphenous nerve entrapment of the adductor canal. Am J Sports Med 1989;17(4):478.
35. Rask M. Superior gluteal nerve entrapment syndrome. Muscle Nerve 1980;3:304–7.
36. Pecina M, Krmpotic-Nemanic J, Markiewitz A. Tunnel Syndromes: Peripheral Nerve Compression Syndromes. 2nd ed. Boca Raton, FL: CRC Press; 1997.
37. LaBan M, Meerschaert J, Taylor R. Electromyographic evidence of inferior gluteal nerve compromise; an early representation of recurrent colo-rectal carcinoma. Arch Phys Med Rehabil 1982;63:33–5.
38. Pecina M. Contribution to the etiological explanation of the piriformis syndrome. Acta Anat 1979;105:181–7.
39. Stoehr M. Traumatic and postoperative lesions of the lumbosacral plexus. Arch Neurol 1978;35:757–60.
40. Sunderland S. Nerves and Nerve Injuries. 2nd ed. Edinburgh: Churchill Livingstone; 1978.
41. Spencer PS. Acute traumatic lesions of nerve. In: Schaumburg HH, Thomas PK, Spencer PS, eds. Disorders of Peripheral Nerves. Baltimore: Davis; 1983:257–80.
42. Puranen J, Orava S. The hamstring syndrome: a new diagnosis of gluteal sciatic pain. Am J Sports Med 1988;16:517–21.
43. Robinson D. Pyriformis syndrome in relation to sciatic pain. Am J Surg 1947;73:335–58.
44. Beaton LE, Anson B. The sciatic nerve and the pyriformis muscle: their interrelation as a possible cause of coccygodynia. J Bone Joint Surg 1938;20:686–8.
45. Papadopoulos EC, Khan SN. Piriformis syndrome and low back pain: a new classification and review of the literature. Orthop Clin North Am 2004;35:65–71.
46. Ripani M, Continenza MA, Cacchio A, et al. The ischiatic region: normal and MRI anatomy. J Sports Med Phys Fitness 2006;46(3):468–75.
47. Fishman LM, Zybert PA. Electrophysiologic evidence of piriformis syndrome. Arch Phys Med Rehabil 1992;73(4):359–64.
48. Fishman LM, Anderson C, Rosner B. Botox and physical therapy in the treatment of piriformis syndrome. Am J Phys Med Rehabil 2002;81(12):936–42.
49. Mayrand N, Fortin J, Descarreaux M, et al. Diagnosis and management of posttraumatic piriformis syndrome: a case study. J Manipulative Physiol Ther 2006;29(6): 486–91.
50. Julsrud ME. Piriformis syndrome. J Am Podiatr Med Assoc 1989;79(3):128–31.
51. D'Ambrosia C, Akuthota V, Tobey J, Sullivan W. Cluneal neuropathy: case report and cadaveric correlation. Poster Presentation at the American Academy of Physical Medicine and Rehabilitation Annual Assembly, October 8, 2004.
52. Maigne JY, Doursounian L. Entrapment neuropathy of the medial superior cluneal nerve: nineteen cases surgically treated, with a minimum of 2 years' follow-up. Spine 1997;22(10):1156–9.
53. Aly T, Tanaka Y, Aizawa T, et al. Medial superior cluneal nerve entrapment neuropathy in teenagers: a report of two cases. Tohoku J Exp Med 2002;197: 229–31.
54. Hofman A, Jones R, Schoenvogel R. Pudendal nerve neuropraxia as a result of traction on the fracture table. J Bone Joint Surg Am 1982;64:136–8.
55. Goodson J. Pudendal neuritis from biking [letter]. N Eng J Med 1981;304:365.
56. Desai K, Gingell J. The hazards of long distance cycling. BMJ 1989;298:1072–3.
57. Weiss BD. Clinical syndromes associated with bicycle seats. Clin Sports Med 1994;13(1):175–86.
58. Silbert PL, Dunne JW, Edis RH, et al. Bicycling induced pudendal nerve injury pudendal pressure neuropathy. Clin Exp Neurol 1991;28:191–6.
59. Weiss BD. Nontraumatic injuries in amateur long distance bicyclists. Am J Sports Med 1985;13(3):187–92.
60. Oberpenning F, Roth S, Leusmann DB. The Alcock syndrome: temporary penile insensitivity due to compression of the pudendal nerve within the Alcock canal. J Urol 1994;151(2):423–5.
61. Andersen KV, Bovim G. Impotence and nerve entrapment in long distance amateur cyclists. Acta Neurol Scand 1997;95(4):233–40.
62. LaSalle MD, Salinupour P, Adelstein M. Sexual and urinary tract dysfunction in female bicyclists. Presented at the 94th Annual Meeting of the American Urologic Asociation, 1997;12:17.

Chapter 12
Lumbar Radicular and Referred Pain in the Athlete

Jonathan T. Bravman, Hector Mejia, Vikas V. Patel, and Venu Akuthota

Introduction

Often numbness and tingling in athletes results from radicular or referred pain from the spine. Low back pain conditions are extremely common in athletes. Most spinal disorders cause axial low back pain, such as pain generated from facet and sacroiliac joints, muscles, and the disc itself. These structures may also cause somatic referred pain into the legs, usually above the knee. Somatic referred pain is typically described as a vague, dull pain in the leg, yet it can be confused with nerve-generated paresthesias. Radicular pain, on the other hand, is less common and is characterized by numbness and tingling that follows a particular dermatome. Radicular pain is exacerbated with dural tension maneuvers, such as straight-leg raising (SLR), seated slump test, and femoral nerve stretch test (FNST). Making the distinction between radicular and referred entities is important when initiating proper treatment. In sports, the following spinal conditions are seen with more frequency:

- Disc herniation
- Spondylolysis (stress fracture of the pars interarticularis)
- Spondylolisthesis
- Lumbar muscle strain
- Piriformis syndrome
- Greater trochanteric pain
- Facet-mediated pain
- Sacroiliac joint (SIJ) pain
- Pelvic stress fractures

J.T. Bravman (✉)
Resident Physician in Orthopaedic Surgery, Department of Orthopaedics, University of Colorado, Aurora, CO, USA

Diagnosis

History

A complete history can help guide the clinician to an accurate diagnosis. For example, back pain in a gymnast mainly on extension is typically related to spondylolysis, while the football player's radicular pain down one leg is more likely related to nerve compression or irritation. Once a preliminary differential diagnosis is developed from the history, the clinician can perform a physical examination to aid in refining the differential diagnosis. Often, acute low back pain from a specific stretch or torque injury in an athlete is due to muscle strain. Low back pain (particularly with radiation into the leg) that does not resolve within the initial 4–6 weeks should be investigated for an underlying cause.

Delineating low back pain from true radicular symptoms should be the clinician's first objective. The interview should address the time frame and pattern of pain, including the rate of onset of symptoms, location, quality, and distribution of pain. It should be determined if activities or positions exacerbate or alleviate symptoms. Mechanism of injury, including the position of the spine at the time of injury and the amount of force applied must be explored. The patient's background in sports participation should be addressed. The type of sport and duration of participation can be helpful in an appropriate diagnosis. For example, Gerbino and d'Hemecourt[1] reported more common involvement of herniated lumbar discs in football players and weightlifters, with spondylolysis more common in gymnasts.

V. Akuthota, S.A. Herring (eds.), *Nerve and Vascular Injuries in Sports Medicine*,
DOI 10.1007/978-0-387-76600-3_12, © Springer Science+Business Media, LLC 2009

Other interrogatives relate to a history of prior lumbar spine injury or surgery. As reported by Green et al.,[2] athletes who reported a history of prior lumbar injury had three times greater risk for injury. In a prospective cohort of 679 varsity athletes, a history of prior lumbar spine injury was found to be the most predictive risk factor for further injury. Specific inquiries of present conditioning, improper play techniques, excessive loading, and abrupt increases in training should be asked, as these items have been previously described as risk factors for lumbar injuries in athletes.[3]

Questions concerning prior or current treatment should also be addressed, including treatment by providers such as a physical therapists and chiropractors. Finally, a thorough review of systems should be performed, especially addressing symptoms, such as unexplained weight loss or night pain. These may be indications of systemic diseases such as infection or tumor.

Finally, possible cauda equina must also be ruled out as this is a surgical emergency. The patient presents with saddle anesthesia, bowel or bladder dysfunction, and possible bilateral lower extremity weakness or decreased sensation. Suspicion of possible cauda equina should be promptly worked up with proper imaging and a surgical spine consultation.[3]

Physical Examination

The physical examination of the athlete should be systematic and used as an adjunct to the history. The examination begins with complete exposure of the spine and lower extremities. The spine should be inspected while the patient is standing to assess for postural abnormalities or asymmetry, which would be suggestive of core musculature weakness or scoliosis. Range of motion, in all cardinal planes, should be recorded. Palpation of paraspinal musculature, greater trochanters, sacroiliac joints, and spinous processes can be useful for identifying areas of focal tenderness.[4]

Motor strength testing should include all major lower extremity muscle groups to assess possible L2 to S1 lower motor root injury. Testing should be performed in maximum stretch of each muscle group and recorded in a scale of 0–5.

Sensory examination of the back and lower extremity dermatomes is helpful but can be variable, as the distributions of dermatomes commonly overlap. The sensory examination should include the sacral dermatomes, as isolated injuries may otherwise be missed. Assessment of the reflexes can aid in differentiating upper versus lower motor neuron injury (e.g., spinal cord injury versus disc herniation). Reflex assessment includes Babinski and clonus evaluation.

Provocative maneuvers such as dural tension tests, FABER (flexion abduction external rotation of the hip), and FADIR (flexion adduction internal rotation of the hip) tests can be invaluable for identifying a specific pain generator. Dural tension tests include a supine SLR (L4–S1) and an FNST (L2–4). An irritated dura can cause pain when stretched by these provocative maneuvers, aiding in the diagnosis of a compressed nerve root. An SLR test is performed with the patient supine while the examiner raises the affected extremity. A positive test is the reproduction of radicular pain when the leg is raised less than 60°. The examiner can increase the sensitivity of the SLR test by dorsiflexing the ankle.[5]

A FABER test is performed with the patient supine and the affected extremity placed in flexion, abduction, and external rotation (Fig. 12.1). If positive, the pain is reproduced in the affected extremity, suggesting sacroiliac joint pathology. The FADIR test can be performed when piriformis syndrome is suspected. The patient is placed in a lateral decubitus position; and the affected hip is flexed, adducted, and internally rotated (Fig. 12.2). This again, if positive, should reproduce the symptoms associated with piriformis compression of the sciatic nerve.

Imaging

Imaging studies should be used in a targeted fashion based on the history and physical examination to identify abnormal anatomy. The clinician should always correlate anatomic findings with the history and physical examination, as it is common to have abnormal anatomic findings in asymptomatic patients. Recommendations from the Agency for Health Care Policy and Research state that plain

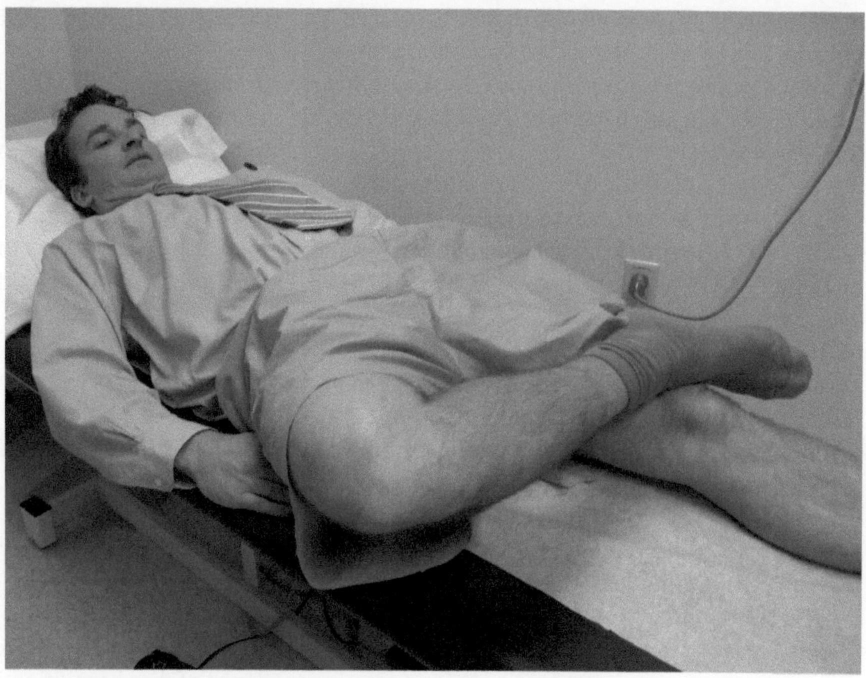

Fig. 12.1 Flexion abduction, external rotation (FABER) test

radiography should be undertaken only when symptoms persist longer than a month unless *red flag* symptoms-recent trauma, history of prolonged steroid use, osteoporosis, constitutional symptoms-are present.[6] Radiographs, although frequently normal in athletes, may be indicated with persistent symptoms. Anteroposterior (AP) and lateral films are sufficient for screening radiographs. If

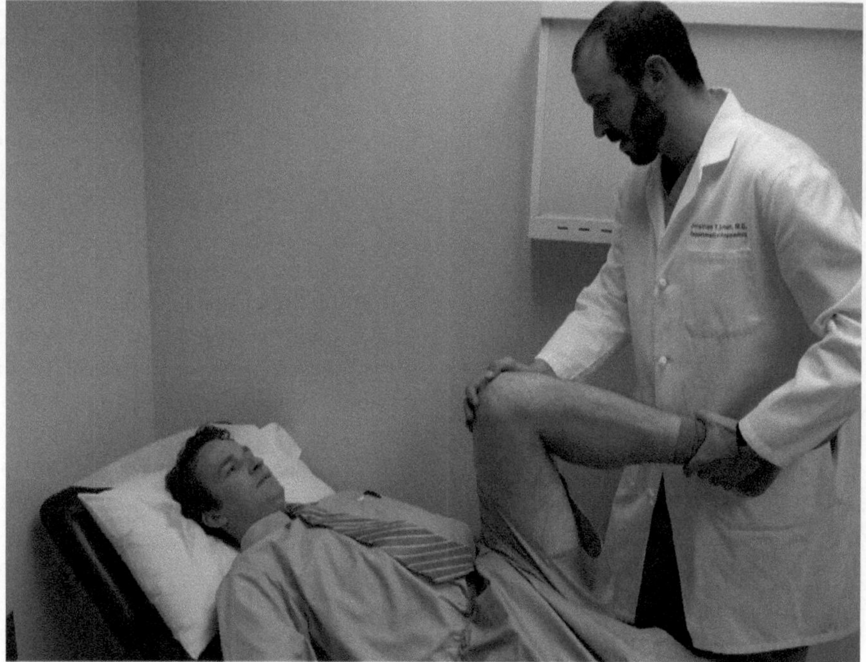

Fig. 12.2 Flexion adduction, internal rotation test (FADIR)

spondylolysis or spondylolisthesis is suspected, oblique radiographs should be obtained, although this doubles the radiation and the cost. In addition, pars defects can often be seen on AP and lateral films.

Computed tomography (CT) scans allow the clinician to see the bony anatomy with greater detail than plain radiography, and magnetic resonance imaging (MRI) provides better soft tissue detail. The decision on when to order a CT scan versus MRI or both can be difficult. CT scans should be obtained when abnormal bony anatomy is seen on radiographs or a fracture is suspected. Thin-cut CT scans can also be helpful for grading the healing of a pars stress fracture. MRI is indicated when cauda equina, disc herniation (Fig. 12.3), disc disease, or a neoplasm is suspected. It is also indicated when radicular symptoms and objective neurologic findings are present. Stress fractures, spondylolytic defects, and neoplastic lesions can also be seen on bone scans or single photon emission computed tomography (SPECT). It has been suggested that anatomic abnormalities or injury patterns seen in these imaging studies may be sport-specific. For example, it has been reported that the prevalence of anatomic lumbar abnormalities seen on MRI are greater in gymnasts than in swimmers. This may be due to the repetitive loading pattern in gymnastics.[3]

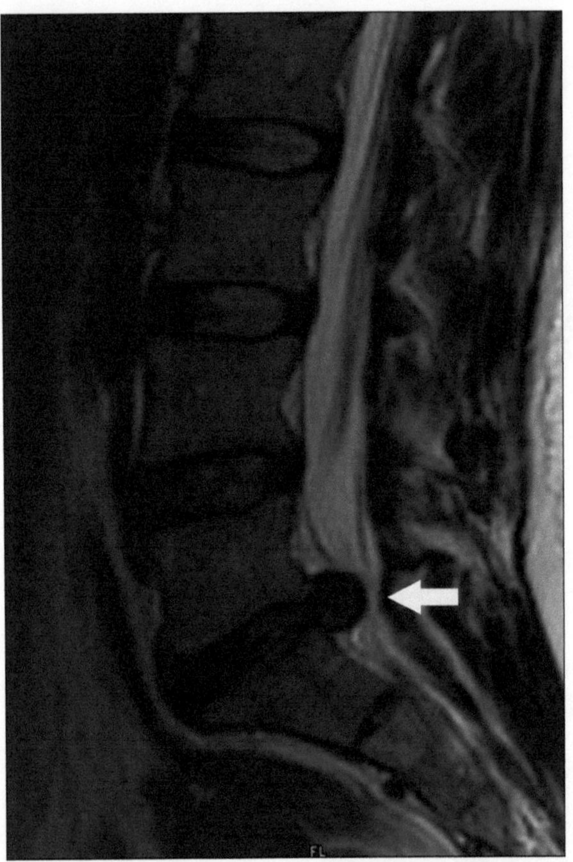

Fig. 12.3 Herniated disc. *Arrow* indicates retropulsed disc material

Specific Conditions

Disc Herniation

Disc herniation is described as the extrusion of nucleus pulposis in the epidural space through an annular tear. This may or may not compress a nerve or the spinal cord and cause symptoms. The incidence of disc herniation in athletes is unknown. The medical literature yields conflicting reports on the prevalence of disc herniation in athletes relative to the general population. Ong et al.,[7] in a pilot study, reported a decrease in disc signal intensity and disc height as well as increased disc displacement in Olympic athletes versus the general population. A total of 31 Olympic athletes who presented to the Olympic Polyclinic with low back pain and/or sciatica were examined with MRI. In contrast, Mundt, in a case-controlled epidemiologic study, failed to show an increase in disc herniation in athletes when compared to the general population.[8]

Disc herniations are classified as central, lateral, and far lateral, describing the direction of the extruded nucleus pulposus. The clinical significance is that the direction can indicate whether the herniation is compressing the exiting or traversing nerve root. For example, a far lateral L4/5 disc herniation typically affects the exiting nerve root L4. In contrast, a paracentral herniation could affect the L5 and possibly S1 traversing nerve roots. Compression of a nerve root can present as pain, weakness, or numbness.

Disc herniation in the lumbar region has clinical presentations that are different from those of other spine areas as the anatomy changes. Specifically, the spinal cord typically ends around L1/2. Compression of the conus and/or cauda equina presents with its own unique symptoms: polyradicular lower limb pain, saddle anesthesia, corresponding motor or sensory changes, and bladder or bowel dysfunction. However, as reported by Ong et al.,[7] in a cohort of athletes L5–S1 was the most common level for disc herniation, followed by L4/5. Patients with L4 nerve root compression can present with anterior thigh radicular pain, sensory changes (usually tingling or numbness), decreased patellar reflex, and tibialis anterior weakness. Patients with disc herniation affecting the L5 nerve root present with pain and sensory changes in the lateral lower leg and foot with possible extensor hallucis longus weakness and medial hamstring reflex change. Patients with S1 nerve root compression can have sensory changes and radicular pain down the posterior thigh to calf and possible plantar flexion weakness and decreased ankle jerk reflex. If the patient has a positive history with concordant objective findings in the physical examination, MRI is warranted after 6 weeks (sooner if surgery is planned). Once the lesion is well defined and correlates with the clinical scenario, treatment modalities can be discussed with the athlete.

The natural history of a herniated disc is favorable and correlates with the resorption of the extruded material. Symptoms usually diminish with resorption of the herniation and relief of the nerve root compression. Conservative management such as a nonsteroidal medication, activity modification, and physical therapy should be the first line of treatment for disc herniation, even in an athlete.[9] If symptoms persist, epidural steroid injections (e.g., transforaminal or selective nerve root injections at the involved level) may help with pain relief. A transforaminal epidural steroid injection consists of an anesthetic and steroid mixture placed at the level involved with the aid of fluoroscopy. The results of the injection can be both therapeutic and diagnostic in nature. The use of these injections in an athlete to benefit continued participation in competition has not been well documented and thus should be used cautiously.

When conservative therapy fails or when cauda equina syndrome is present, surgical intervention is warranted. Surgical outcomes in the general population have shown good results. Overall, microdiscectomy has produced results similar to those achieved with open discectomy, with smaller operative exposure.[10] The athlete's demand during physical activity, return to play, and high expectations pose an increased theoretical risk of failure postoperatively, although no randomized controlled trials have documented this phenomenon. In fact, several prospective and retrospective studies have suggested otherwise. A retrospective study of professional and Olympic athletes showed a return to sport for 53 of the 60 athletes with the return within an average of 5.2 months.[11] Wang et al.[12] reported excellent results in a prospective study of 14 athletes. They compared 14 elite athletes with age-matched general population controls using the SF-36 questionnaire after one- or two-level microdiscectomy. In all, 90% of the one-level microdiscectomy group returned to play whereas the two-level group did not. Although not statistically significant, all athletes scored improved values over the control group for bodily pain, physical role, general health, and social function.

Spondylolysis and Spondylolisthesis

The condition termed *spondylolysis* refers to a defect in the pars interarticularis.[13] In the athletic population, this is typically the result of repetitive hyperextension activity, such as that occurring in gymnasts, football linemen, weightlifters, javelin throwers, and pole vaulters. This condition is often accompanied by the presence of *spondylolisthesis* (forward displacement of one vertebra on its adjacent vertebra). There are multiple identified causes of spondylolisthesis, which has a reported incidence of 4.4% at age 6 and 6.0% in adults. In the athlete, the most common type is spondylolytic spondylolisthesis.[14,15] In adult athletes, spondylolysis is often a preexisting condition but may represent as a stress fracture in adolescent athletes. Although spondylolysis is asymptomatic in most individuals, as many as 13% of patients report long-term pain.[16]

Radicular symptoms are seen after repetitive extension trauma due to nerve root irritation as the root courses under the inflamed tissue of the resultant pars defect. The L5 level is most commonly affected, with 85%–95% incidence at this level in cases with bilateral pars defects.[16] The pathophysiologic mechanism is thought to be a combination of repetitive axial loading in the presence of extreme spine extension, overloading the posterior elements and leading to pars stress fracture and back pain.

Patients typically present with low back pain and radicular pain worsened by activity. With spondylolysis accompanied by a severe slip, the presence of a stiff-legged gait is often identified due to hamstring spasm and decreased forward flexion. Palpation may reveal paraspinal tenderness; and in patients with severe spondylolisthesis a palpable step-off may be present. Pain is often provoked by hyperextending and ipsilaterally rotating the lumbar spine.

Radiographic diagnosis is most often made utilizing upright lateral or oblique plain radiography. The classic finding of *a collar on the neck of the Scotty dog* (Fig. 12.4) is pathognomonic for a pars defect. Stability may be assessed using flexion/extension radiography. In cases where plain films are inconclusive, CT scans may be used to delineate the bony anatomy; these scans show disruption of the posterior arch at the level of the basivertebral vein. Thin-cut CT scans can also grade pars stress fractures into acute (early), healing (progressive), and chronic sclerotic (terminal) lesions. MRI is an

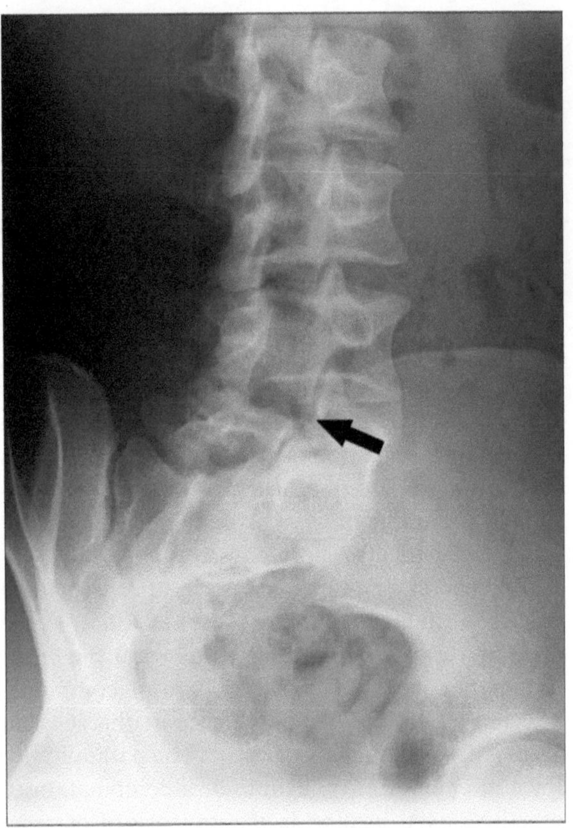

Fig. 12.4 Spondylolysis. *Arrow* denotes fracture (the "break in the collar of the Scotty dog")

Table 12.1 Grading of Spondylolisthesis

Grade	% Displacement
I	< 25
II	< 50
III	< 75
IV	< 100

additional useful adjunct for assessing neural compression and disc status in these patients. The most sensitive study to evaluate these stress reactions and impending fractures is SPECT.[17]

Mainstays of treatment focus on restriction of activity and extension-block bracing. Indications for bracing include symptomatic spondylolysis, low-grade spondylolisthesis (Table 12.1), and unilateral pars defects. Outcomes of bracing have been correlated negatively with age and delay in diagnosis[18] and positively with acute, unilateral lesions guided by SPECT imaging.[19,20] These studies reported good or excellent results in 78% of patients despite a union rate of only 25%, with 89% able to return to competitive sports within an average of 5.5 months after onset of treatment. Additional components of functional rehabilitation must focus on lumbar abdominal muscle and lower extremity strengthening and range of motion. Patients with higher-grade spondylolisthesis must be treated with more aggressive rehabilitation and must be followed more closely until skeletal maturation because of the potential for progression of their slip during adolescence.

Surgical treatment is indicated in patients with progressive listhesis or listhesis greater than grade 3, back pain resistant to conservative measures, or a neurologic deficit. Repair techniques include posterior transverse and spinous process wiring, translaminar screws, or pedicle screw-hook constructs. Fusion may be considered in the presence of disc degeneration or advanced spondylolisthesis. This may be accomplished by various standard techniques, although no outcome data focusing specifically on the athletic population are available to evaluate outcomes in these unique patients.

Piriformis Syndrome

At the turn of the previous century, a lack of understanding of herniation of the nucleus pulposis in the pathogenesis of sciatica symptoms led to the wide belief that this radicular pain was generated by *periarthritis* at the sacroiliac joint, involving the piriformis muscle and the sciatic nerve owing to their close anatomic relations.[21] Once Mixter and Barr[22] described nerve root compression by a herniated disc as the most common cause of sciatica, ideas of the piriformis as a pathophysiologic actor in this process fell out of favor. The term *piriformis syndrome* was subsequently introduced by Robinson[23] in 1947 and encompassed the diagnostic paradigm we attribute to the syndrome to this day. He recognized sciatica as a symptom and described piriformis syndrome as a specific type of sciatica arising from an abnormal condition of the piriformis muscle, typically traumatic in origin, with several cardinal features:

- History of trauma to the sacroiliac and gluteal regions
- Pain in the region of the sacroiliac joint, greater sciatic notch, and piriformis muscle that usually extends down the limb and causes difficulty with walking
- Acute exacerbation of pain caused by stooping or lifting (and moderate relief of pain by traction on the affected extremity with the patient in the supine position)
- Palpable sausage-shaped mass, tender to palpation, over the piriformis muscle on the affected side
- Positive lasegue (SLR with dorsiflexion) sign (Fig. 12.5)
- Gluteal atrophy, depending on the duration of the condition

The mechanism of piriformis syndrome continues to be controversial, as is the diagnosis itself. It remains a diagnosis of exclusion owing to a lack of consensus regarding diagnostic criteria, findings, studies, and treatment. Three hypotheses of pathophysiologic mechanisms have been proposed. The first, proposed by Robinson, attributes symptoms to sciatic nerve entrapment within adhesions of the

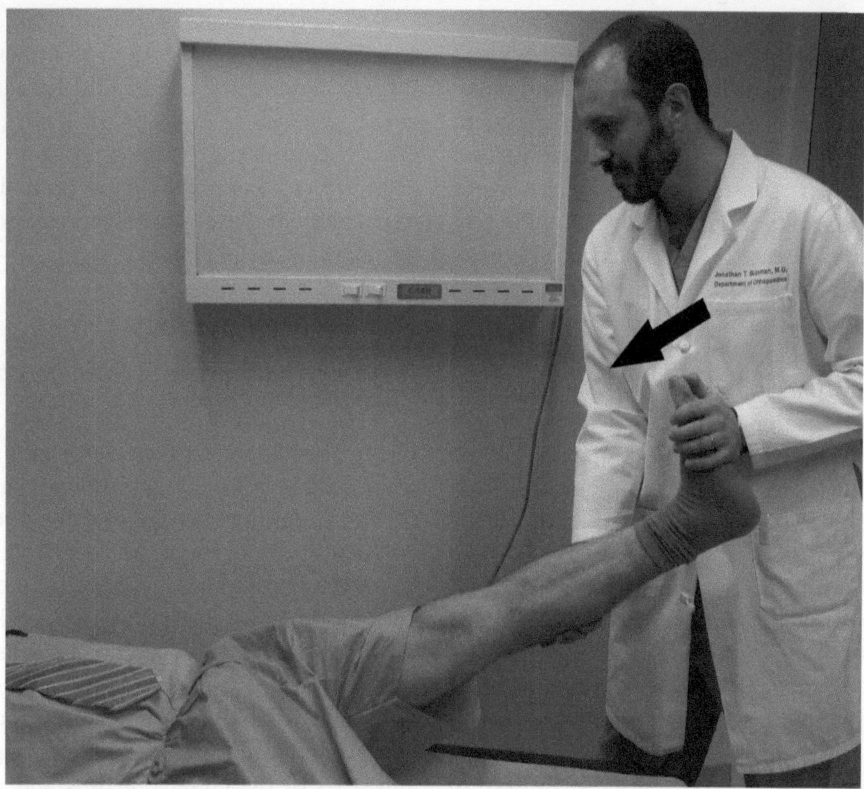

Fig. 12.5 Straight-leg raise with the foot passively dorsiflexed, eliciting the "Lasegue sign." *Arrow* denotes dorsiflexion of the ankle, increasing the diagnostic specificity of this test

piriformis muscle caused by the initial injury. Pecina proposed that compression of the nerve through the tendinous portion of the piriformis with internal hip rotation causes symptoms,[24] and Pace and Nagle believed that local muscle irritability caused by trauma result in a myofascial pain syndrome (treatable by trigger point injection) to be the etiologic cause of the piriformis syndrome.[25]

The incidence has been reported from 0.33% to 6.0% in patients with low back or lower extremity pain and sciatic symptoms.[25–28] Most patients present at 30–40 years of age, although the diagnosis has been made sporadically in patients less than 20 years of age with a male to female ratio of 6:1.[25]

The typical patient with piriformis syndrome complains of deep buttock pain with radiation down the back of the leg, at times to the calf, and rarely with weakness or numbness distally. The athlete may complain of hamstring tightness or a feeling of imminent tearing and back pain in addition to buttock pain.[27,29] The diagnosis is strongly suggested from a history of blunt trauma (even remote) to the gluteal area, although it may be exacerbated by overactivity of the hip rotators or from prolonged sitting on hard surfaces. Athletes involved in skiing, skating, gymnastics, and dance are particularly prone to this problem owing to the frequent hip flexion, internal rotation, and adduction required for their sport. Athletes involved in motor sports or cycling may become unable to continue activity because of prolonged sitting intolerance. Due to referred pain, athletes may additionally complain of pain with bowel movements, dyspareunia in females, and pain or paresthesia in the labia or scrotum.[27,29,30]

The physical examination often shows spasm and localized buttock pain with pain at the sciatic notch. Atrophy of the gluteus may be noted. Pain with the Lasegue sign may be positive, although it has been shown to be inconsistent.[31–34] The Frieberg sign (pain with forced internal rotation of the extended thigh) and Pace sign (pain with resisted external rotation and abduction of the thigh) may or may not be positive. The most consistent finding is a positive FADIR maneuver, which has been shown to be present in 100% of surgically proven cases.[35] The foot examination should also look for the presence of a Morton foot. Due to the presence of a prominent second metatarsal head, instability during push-off leads to foot pronation with compensatory hip and knee internal rotation. The hip external rotators contract to counteract this motion, which may lead to piriformis syndrome.[25,27,30,31,35–37]

Imaging is largely used to rule out other causes of similar presentation including herniated nucleus pulposus, tumor, abscess, spinal stenosis, posterior facet syndrome, and lateral recess stenosis.[38] The authors consider the diagnosis of piriformis syndrome one of exclusion.

The mainstays of management are nonoperative modalities. First, any biomechanical imbalance must be corrected, including leg-length discrepancy, pelvic obliquity, postural aberrance, and foot and ankle pathology. Nonsteroidal antiinflammatory drugs (NSAIDs) and other medications may be used acutely[30,34,39] and physical therapy instituted focusing first on stretching and then strengthening.[27,31,34] Ultrasound and massage have also been successfully used in this condition. Anesthetic and corticosteroid injections may be attempted if these modalities fail.[23,25,32,37,39–43]

Surgical treatment is reserved for patients who have failed all nonoperative treatments, although surgery may be indicated as the first-line treatment in the presence of myositis ossificans, infection, or pseudoaneurysm causing symptoms.[38] Open and arthroscopic techniques have been described and have been reported to give overall satisfactory results in refractory cases.[44,45]

Greater Trochanteric Pain Syndrome

Greater trochanteric pain syndrome (GTPS) is a common regional pain syndrome characterized by chronic, intermittent pain over the buttock and lateral aspect of the thigh that may radiate down the leg to the lateral knee.[4,46] Because the lumbar dermatomes overlap that of the iliotibial tract, GTPS may have symptoms similar to those of lumbar radiculopathy.

Trochanteric bursitis is the most common mechanism leading to GTPS, although tendinosis and tears of the gluteus medius and minimus may contribute to pain in this area.[4,47] GTPS was present in 20% of patients presenting to a tertiary referral spine clinic for evaluation of low back pain[4] and has been shown to be associated with low back pain in patients referred to medical, occupational health, and rheumatology clinics.[48] In the athletic population, GTPS is frequently seen in dancers who adduct beyond the midline, runners with a crossover gait, and runners who train in a single direction on sloped surfaces.[49,50]

Patients typically present with localized pain, with or without radicular symptoms. Often there is discomfort when sleeping on the affected side and a complaint of increased pain in this region when arising. The bursa is directly tender to palpation in most instances. The diagnosis is confirmed if there is no snapping sensation after passively internally rotating and adducting the hip and then abducting it.[49,51,52] Diagnostic injection with local anesthetic and corticosteroid may be undertaken.[4] Although typically a clinical diagnosis, a recent report by Walker et al.[53] demonstrated the utility of MRI and bone scintigraphy for the diagnosis and for determining the response to local injection. They demonstrated a correlation between lumbar degenerative disease, gluteus medius tendinopathy, and trochanteric bursitis and showed that the major risk factor for relapse after therapeutic injection was the presence of moderate to severe lumbar degenerative disease as seen on scintigraphic imaging.

Treatment is largely conservative for 6–8 weeks, focusing on rest, NSAIDs, stretching and strengthening, ice and/or warm packs, and ultrasound. Athletes who do not respond to these modalities are candidates for local injection of anesthetic and corticosteroid directly into the bursa.[49,51,54–56] Patients who fail these conservative measures may be candidates for surgical treatment. Several techniques have been described-including open and arthroscopic bursectomy and iliotibial band resection or release-with satisfactory results.[51,54]

Facet-Mediated Pain

Pain emanating from the lumbar Z-joints (or facet joints) has been estimated to occur in 15% of patients with chronic low back pain.[57] Anatomically, the lumbar facets are synovial, knuckle-sized joints innervated by two adjacent medial branches of the lumbar posterior rami. They serve mainly to limit motion. The sagittally oriented facets prevent axial rotation, and coronally oriented facets limit anteroposterior shear. The lumbar facets also provide 15% of the axial weight bearing of the spinal three-joint complex. This percentage rises in extension and falls in flexion.

Facet-mediated pain usually presents as localized paravertebral pain provoked by extension and/or rotation of the lumbar spine.[58] Theoretically, facet-mediated pain may also be provoked with forward bending because of stretching of sensitized nocioceptors in the facet capsule. Facet-mediated pain may also extend into the lower limb in a sclerotomal distribution. The causes of facet-mediated pain are uncertain but include hyperextension of the lumbar spine, arthropathies, meniscoid entrapment, microtrauma, and synovial cysts.[59] This uncertainty is compounded by several prospective trials demonstrating a lack of correlation between the history and physical examination findings and significant pain relief with anesthetic facet blocks.[57,60,61] The history and physical examination cannot definitively distinguish facet-mediated pain from other sources of low back pain. Imaging studies are also poor in identifying facet-mediated pain. Facet degeneration is seen commonly on CT scans and plain films of asymptomatic individuals.[59,62] There remains no noninvasive gold standard test for diagnosing facet-mediated pain. The current diagnostic gold standards are facet intraarticular anesthetic injections and/or two-level medial branch blocks. These interventional tests can be used if conservative treatment fails and if more specific treatment is contemplated.

An interdisciplinary treatment plan is employed with facet-mediated pain. An exercise program for facet pain should include a flexion-biased lumbar dynamic stabilization program. The goal of any lumbar stabilization is to maximize motor control of all the muscles that influence spinal movement. The exercise program should also be designed to unload the posterior elements. Eliminating excess anterior pelvic tilt prevents compensatory lumbar spine extension. Manual therapy or manipulation appears to work best for acute facet pain, and the treatment effect is often short-lived.[59] There is considerable controversy about manipulation for chronic facet-mediated pain but little compelling research. Facet corticosteroid injections may work to reduce pain, but their efficacy has not been borne out by randomized controlled trials.[63,64] Radiofrequency neural ablation of the medial branches of the lumbar posterior rami may be an option.[65] Surgical fusion does not appear to be that useful.[59]

Sacroiliac Joint

The SIJ has been implicated as a pain generator in young athletes. Critics argued that with a scant 4° of movement and 1.6 mm of total translation the SIJ was unlikely to be a pain source.[66] The SIJ syndrome is difficult to examine, diagnose, and treat. Recent injection studies confirm the SIJ as a pain generator.[67,68] The surrounding ligaments likely also have pain-generating capability. Furthermore, the SIJ has been a known and accepted source of pain in the seronegative spondyloarthropathies (e.g., ankylosing spondylitis) and in third trimester pregnant females, in whom the hormone relaxin causes ligamentous laxity and gapping of the SIJ.

Anatomically, the SIJ is an auricular or C-shaped diarthrodial synovial joint containing both hyaline and fibrocartilage that serves to transmit and dissipate upper trunk loads to the lower limbs during weight bearing. The SIJ is arguably innervated from the anterior and posterior rami of L4–S4.[66] Grob et al., in a cadaveric histologic study, demonstrated that the innervation was exclusively from the posterior rami of S1–4.[67] A potentially wide range of segmental innervation may account for the wide range of referred pain, even distal to the knee.

As with the diagnosis of facet-mediated pain, there is no completely validated method to diagnosis a painful SIJ using the history, physical examination, or radiography. The history and physical examination often lead the clinician in the correct direction. Patients frequently point to their posterosuperior iliac spine (PSIS) as the site of maximum tenderness.[68,70] The pain may be referred in a variable distribution, but the core referral zone is from the PSIS to the greater trochanter.[68,69] Typically, the pain is worsened with transitional maneuvers such as going from sit to stand positions. The physical examination includes quality of motion assessment (Gillet test) and provocative maneuvers (Patrick, Gaenslen, sacral thrust test).[71] Bone scans may be beneficial in runners as they can rule out pelvic stress fractures, which may present similarly to SIJ pain.

The treatment of SIJ dysfunction is based on the etiology; thus, an integrated approach using osteopathic medicine, chiropractic knowledge, manual physical therapy, and medical management is best. Usually, a focused exercise program is started to correct muscle imbalances. Inhibited muscles such as the gluteus maximus, gluteus medius, and hip external rotators are facilitated; and tight muscles, such as the hip flexors and the hamstrings, are stretched. These tight muscles may cause secondary myofascial pain, which may also need to be addressed. Others also advocate manipulation to correct pelvic girdle dysfunctions observed on an osteopathic or segmental examination. In addition, medications, education, and sacroiliac belts all may have roles in the treatment of SIJ dysfunction. In particular, SIJ injections have been used not only to treat SIJ pain but also to diagnose it. These injections should be performed under fluoroscopic guidance to confirm entry into the joint. Unproven methods of treatment include SIJ fusion, SIJ denervation, and prolotherapy. Acupuncture has also been tried with anecdotal success.

Conclusion

The athlete with radicular pain presents a challenge for the clinician. With the aid of an appropriate history, physical examination, and diagnostic studies, an accurate diagnosis is readily attainable. Most of these patients do well with appropriate conservative management, which serves as the mainstay of treatment for most of the aforementioned conditions. However, surgical interventions have proved to produce satisfactory results in recalcitrant cases.

References

1. Gerbino PG, d'Hemecourt PA. Does football cause an increase in degenerative disease of the lumbar spine? Curr Sports Med Rep 2002;1(1):47–51.
2. Greene HS, Cholewicki J, Galloway MT, et al. A history of low back injury is a risk factor for

recurrent back injuries in varsity athletes. Am J Sports Med 2001;29(6):795–800.
3. Lawrence JP, Greene HS, Grauer JN. Back pain in athletes. J Am Acad Orthop Surg 2006;14(13):726–35.
4. Tortolani PJ, Carbone JJ, Quartararo LG. Greater trochanteric pain syndrome in patients referred to orthopedic spine specialists. Spine J 2002;2(4):251–4.
5. Slipman CW, Sternfeld E. The predictive value of provocative sacroiliac joint stress maneuvers in the diagnosis of sacroiliac joint syndrome. Arch Phys Med Rehabil 1998;79(3):288–92.
6. Bigos S, Bowyer O, Braen G, et al. Acute Low Back Problems in Adults: Clinical Practice Guideline. Agency for Health Care Policy and Research. Vol 14. Rockille, MD: U.S. Department of Health and Human Services; 1994.
7. Ong A, Anderson J, Roche J. A pilot study of the prevalence of lumbar disc degeneration in elite athletes with lower back pain at the Sydney 2000 Olympic Games. Br J Sports Med 2003;37(3):263–6.
8. Mundt DJ. An epidemiologic study of sports and weight lifting as possible risk factors for herniated lumbar and cervical discs; the Northeast Collaborative Group on Low Back Pain. Am J Sports Med 1993;21(6):854–60.
9. Dec KL. Nonoperative versus operative treatment of acute disc injuries in athletes. Curr Sports Med Rep 2002;1(1):35–42.
10. Gibson JN, Waddell G. Surgical interventions for lumbar disc prolapse. Cochrane Database Syst Rev 2007;(2):1350.
11. Watkins RG, Williams LA, Watkins RG 3rd. Microscopic lumbar discectomy results for 60 cases in professional and Olympic athletes. Spine J 2003;3(2):100–5.
12. Wang JC, Shapiro MS, Hatch JD, et al. The outcome of lumbar discectomy in elite athletes. Spine 1999;24(6):570–3.
13. D'Hemecourt PA, Gerbino PG, Micheli LJ. Back injuries in the young athlete. Clin Sports Med 2000;19(4):663–79.
14. Fredrickson BE, Baker D, McHolick WJ, et al. The natural history of spondylolysis and spondylolisthesis. J Bone Joint Surg Am 1984;66(5):699–707.
15. Wiltse LL, Newman PH, Macnab I. Classification of spondylolysis and spondylolisthesis. Clin Orthop 1976;117:23–9.
16. Saraste H. Long-term clinical and radiological follow-up of spondylolysis and spondylolisthesis. J Pediatr Orthop 1987;7(6):631–8.
17. Bellah RD, Summerville DA, Treves ST, et al. Low-back pain in adolescent athletes: detection of stress injury to the pars interarticularis with SPECT. Radiology 1991;180(2):509–12.
18. Steiner ME, Micheli LJ. Treatment of symptomatic spondylolysis and spondylolisthesis with the modified Boston brace. Spine 1985;10(10):937–43.
19. Anderson K, Sarwark JF, Conway JJ, et al. Quantitative assessment with SPECT imaging of stress injuries of the pars interarticularis and response to bracing. J Pediatr Orthop 2000;20(1):28–33.
20. Sys J, Michielson J, Bracke P, et al. Nonoperative treatment of active spondylolysis in elite athletes with normal X-ray findings: literature review and results of conservative treatment. Eur Spine J 2001;10(6):498–504.
21. Yeoman W. The relation of arthritis of the sacro-iliac joint to sciatica. Lancet 1928;2:119–22.
22. Mixter WJ, Barr JS. Rupture of the intervertebral disc with involvement of the spinal canal. N Engl J Med 1934;211:210–5.
23. Robinson D. Pyriformis syndrome in relation to sciatic pain. Am J Surg 1947;73:355–8.
24. Pecina M. Contribution to the etiological explanation of the piriformis syndrome. Acta Anat Basel 1979;105(2):181–7.
25. Pace JB, Nagle D. Piriformis syndrome. West J Med 1976;124(6):435–9.
26. Bernard TN, Kirkaldy-Willis WH. Recognizing specific characteristics of nonspecific low back pain. Clin Orthop 1987; 217:266–80.
27. Parziale JR, Hudgins TH, Fishman LM. The piriformis syndrome. Am J Orthop 1996;25(12):819–23.
28. Goldner JL. Piriformis compression causing low back and lower extremity pain. Am J Orthop 1997;26(5):316–8.
29. McCrory P, Bell S. Nerve entrapment syndromes as a cause of pain in the hip, groin and buttock. Sports Med 1999;27:261–74.
30. Barton PM. Piriformis syndrome: a rational approach to management. Pain 1991;47(3):345–52.
31. Hughes SS, Goldstein MN, Hicks DG, et al. Extrapelvic compression of the sciatic nerve: an unusual cause of pain about the hip-report of five cases. J Bone Joint Surg Am 1992;74(10):1553–9.
32. Jankiewicz JJ, Hennrikus WL, Houkom JA. The appearance of the piriformis muscle syndrome in computed tomography and magnetic resonance imaging: a case report and review of the literature. Clin Orthop 1991;262:205–9.
33. Solheim LF, Siewers P, Paus B. The piriformis muscle syndrome: sciatic nerve entrapment treated with section of the piriformis muscle. Acta Orthop Scand 1981;52(1):73–5.
34. Vandertop WP, Bosma NJ. The piriformis syndrome: a case report. J Bone Joint Surg Am 1991;73(7):1095–7.
35. Benson ER, Schutzer SF. Posttraumatic piriformis syndrome: diagnosis and results of operative treatment. J Bone Joint Surg Am 1999;81(7):941–9.
36. Freiberg A. Sciatic pain and its relief by operations on muscle and fascia. Arch Surg 1937;34:337–49.
37. Hallin RP. Sciatic pain and the piriformis muscle. Postgrad Med 1983;74(2):69–72.
38. Melamed HM. Soft tissue problems of the hip in athletes. Sports Med Arthrosc 2002;10:168–75.
39. Rich B. When sciatica is not disc disease. Phys Sports Med 1992;20:105–15.
40. Beaton L. Relation of sciatic nerve and subdivision to piriformis muscle. Anat Rec 1937;70:1–3.
41. Melzack R. Prolonged relief of pain by brief, intense transcutaneous somatic stimulation. Pain 1975;1(4):357–73.
42. Wyant GM. Chronic pain syndromes and their treatment. III. The piriformis syndrome. Can Anaesth Soc J 1979;26(4):305–8.

43. Kirkaldy-Willis WH, Hill RJ. A more precise diagnosis for low-back pain. Spine 1979;4(2):102–109.
44. Dezawa A, Kusano S, Miki H. Arthroscopic release of the piriformis muscle under local anesthesia for piriformis syndrome. Arthroscopy 2003;19(5):554–7.
45. Mullin V, de Rosayro M. Caudal steroid injection for treatment of piriformis syndrome. Anesth Analg 1990;71(6):705–7.
46. Shbeeb MI, Matteson EL. Trochanteric bursitis (greater trochanter pain syndrome). Mayo Clin Proc 1996;71(6):565–9.
47. Kingzett-Taylor A, Tirman PF, Feller J, et al. Tendinosis and tears of gluteus medius and minimus muscles as a cause of hip pain: MR imaging findings. AJR Am J Roentgenol 1999;173(4):1123–6.
48. Collee G, Dijkmans BA, Vandenbroucke JP, et al. Greater trochanteric pain syndrome (trochanteric bursitis) in low back pain. Scand J Rheumatol 1991;20(4):262–6.
49. Arendt E. Growing pain in the athlete. In: Griffin L, ed. Orthopaedic Knowledge Update: Sports Medicine. Rosemont, IL: AAOS; 1998:281–9.
50. Generini S, Matucci-Cerinic M. Iliopsoas bursitis in rheumatoid arthritis. Clin Exp Rheumatol 1993;11(5):549–51.
51. Slawski DP, Howard RF. Surgical management of refractory trochanteric bursitis. Am J Sports Med 1997;25(1):86–9.
52. Hays M. The trochanteric syndrome. J Bone Joint Surg Am 1963;45:657–61.
53. Walker P, Kannangara S, Bruce WJ, et al. Lateral hip pain: does imaging predict response to localized injection? Clin Orthop 2007;457:144–9.
54. Little H. Trochanteric bursitis: a common cause of pelvic girdle pain. Can Med Assoc J 1979;120(4):456–8.
55. Clancy WG. Runners' injuries. Part 2: Evaluation and treatment of specific injuries. Am J Sports Med 1980;8(4):287–9.
56. Broadhurst N. Iliopsoas tendinitis and bursitis. Aust Fam Physician 1995;24(7):1303.
57. Schwarzer AC, Aprill CN, Derby R, et al. The relative contributions of the disc and zygapophyseal joint in chronic low back pain. Spine 1994;19(7):801–6.
58. Helbig T, Lee CK. The lumbar facet syndrome. Spine 1988;13(1):61–4.
59. Dreyer SJ, Dreyfuss PH. Low back pain and the zygapophysial (facet) joints. Arch Phys Med Rehabil 1996;77(3):290–300.
60. Schwarzer AC, Derby R, Aprill CN, et al. Pain from the lumbar zygapophysial joints: a test of two models. J Spinal Disord 1994;7(4):331–6.
61. Revel ME, Listrat VM, Chevalier XJ, et al. Facet joint block for low back pain: identifying predictors of a good response. Arch Phys Med Rehabil 1992;73(9):824–8.
62. Schwarzer AC, Wang SC, O'Driscoll D, et al. The ability of computed tomography to identify a painful zygapophysial joint in patients with chronic low back pain. Spine 1995;20(8):907–12.
63. Carette S, Leclaire R, Marcoux S, et al. Epidural corticosteroid injections for sciatica due to herniated nucleus pulposus. N Engl J Med 1997;336(23):1634–40.
64. Lilius G, Laasonen EM, Myllynen, et al. Lumbar facet joint syndrome: a randomised clinical trial. J Bone Joint Surg Br 1989;71(4):681–4.
65. Bogduk N. Evidence-informed management of chronic low back pain with facet injections and radiofrequency neurotomy. Spine J 2008;8(1):56–64.
66. Bernard TN, Cassidy D. The sacroiliac joint syndrome: pathophysiology, diagnosis, and management. In: Frymoyer JW, ed. The Adult Spine: Principles and Practice. Philadelphia: Lippincott-Raven; 1997:2343–66.
67. Grob KR, Neuhuber WL, Kissling ROI. Innervation of the sacroiliac joint of the human. Z Rheumatol 1995;54(2):117–22.
68. Fortin JD, Aprill CN, Ponthieux B, et al. Sacroiliac joint: pain referral maps upon applying a new injection/arthrography technique. Part I: Asymptomatic volunteers. Spine 1994;19(13):1475–82.
69. Fortin JD, Dwyer AP, West S. Sacroiliac joint: pain referral maps upon applying a new injection/arthrography technique. Part II: Clinical evaluation. Spine 1994;19(13):1483–9.
70. Fortin JD, Falco FJ. The Fortin finger test: an indicator of sacroiliac pain. Am J Orthop 1997;26(7):477–80.
71. Hancock MJ, Maher CG, Latimer J, et al. Systematic review of tests to identify the disc, SIJ or facet joint as the source of low back pain. Eur Spine J 2007;16(10):1539–50.

Chapter 13
Vascular Injuries in the Lower Limb of Athletes

Ellen Casey, Paul H. Lento, Joseph M. Ihm, and Heron Rodriguez

Introduction

Athletes are susceptible to a wide variety of traumatic and nontraumatic vascular injuries to the lower limb. The incidence of vascular injuries in the athletic population is rising, particularly in sports characterized by repetitive motion or high-speed collisions.[1]

Despite the increasing incidence, vascular injuries are often unrecognized in the athletic population. There are several contributing factors that make the diagnosis of sports-related vascular injuries difficult. One factor is the lack of obvious abnormalities during the routine physical examination; therefore, without provocative testing or appropriate imaging, the athlete's exercise-induced symptoms may be undetected. Another reason is the lack of suspicion of vascular injury in athletes. This is not only because lower limb complaints in an athlete are most likely to be due to musculoskeletal pathology but also that physicians may not be accustomed to considering vascular pathology in a young, otherwise healthy athlete. Finally, sports medicine physicians may be delayed in diagnosing vascular injuries due to decreased familiarity with the vascular anatomy of the lower limb or with the typical presentation of vascular pathology. This is partly due to the relatively low incidence of vascular injuries within the realm of sports medicine as well as the paucity of sports medicine literature dedicated to vascular injuries in sports. Regardless of the reason, the failure to diagnosis a vascular injury in the lower limb can lead to devastating consequences, including retirement from sport, loss of limb function, or loss of the limb itself. The relevant arterial anatomy of the lower extremity is detailed in Figure 13.1.

The intent of this chapter is to present a review of vascular injuries and to provide sports medicine practitioners with a reference for the presentation, evaluation, and management of the lower extremity sports-related vascular injuries, including a guide to return to sport where appropriate.

Traumatic Injuries

Trauma to the lower extremities is classified as penetrating or blunt. It occurs in a variety of sports, particularly those with a risk of high-velocity contact. The management of penetrating injuries to the lower extremities is beyond the scope of this article but a variety of excellent references are available in the current literature, including *Vascular Trauma* by Rich et al.[2] Nonpenetrating or blunt trauma most commonly affects the popliteal artery, followed by the common femoral, superficial femoral, and anterior tibial arteries.[3] Patients with this type of injury can seek medical attention hours to days after their injury and may present with a history of lower extremity trauma resulting in pain, swelling, and sensorimotor deficits due to occlusion, dissection, or aneurysm of the involved artery.

E. Casey (✉)
Resident Physician, Department of Physical Medicine and Rehabilitation, Rehabilitation Institute of Chicago/ Northwestern Memorial Hospital, Chicago, IL, USA

V. Akuthota, S.A. Herring (eds.), *Nerve and Vascular Injuries in Sports Medicine*,
DOI 10.1007/978-0-387-76600-3_13, © Springer Science+Business Media, LLC 2009

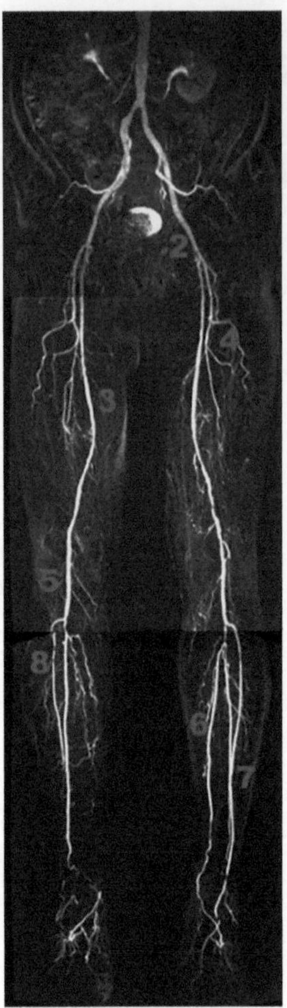

Fig. 13.1 Magnetic resonance angiography (MRA) of the lower limb arterial anatomy. (1) External iliac artery; (2) common femoral artery; (3) superficial femoral artery; (4) deep femoral artery; (5) popliteal artery; (6) anterior tibial artery (not visualized on the right leg); (7) posterior tibial artery; (8) peroneal artery. Courtesy of Dr. Heron Rodriguez

Traumatic Arterial Injuries

External Iliac Artery/Common Femoral Artery

The incidence of trauma to the external iliac artery or common femoral artery has been reported to be as low at 0.4%–7.0% of all vascular injuries.[4] These injuries are rare because the external iliac and femoral arteries are generally well protected by the bony pelvis and femoral sheath. However, the portion that is least protected and most frequently injured is where the external iliac artery travels between the superior pubic ramus and the inguinal ligament and femoral artery within the femoral canal. The sports medicine literature contains several case reports of blunt trauma to the external iliac or common femoral artery injury, most often due to bicycle handlebar trauma (Fig. 13.2). The proposed mechanism of injury includes compression of the artery against underlying osseous structures, leading to intimal disruption, luminal fibrosis, subintimal fibrosis, or intramural hematoma.[5,6]

Patients with blunt trauma to the external iliac or common femoral artery can present hours to months after the initial inciting event. They may have gradually worsening symptoms of lower limb claudication or develop acute lower limb ischemia. These patients are most commonly children, and they may complain of abdominal, pelvic, or lower extremity pain, paresthesias, or weakness.[6] The examination may be

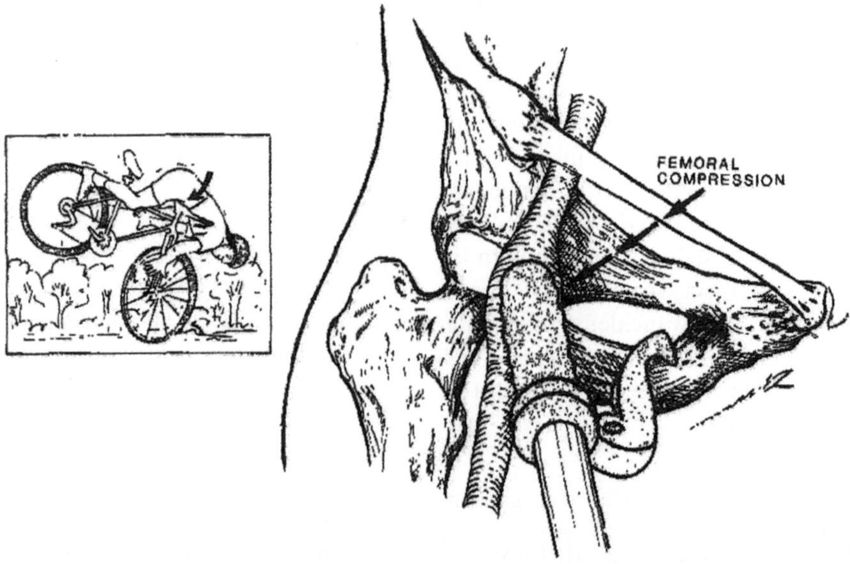

Fig. 13.2 Compression injury to the common femoral artery from handle bars impact during a fall. From Sarfati MR, Galt SW, Treiman GS, et al.[6] With permission of Elsevier Limited

within normal limits or there may be evidence of the classically described 5 P's of arterial occlusion: pain, pallor, paresthesias, pulselessness, and paralysis. Because as many as 25% of patients have an arterial injury despite normal distal pulses,[7] a patient with a history of blunt trauma and any of the above signs or symptoms deserves further evaluation. A thorough physical examination should include measurement of ankle pressures, and those with a more than 10–20 mm Hg side-to-side difference should undergo noninvasive evaluation, including Doppler ultrasonography, duplex scanning, and/or arteriography (Strength of recommendation = A).[8] Treatment options for patients are almost always surgical, including repair, resection, graft placement, bypass, or ligation of the damaged portion of the artery. According to various review articles, the preferred interventions are repair and resection (Strength of recommendation = C).[9]

Popliteal Artery

Popliteal artery injury is a well documented complication of trauma to the knee. The popliteal artery is relatively immobile as it is tethered between the adductor hiatus and the soleus arch, which increases its susceptibility to injury during trauma. There are reports of popliteal artery injury due to blunt trauma, hyperextension, dislocation, periarticular fractures, and ligamentous rupture in martial arts, football, rugby, kayaking, weight lifting, wind surfing, and cycling.

Popliteal artery injury occurs in 30%–50% of cases of complete knee dislocation,[10] but clinicians should also have a high index of suspicion of arterial injury with knee hyperextension or ligamentous rupture. Kennedy[11] showed that only 50° of hyperextension is needed to tear the popliteal artery, and Varnell et al.[12] demonstrated that there is no significant difference in the incidence of arterial injury with ligamentous instability with dislocation versus ligamentous instability without dislocation.

The types of arterial damage sustained during these injuries include intimal injury, avulsion, occlusion, or aneurysm formation that may be complicated by rupture or the formation of thrombosis or emboli. Popliteal artery trauma is usually obvious in open knee injuries, but recognition of arterial injury after blunt knee injuries is usually delayed. If the extent of the injury causes flow interruption in the popliteal artery, patients may complain of pain, paresthesias, or loss of sensation or motor function distal to the knee. More commonly, injury creates an intimal flap with initial preservation of flow and complete lack of symptoms. As the abnormalities in the arterial wall progress, flow becomes compromised. Because of this, and given the frequency at which arterial injury occurs after knee dislocations, all patients diagnosed or suspected to have a knee dislocation require immediate evaluation by an experienced vascular specialist (SOR = C). In most cases, an angiogram—obtained with conventional angiography, commuted tomography angiography (CTA), or magnetic resonance angiography (MRA) is needed to rule out an intimal injury effectively. Alternatively, experienced vascular specialists have shown that serial measurement of the ankle brachial index (ABI) and the use of duplex ultrasonography are effective management strategies. It must be emphasized that this noninvasive strategy is advocated only for centers with significant experience in the management of these injuries and that the prompt use of angiography frequently prevents catastrophic delays in the diagnosis of this arterial injury that can result in limb loss. If there are obvious signs of limb ischemia, immediate surgical intervention is needed because ischemia for more than 4–6 hours can cause irreversible neurologic damage and muscle necrosis; this in turn has been shown to correlate with adverse outcomes, including limb loss.[13] In the presence of acute limb ischemia, any delay to obtaining imaging studies could prove catastrophic. Standard management includes surgical exploration with definitive treatment being primary repair or, more commonly, a short bypass with a saphenous vein graft.[14] If ischemia is present for several hours, fasciotomies to treat or prevent compartment syndrome are mandatory. Most patients in the case studies underwent outpatient physical therapy after their surgical sites were healed and were gradually transitioned back into sport. It is standard of practice to perform regular follow-up to assess graft patency with Doppler ultrasonography several weeks postoperatively and then one or two times per year thereafter (SOR = B).[15]

Anterior Tibial Artery

The anterior tibial artery branches off the popliteal artery at the distal border of the popliteus muscle and provides blood to the anterior compartment of the lower limb and the dorsum of the foot. The anterior tibial artery is particularly susceptible to injury with trauma of the anterolateral knee, shin, or ankle (Fig. 13.1). Arterial injury can lead to extravasation of blood into the surrounding soft tissues, which acts as a false wall, or pseudoaneurysm. This false aneurysm is inherently unstable and therefore highly predisposed to expansion, rupture, or the development of thromboses. Such an injury is not only described in the context of high-velocity blunt trauma to the knee or proximal shin; it has also occurred in the setting of severe hyperplantar flexion and inversion ankle injury.

The clinical presentation of anterior tibial artery pseudoaneurysm is variable. There are limited case studies in the literature: One described a patient who was kicked in the anterior lower leg during Tae Kwon Do and developed distal microemboli over the course of months and another was a baseball player who sustained a lateral ankle sprain during a slide who presented with a pulsatile hematoma secondary to a distal aneurysm (Fig. 13.3).[16] In general, patients with injury to the anterior tibial artery present with lower extremity injury or trauma with gradually worsening swelling, pain, or sensorimotor impairment distal to the knee. Depending on the size, location, or presence of thrombus, patients with an anterior tibial artery pseudoaneurysm may have decreased pulses, hematoma, or evidence of ischemia (from microembolization or thrombus occlusion) on examination. They can also be completely asymptomatic.

Evaluation of a patient with a suspected anterior artery pseudoaneurysm should include ultrasonography, CTA, MRA, or conventional angiography to confirm the diagnosis (SOR = B). In all cases documented in the literature, direct surgical correction is the preferred treatment; this includes exploration, thrombectomy, and ligation of the affected portion of the artery. Alternatively, percutaneous interventions (e.g., stenting, coiling) are available, but some have found them inferior to surgical repair due to increased risk for embolization and digital ischemia.

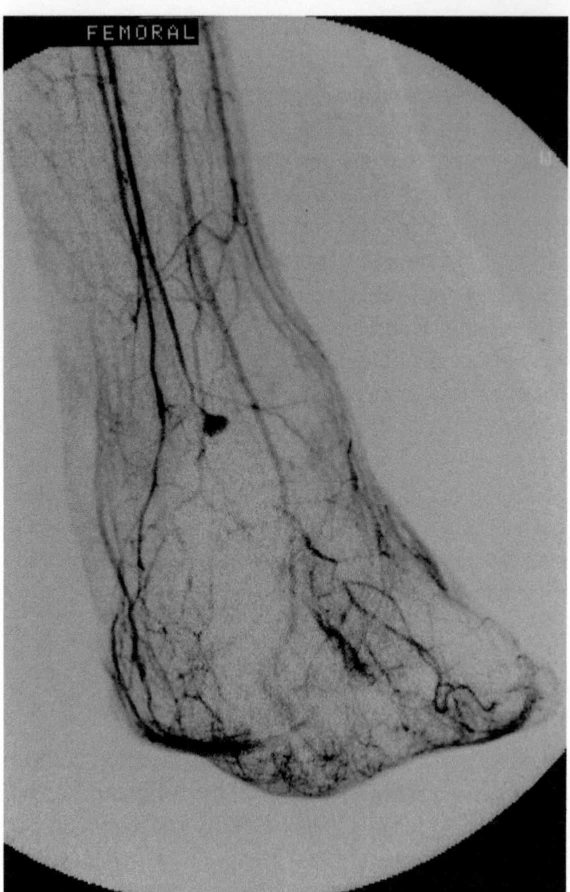

Fig. 13.3 Anterior tibial artery pseudoaneurysm from an inversion ankle injury. From Dhawan A, Doukas WC. Acute compartment syndrome of the foot following an inversion injury of the ankle with disruption of the anterior tibial artery: a case report. J Bone Joint Surg Am 2003;85:528–32. Used with permission from JBJS, Inc.

Traumatic Compartment Syndrome

There are at least 20 reported cases of acute compartment syndrome due to blunt trauma in sports. In order of decreasing incidence, they are handball, soccer, rugby, cycling, kickboxing, karate, lacrosse, baseball, and football.[17] Compartment syndrome of the lower extremities can occur in the thigh as well as the calf, but the larger fascial compartments of the thigh make this syndrome much less common there than below the knee. The anterior compartment is the most frequently affected compartment in the thigh, and the most frequent etiology in athletes is contusion.[18] Other causes include acute muscle overuse,[19] blunt trauma, fractures, and underlying coagulopathy.

A typical presentation is a patient with a history of lower extremity trauma with acute, excessive thigh or calf pain out of proportion to the pain expected from the inciting event. The examination is notable for a tense, edematous thigh or calf, increased pain with passive stretch of the muscles in the affected compartment, paresthesias, paralysis, distal hypothermia, and diminished or absent pulses.[20]

In most cases, acute compartment syndrome is a clinical diagnosis. However, interstitial pressure monitoring can be included, particularly when the clinical presentation is complicated by a patient with decreased mental status or altered sensorium. Measurement of compartment pressures is controversial because of the wide range of values thought to be diagnostic (normal is 0–8 mm Hg; abnormal is anywhere from > 30 to 55 mm Hg),[21] which contributes to the low sensitivity and specificity of intracompartmental pressures. Magnetic resonance imaging (MRI) can also be used in the diagnostic workup as it can show edema, hemorrhage, hematoma, vessel injury, and inflammation. Laboratory data, including creatine phosphokinase and myoglobinuria assays, coagulation parameters, and a complete blood count are also helpful. At our institution and many others, intracompartmental pressures and other studies are rarely obtained; we advocate the liberal use of fasciotomies when the history and physical examination findings are suggestive of compartment syndrome (SOR = C).

The standard management for patients with acute compartment syndrome is emergent fasciotomy and hematoma evacuation (SOR = A). Longer intervals from injury to decompression are associated with increased complications including bleeding, myonecrosis, wound infection, amputation, sepsis, and death. Fortunately, these complications have not been documented in the athletic population; they are most often associated with polytrauma from motor vehicle accidents.

Thigh contusion without the development of acute compartment syndrome is a less severe manifestation within a spectrum of traumatic vascular injuries due to sports-related blunt trauma. Although there are no true guidelines to distinguish between these two entities, a multicenter analysis of 28 patients with documented compartment syndrome of the thigh showed that pain with passive stretch was the most sensitive sign, and a lack of distal pulses was the least sensitive finding among conscious patients with documented compartment syndrome.[21] If there is any question of the presence of compartment syndrome, immediate workup and management as described above is mandatory (SOR = A).

Traumatic Venous Injuries

Deep Vein Thromboses

Deep vein thromboses (DVTs) can occur as a direct result of sports-induced trauma or as a complication of other sports-related behaviors. Virchow's triad describes the pathophysiology of a DVT: venous stasis, intimal injury, and coagulation diathesis. Risk factors in the general medical population include immobility, pregnancy, surgery, cancer, hormone replacement therapy, and smoking. Risk factors with particular relevance to the athletic population include immobilization (during prolonged travel or due to healing from another injury), coagulopathy (equal prevalence in elite athletes and the general population),[22] intense exercise, fracture, surgery, polycythemia and hemoconcentration due to dehydration or blood doping, and anabolic steroid abuse.[23,24] Traumatic DVTs in athletes have been reported in the popliteal, posterior tibial, and peroneal veins from direct, compressive, or shearing forces due to rapid knee hyperextension, knee dislocation, or lower extremity torsion while kicking or tackling.[25]

Athletes with a DVT may or may not report a history of trauma; and they often have the same classic complaints of leg swelling and pain as are described in the general population. Additional signs include ecchymoses, positive Homan's sign (pain with passive ankle dorsiflexion), and a palpable mass or chord. Unfortunately, the unreliability of physical examination alone for diagnosing or excluding DVT has been largely documented.[26] One meta-analysis illustrated the limitations of a variety of physical examination maneuvers; a positive Homan's sign has a sensitivity and specificity for DVT of 11%–56% and 11%–61%, respectively, and corresponding figures regarding the presence of edema on physical examination was found to be 42%–78% and 26%–67%, respectively.[27] Duplex ultrasonography is the modality of choice for evaluating patients suspected to have DVT. A positive test demonstrates thrombus-filled veins that have lost their normal compressibility. In rare occasions, venography is needed for cases when ultrasonography fails to define the presence of a thrombus.[28]

Controversy exists regarding the extent of the workup needed to rule out an underlying hypercoagulable state in a young, otherwise healthy athlete diagnosed with a DVT in whom no additional risk factors for thromboembolism are present. Such a workup may include evaluation of the patient's complete blood count (CBC), erythrocyte sedimentation rate (ESR), C-reactive protein (CRP), activated partial thromboplastin time (aPTT), prothrombin time (PT), international normalized ratio (INR), proteins C and S, lupus anticoagulant, antithrombin III, factor V Leiden, prothrombin gene mutation, rapid plasma regain (RPR), and antinuclear antibody (ANA). Our current practice is to refer young patients with idiopathic DVT for hematologic consultation, and the consulting hematologist determines the extent of the investigation.[29]

The mainstay of treatment for a DVT is anticoagulation and compression therapy to prevent pulmonary embolism, postthrombotic syndrome (PTS), and lower extremity pain. Initial anticoagulation is achieved with therapeutic heparin or low-molecular-weight heparin with transition to Coumadin (warfarin) with a goal INR of 2–3. Coumadin is continued for 3–6 months. Potential long-term sequelae include chronic venous insufficiency, or PTS. PTS is characterized by a spectrum of symptoms: heavy or achy limbs, edema, dermatitis, hyperpigmentation, ulceration, paresthesias, gait dysfunction, and chronic pain. It occurs in 20%–50% of patients with a DVT who do not have complete clot resolution, and there is some concern that return to play too early in athletes with a DVT might also predispose them to PTS.[30]

The sole return-to-play protocol in the literature on sports medicine was developed for a triathlete by Roberts and Christie.[23] Their approach includes a gradual return to training once the patient has a stable, therapeutic INR as well as full resolution of symptoms. They discouraged impact loading activities until 6 weeks after the initiation of anticoagulation based on hematologic data showing that clot lysis takes 4–6 weeks. Their patient began running just 3 weeks after starting anticoagulation and unfortunately developed PTS. However, there is a subsequent case report of a football player who waited to start high-impact activity until he had completed his anticoagulation course (approximately 3 months) and was able to return to play without any complications.[31] These examples support refraining from high impact or high intensity activity until the patient has completed anticoagulation, but clearly more research is indicated to develop a more specific return-to-play protocol.

Common Femoral Vein Pseudoaneurysm

Yet another possible etiology of posttraumatic thigh pain is a pseudoaneurysm of the common femoral vein. This rare complication has been described in a case report of a soccer player who suffered a kick to the anterior thigh during a game.[32] He presented 2 weeks after the injury complaining of progressively worsening exercise-induced thigh pain. His examination was notable only for mild thigh tenderness and edema. Postexercise Doppler ultrasonography and digital subtraction angiography showed a pseudoaneurysm of the left superficial femoral artery, and MRI showed surrounding hematoma and edema. The patient was taken to the operating room for surgical correction but was found to have a common femoral vein pseudoaneurysm rather than arterial injury. His postoperative course included anticoagulation for several months and gradual return to physical activity, progressing from isometric exercises to more dynamic movements. This is clearly not the most likely cause of thigh pain in sports-related trauma; but because of the potential complications of DVT and pulmonary embolism, it should be considered in athletes with thigh trauma.

Nontraumatic Injuries

Introduction

Repetitive stress in the high-level athlete not only affects the musculoskeletal system but can lead to breakdown of the vascular system as well. Arterial stenosis, kinking, dissection, and entrapment are just a few of the vascular injuries that are due to excessive hemodynamic and biomechanical stress placed on the body during training. Any athlete exposed to repetitive movements and rigorous training is susceptible to these disorders; however, there are sport-specific factors that predispose athletes to certain types of vascular injuries. For example, the hemodynamic and biomechanical demands associated with high-intensity cycling can lead to stenosis of the external iliac artery.

The general presentation includes exercise-induced lower extremity claudication and cramping (unilateral or bilateral) as well as complaints of reduced power that occurs at defined exercise intensity and abates with rest.[33] Unfortunately, vascular pathology often mimics musculoskeletal pathology affecting the lower extremities, including lumbar radiculopathy, sacroiliac dysfunction, medial tibial stress syndrome (MTSS), or stress fracture. The diagnosis is further complicated by a fairly unremarkable examination at rest, often requiring testing after high intensity exercise coupled with repetitive, sport-specific maneuvers to diagnosis this obscure problem.[34] If vascular disease is suspected, it is also important to rule out non-sports-related causes of peripheral vascular disease, including premature accelerated atherosclerosis, collagen vascular disease, Takayasu's arteritis, and thromboangiitis obliterans. However, these disorders can cause symptoms at rest and would lead to more systemic disease than exercise-related vascular disease in the lower extremity.

Nontraumatic Arterial Injuries

External Iliac Artery Endofibrosis

The external iliac artery is one of the most commonly affected vessels in atraumatic, sports-related injuries. Chevalier et al. first described external iliac artery endofibrosis (EIAE) in 1986 in 23 competitive male cyclists. These athletes were found to have arterial stenosis, smooth muscle hyperplasia, and collagen deposition in the intima, the innermost layer of the arterial wall (Figs. 13.4, 13.5a).[35] Subsequent studies have confirmed these histologic

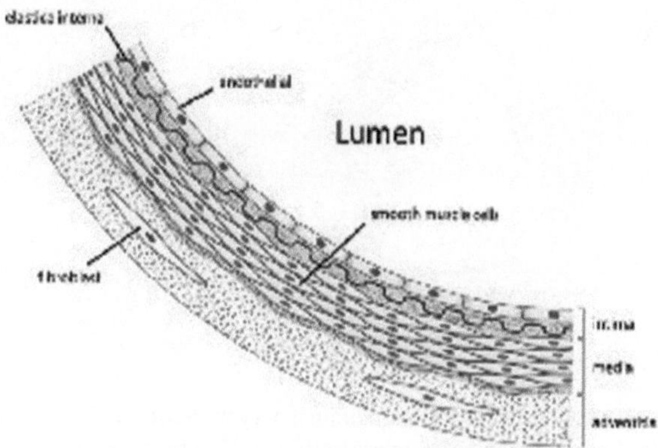

Fig. 13.4 Cross section of a normal artery. Creative commons license

changes in the intima and have demonstrated smooth muscle hyperplasia in the media and adventitia of the external iliac artery of elite female cyclists (Fig. 13.5b,c).[36] The proposed pathophysiology of EIAE is damage from mechanical stress on the vessel secondary to excessive hip flexion coupled with shear stress from the high blood flow during maximum exertion. Other factors postulated to predispose athletes to EIAE are arterial kinking and compression from a hypertrophied psoas muscle and the inguinal ligament.[37]

Elite cyclists are the most common athletes to develop EIAE, which occurs in as many as one in five,[38] and there is a linear relation between mileage of more than 150,000 km and the development of endofibrosis.[39] The predominance of EIAE in cyclists is not surprising owing to the sport-specific biomechanics requiring prolonged, excessive hip flexion and the hemodynamic stress of high cardiac output and local arterial turbulence at maximum intensity. However, EIAE has also been described in athletes not exposed to such extreme hip flexion, including cross-country skiers, runners, rugby players, and weightlifters.[35]

Endofibrosis was initially thought to be the sole cause of external iliac artery flow limitations; however, some more recent studies have shown that arterial kinking without the presence of luminal stenosis can also be a contributor.[40] Kinking is the result of increased tension from arterial branches to hip flexion musculature during repetitive, extreme hip flexion; the external iliac artery becomes elongated and can form sharp curves or loops, impeding blood flow.

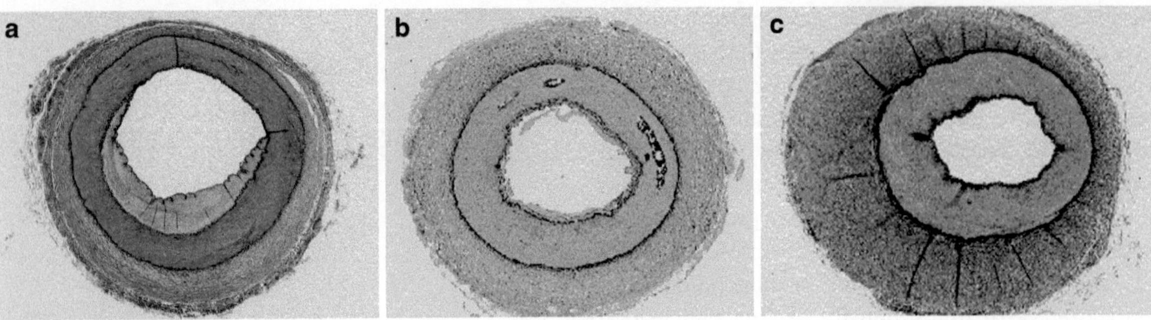

Fig. 13.5 (**a**) Cross section of an artery with intimal hyperplasia from a patient with external iliac artery endofibrosis (EIAE). (**b**) Cross section of an artery with medial hyperplasia from a patient with EIAE. (**c**) Cross section of an artery with adventitial hyperplasia from a patient with EIAE. From Kral et al.[36] With permission from Elsevier Limited

Patients with flow restriction from endofibrosis with or without kinking are young (20–30 years), highly trained, and without any obvious risk factors for atherosclerotic disease. The symptoms usually consist of unilateral pain and lack of power in the lower extremities during intense exercise; however, 15% of patients present with bilateral symptoms.[41] Occasionally, patients also report a subjective sensation of thigh edema, paresthesias, or progressively worsening symptoms that begin to occur even at rest. The resting vascular, neurologic, and musculoskeletal examinations are usually within normal limits. Some patients have a bruit if checked after exercise or in extreme hip flexion.

Noninvasive testing for EIAE includes the ankle brachial pressure index (ABPI), duplex ultrasonography, and MRA. The ABPI is usually normal at rest but may drop significantly during the first 4–5 minutes after exercise. Unfortunately, even a reduction in the postexertional ABPI to < 0.5 only has a sensitivity of 85% in EIAE.[42] One reason for this may be that most protocols use treadmill exercise testing rather than sport-specific cycle ergometer testing. In addition, most studies using ABPI to diagnose EIAE do not use simultaneous pressure recordings from all four limbs; this may affect the results as small differences in time for blood pressure measurements (even less than a minute) result in important differences in the measured values.[43]

Resting duplex ultrasonography is reportedly diagnostic in 80% of patients with EIAE,[44] but the addition of postexercise testing or the use of intravascular ultrasonography can increase the sensitivity.[45] MRA with gadolinium is most useful for distinguishing kinking with luminal stenosis from kinking alone.[35] Echo-Doppler has high sensitivity and specificity for visualizing intravascular lesions, but the results can be operator dependent (Fig. 13.6).[44] Angiography, particularly intraarterial digital subtraction angiography with vasodilatation-induced pressure measurements, is the most useful confirmatory test for EIAE.[38] Unfortunately, in many of the cases described in the literature, the average delay in diagnosis of EIAE in cyclists was 2 years, and many of the athletes were forced to retire from competition during this time.[46]

There is little consensus on the best treatment for EIAE. There is some evidence that conservative management, including activity modification, may lead to improvement in flow limitations over time. However, many highly competitive athletes decide to proceed with surgical intervention rather than risk an early end to their athletic careers. Percutaneous transluminal balloon angioplasty (PTBA) has been successful in athletes with EIAE. This method is attractive because it is minimally invasive and has a shorter recuperation period than surgical intervention. On the other hand, there are concerns about the possibility of initiating arterial dissection with angioplasty and a relative lack of knowledge about the long-term efficacy. If the flow obstruction is due to kinking without luminal stenosis, surgical release of the arterial branches to the hip flexor musculature and partial resection of the elongated artery is a possible option. Definitive treatment for stenosis due to endofibrosis (with or without kinking) is arterial resection and saphenous vein graft or endarterectomy with vein patch angioplasty (SOR = C).[42] Of note, medical therapy for atherosclerosis (e.g., antiplatelet agents or statins) is not

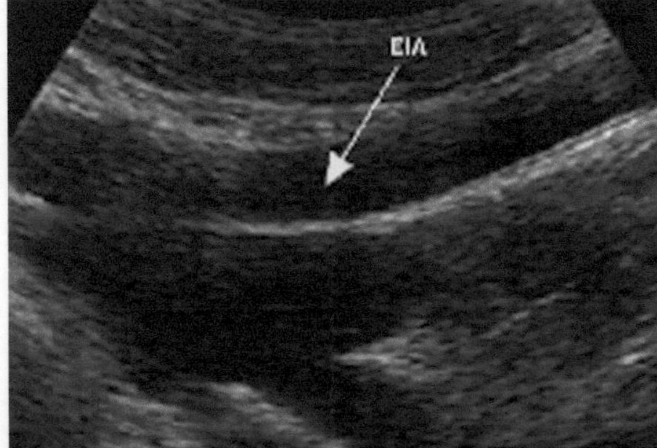

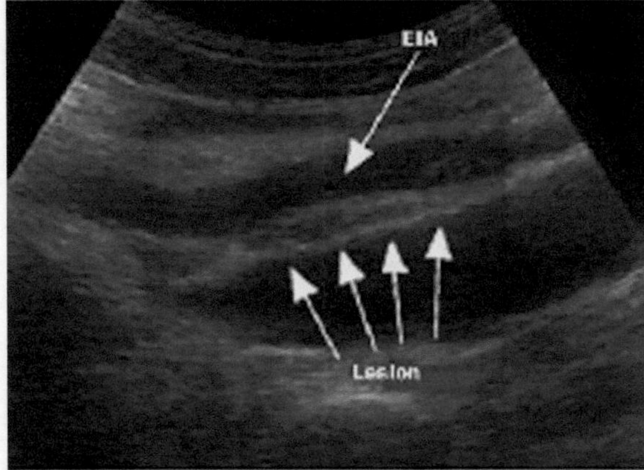

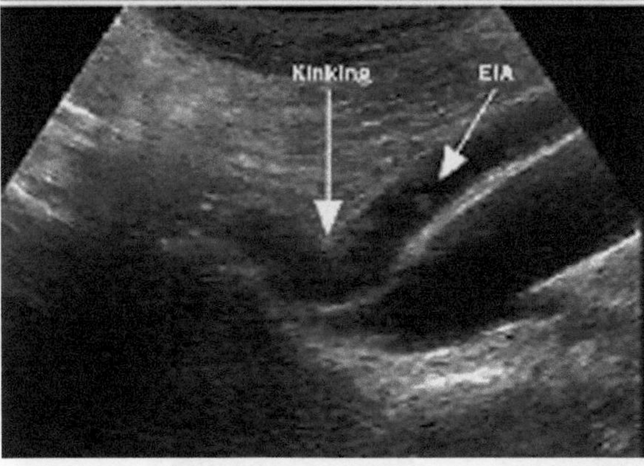

Fig. 13.6 Doppler ultrasonography of a normal external iliac artery, EIAE, and an external iliac artery with kinking. From Schep G, Bender MH, van de Tempel G, et al. Detection and treatment of claudication due to functional iliac obstruction in top endurance athletes: a prospective study. Lancet 2002;359:466–73. By permission of Elsevier Limited

effective management in these patients because the pathophysiology is smooth muscle hyperplasia within the artery, not plaque formation and rupture due to elevated blood pressure, cholesterol, or triglycerides.

Superficial Femoral Artery Stenosis

The superficial femoral artery travels through the middle one-third of the thigh in the adductor canal, an aponeurotic tunnel that is bordered by the vastus medialis anterolaterally, adductor longus and magnus posteriorly, and the sartorius medially. During its course through the adductor canal, the femoral artery is susceptible to compression from either an anomalous musculotendinous band or hypertrophied surrounding musculature.[47] This femoral artery compression, otherwise known as adductor canal syndrome (or Hunter's canal syndrome), usually results in stenosis, but thrombosis and dissection can also occur.

Adductor canal syndrome is most frequently reported in runners and skiers who present with complaints of exercise-induced calf pain and paresthesias (especially numbness of the toes). The symptoms usually progress gradually; however if complete arterial occlusion occurs, they may present with rapid progression of pain, paralysis, paresthesias, pallor, and pulselessness.

The examination of a patient with superficial femoral artery stenosis may be within normal limits at rest, although the athlete may have decreased distal pulses, presence of a bruit, or a decreased resting ABI if the lesion is reaching the critical threshold of luminal narrowing. If the resting examination is unremarkable, the patient should undergo determination of the postexertional ABI of both limbs, with the expectation that the affected limb will have a reduced ABI. Arteriography can establish the diagnosis in patients without evidence of critical ischemia on physical examination. Standard treatment includes separation or resection of any abnormal musculotendinous bands plus vein patch angioplasty or bypass of the damaged portion of the artery (Fig. 13.7). Patients with an examination consistent with complete occlusion require emergent revascularization. In both situations, an investigation of the contralateral limb for the presence of subclinical lesions or anatomic abnormalities that may lead to a similar lesion is warranted. The short-term results of these interventions are good, with many athletes returning to their previous level of competition. However, long-term results are lacking.[46]

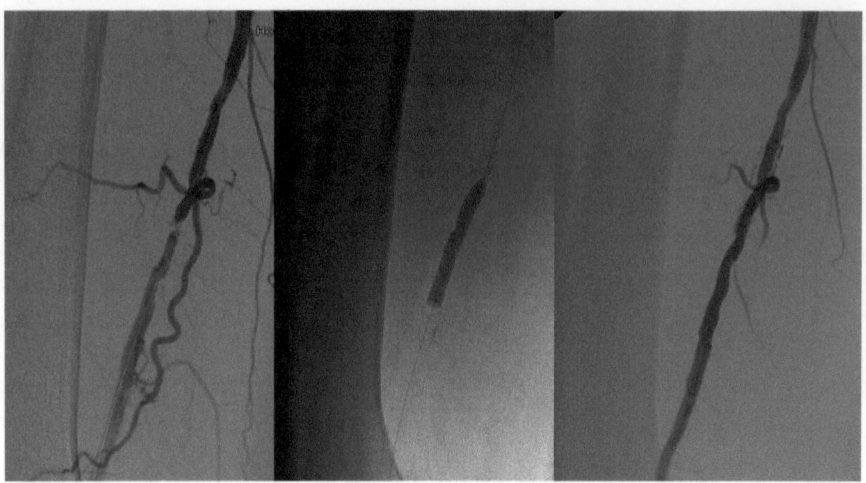

Fig. 13.7 Angiography demonstrating adductor canal syndrome with stent placement and vessel reperfusion. Courtesy of Dr. Heron Rodriguez

Popliteal Artery Entrapment Syndrome

Popliteal artery entrapment syndrome (PAES) is defined as congenital fibromuscular anomalies in the popliteal fossa producing extrinsic compression of the neurovascular bundle (Fig. 13.8).[48] In addition to congenital PAES, the sports medicine literature describes a related syndrome known as functional popliteal artery entrapment syndrome (FPAES). FPAES is due to physiologic impingement of the popliteal artery caused by exercise-induced increased blood flow and muscle hypertrophy of the gastrocnemius, soleus, plantaris, or semimembranosus. Patients with FPAES are usually young and female, and they participate in sports requiring repetitive overuse of the lower extremities. Symptoms include calf claudication, paresthesias, and calf muscle fatigue during exercise; these symptoms are not typically present at rest.[49]

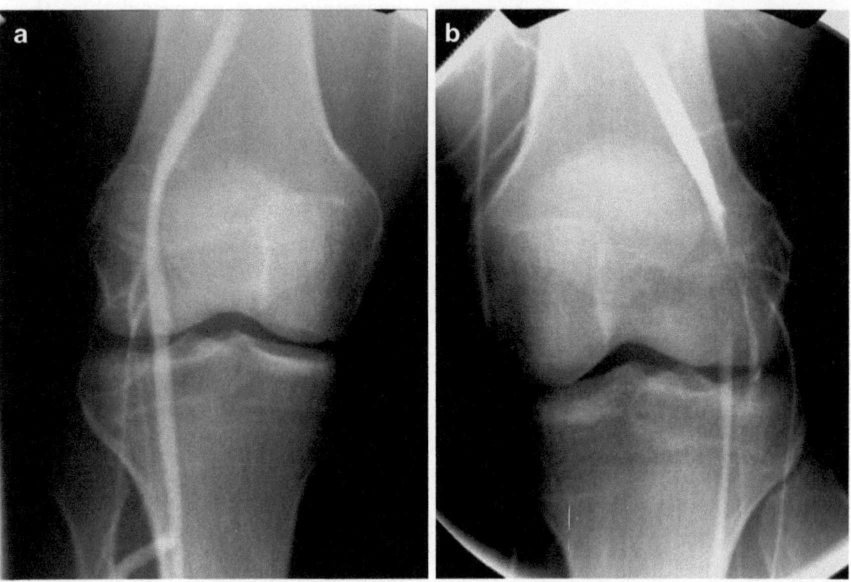

Fig. 13.8 (**a**) Angiography of the right popliteal artery showing lateral displacement of the artery without flow abnormality and (**b**) the left popliteal artery with flow reduction secondary to popliteal artery entrapment

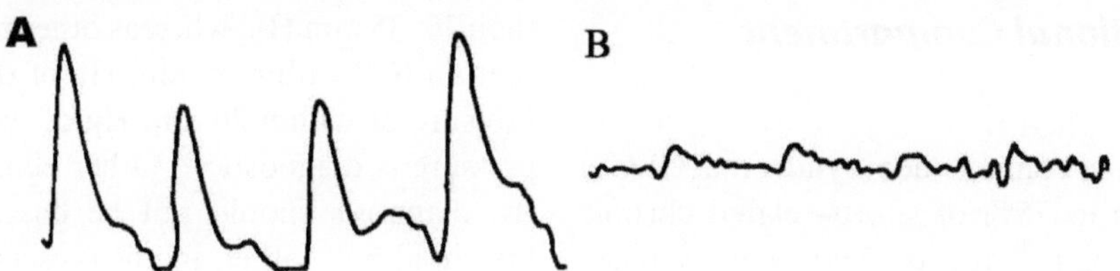

Fig. 13.9 Popliteal artery entrapment syndrome (PAES) demonstrated by normal Doppler waveforms with the patient in neutral lower limb position (**a**) and decreased waveforms with active plantar flexion of the ankle (**b**). Courtesy of Dr. Heron Rodriguez

Although most cases are unilateral, up to 25% of patients experience bilateral involvement.[50]

Most patients have normal peripheral pulses on examination, but occasionally ankle dorsiflexion or plantar flexion coupled with knee extension can cause notable reduction in pedal pulses.[51] Decreased peripheral pulses are not diagnostic, however, as approximately one-half of normal subjects can occlude the popliteal artery temporarily with extension of the knee combined with active plantar flexion.[52] The affected leg may also have a decreased postexercise ABI. Noninvasive vascular testing, including arterial Doppler segmental pressures (Fig. 13.9), CT scan, MRI, and arteriography can be used to confirm the diagnosis. CT scanning is reportedly the most sensitive test for congenital PAES, and photoplethysmography is most sensitive for FPAES. Photoplethysmography, an optically obtained measurement of the volume and vascular perfusion of various organs, can be performed with dynamic ankle plantar flexion and dorsiflexion to show functional arterial occlusion. However, the high false-positive rate for this test must be considered, as 50%–60% of the normal population have transient popliteal artery occlusion with knee extension and plantar flexion.[53]

Functional PAES may be initially treated conservatively (relative rest, compression stockings, lower extremity elevation, and stretching). If symptoms are intolerable or progressive, surgical correction may be indicated. The surgical treatment of congenital PAES includes resecting the popliteal artery from the musculotendinous or fibrous tissue compressing the artery as well as autogenous saphenous vein patch angioplasty with thrombectomy if intimal damage is present.[53] Follow-up for these patients should include periodic duplex scanning and gradual return to activity when they are asymptomatic.

Cystic Adventitial Disease of the Popliteal Artery

Cystic adventitial disease is a rare cause of arterial occlusion, but it causes popliteal artery claudication in 1 in 1200.[54] It is classified as the development of mucin-containing cysts in the adventitial tissue, possibly secondary to repetitive trauma in sports, causing flow limitations that are exacerbated by the increased cardiovascular demands of exercise.

Patients with cystic adventitial disease of the popliteal artery are typically male (5:1), are in their fourth to fifth decade of life, and present with progressive exercise-induced calf claudication. Active and sedentary patients are affected with the same relative frequency, although it is hypothesized that athletic patients are more frequently diagnosed because symptoms are interfering with their sports participation. The examination is usually unremarkable at rest, although occasionally there is loss of pedal pulses with knee flexion (Ishizawa's sign).[55] Cystic adventitial disease of the popliteal artery is often diagnosed by an incidental finding seen on imaging that was performed to evaluate the posterior knee or calf pain.[56] MRI is the diagnostic test of choice to allow visualization of one or multiple (chain formation) cysts in the wall of the popliteal artery. Other imaging options include MRA or Doppler-derived waveform analysis of the popliteal artery. Treatment includes cyst aspiration, evacuation with removal of the cyst wall, vein graft, vein patch, or a synthetic graft. In a review of 98 patients with cystic adventitial disease of the popliteal artery, 56 underwent cyst evacuation and 42 had segmental arterial resection with success rates of 85% and 91%, respectively.[40]

Chronic Exertional Compartment Syndrome

Chronic exertional compartment syndrome (CECS) accounts for up to 75% of sports-related chronic lower extremity pain.[40] It is defined as an exercise-induced increase in pressure in one of the four compartments of the lower extremity, including the anterior, lateral, superficial posterior, and deep posterior compartments. During exercise, muscles swell secondary to increased blood flow and fluid retention; and in some individuals, the inelastic structures (fascia and bone) surrounding the compartments are unable to accommodate this swelling. When interstitial pressure becomes greater than capillary pressure, blood flow is impaired; and tissue ischemia, microhemorrhage, and edema lead to pain and neuromuscular dysfunction.

The CECS is well documented in the sports medicine literature. Most descriptions are about female runners, skiers, and in-line skaters; however, there are case reports in both sexes and other sports, including soccer, rugby, tennis, and basketball. Regardless of the athlete's sport, the general presentation is a young athlete who complains of anterior, lateral, or posterior cramping or squeezing calf pain that occurs at a well defined, reproducible point during the activity and persists until the activity is discontinued. Approximately 70% of patients have bilateral symptoms, but often one limb is more affected than the other. The patient may also develop foot drop or dorsal foot paresthesias if the anterior compartment is affected. If the superficial posterior compartment is affected, the patient might have weak plantar flexion and paresthesias of the lateral foot. Finally, if the compartment syndrome involves the deep posterior compartment, the patient may have decreased toe flexion and ankle inversion with paresthesias of the plantar aspect of the foot.[57]

The examination of a patient with CECS usually demonstrates normal strength, sensation, and distal pulses. Therefore, provocative testing and imaging are required to assist in making the diagnosis. The gold standard for diagnosis is the comparison of intracompartmental pressures (ICP), both at rest and after exercise. Normal ICP is approximately 5–10 mm Hg. However, there is no clear consensus regarding what degree of pressure elevation is required to diagnose CECS. Many advocate assigning the diagnosis if postexercise pressures are greater than 30–35 mm Hg, whereas other research indicates that an ICP within 40 mm Hg of the systolic blood pressure or within 20 mm Hg of the diastolic blood pressure is diagnostic.[58] Other clinicians argue that the diagnosis should not be based on a numeric threshold but, rather, by the presence of both symptoms and pressure elevation during exercise. The best reported sensitivity and specificity for ICP measurement in a large clinical trial that used cutoff point of 35 mm Hg were 93% and 74%, respectively.[59]

Other promising, less invasive diagnostic options include MRI and near-infrared spectroscopy (NIRS). MRI shows an increased signal on T2-weighted images that correlate well with ICP measurements.[60] NIRS is able to indicate the level of intracompartmental ischemia based on the tissue hemoglobin saturation. There are limited data regarding the sensitivity and specificity of MRI and NIRS for diagnosing CECS. One prospective study of 50 patients with CECS showed similar sensitivities for the ICP measurement and NIRS: 77% and 85%, respectively. This study also found MRI to be less sensitive than either ICP or NIRS for diagnosing CECS.[61]

Treatment usually begins with conservative management including relative rest for 2–3 months with gradual return to sports activity. If conservative management fails, surgical decompression via open or subcutaneous fasciotomy is indicated. Many studies have described the importance of resuming activity as soon as possible to prevent fascial closure and recurrence of symptoms. This concept is illustrated in a review of 21 adolescent athletes who underwent fasciotomy for CECS. They began passive range of motion immediately after surgery, started ambulation after 24–46 hours, and resumed loading exercises after 2–4 weeks. They were back to full activity after 4–6 weeks, and no recurrences were reported during the 4-year follow-up period.

Nontraumatic Venous Injuries

Effort-Induced Deep Vein Thrombosis

Effort-induced thrombosis (otherwise known as Paget-Schroetter syndrome) is due to sports participation and is most commonly seen in the axillary or subclavian veins, although there are a few case studies describing effort-induced venous thrombus in the lower extremities in distance runners and skiers. Although exercise is generally thought to be preventative against thrombus formation, high-intensity exercise can lead to impaired venous flow and vessel wall trauma, leading to thrombus formation and occlusion.[62] Unlike the pathophysiology of EIAE, effort-induced DVT includes only intramural thrombus, not histologic changes to the walls of the veins.

Patients with effort-induced DVT in the lower extremities likely present with complaints of lower extremity swelling, aching, stiffness, decreased sensation, and impaired sports performance. The examination may be unremarkable but may be significant for asymmetrical lower extremity circumference due to swelling, pitting edema, and discoloration. Pain may be elicited with passive dorsiflexion of the ankle known as Homan's sign; but as mentioned for trauma-induced DVT, physical examination signs have limited sensitivity and specificity in the diagnosis of DVT. Doppler ultrasonography is the gold standard for this diagnosis. Any patient with suspected effort-induced DVT should undergo evaluation for coagulation diathesis, as both the factor V Leiden mutation and hereditary thrombophilia have been shown to increase the risk of venous thrombus in both athletes and the general population (SOR = C).[63]

Case Presentation

23-Year-Old Man With Bilateral Calf Claudication

A 23-year-old man presented with bilateral calf pain during running. He started a marathon-training

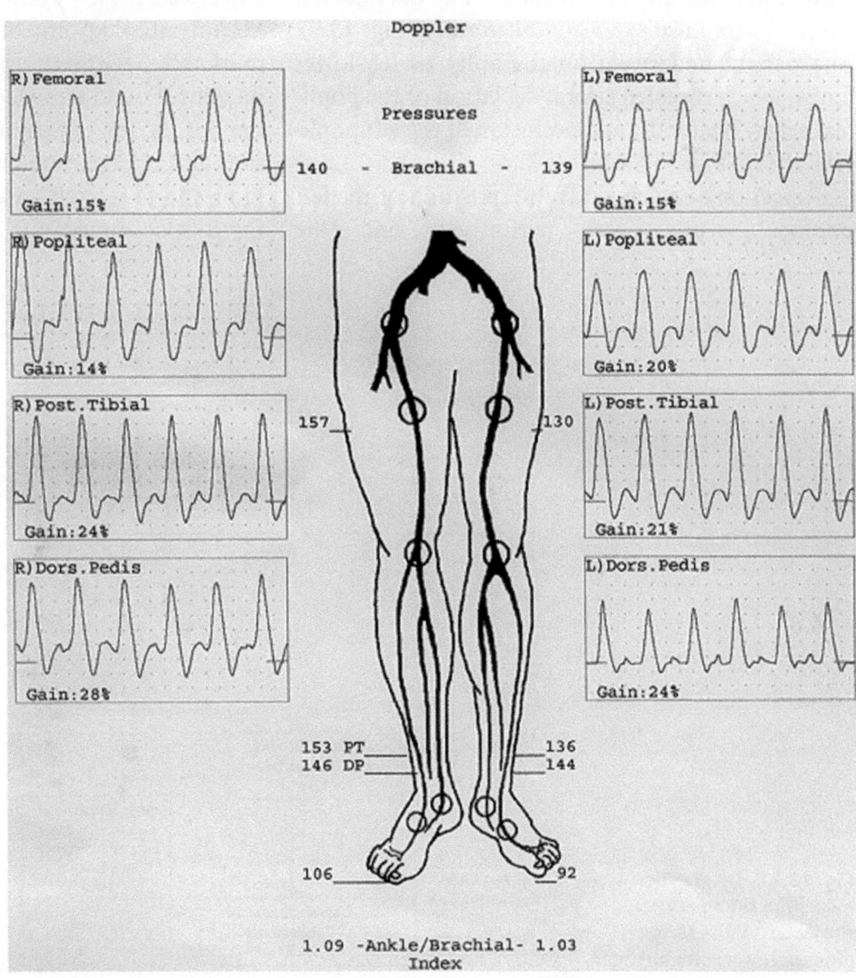

Fig. 13.10 Ankle brachial index (ABI). Courtesy of Dr. Heron Rodriguez

program 2 months previously and gradually increased his weekly mileage to approximately 30 miles. The pain occurred only after he had run about 8–10 miles; and it was alleviated by rest. In addition to the pain, he had also felt numbness and tingling in his calves (the left calf more than the right one) when he ran 15 miles and once during sleep. He noted that the other runners in his training program thought that they were getting stronger, but he felt like his legs were getting weaker, particularly his calf muscles. He denied any other pain or paresthesias throughout the rest of his body. His past medical history, family history, and social history were unremarkable.

The patient's resting physical examination was unremarkable, including distal pulses (2 + and symmetrical) and an ABI that was within normal limits (Fig. 13.10). However, provocative measurements of his pedal pulses were significant because of a reduction with plantar flexion and dorsiflexion coupled with knee extension bilaterally (Fig. 13.9). The patient underwent angiography of his lower limbs, which revealed lateral deviation of the popliteal artery bilaterally and occlusion of the left popliteal artery (Fig. 13.8a,b).

Resection and vein graft interposition of the left popliteal artery were performed, and the fibromuscular bands in the popliteal fossa leading to lateral deviation of the popliteal arteries were removed. This procedure was done on the right side, as the patient was symptomatic despite the lack of occlusion seen on angiography.

The patient gradually returned to running after receiving clearance from his vascular surgeon, and he has been asymptomatic despite continuing to train for distance races, including a marathon.

Conclusion

A variety of lower limb vascular injuries can occur in the athletic population. These injuries can be due to a traumatic event or repetitive stress over time. The diagnosis of lower limb vascular injuries in athletes is not always straightforward, as these injuries have a presentation similar to that of musculoskeletal pathology and often the examination is unremarkable without postexertional testing or imaging. Sound knowledge about the vascular anatomy of the lower extremity as well as the presentation and appropriate evaluation of the most common sports-related vascular injuries is imperative for a sports medicine practice (Fig. 13.11). The

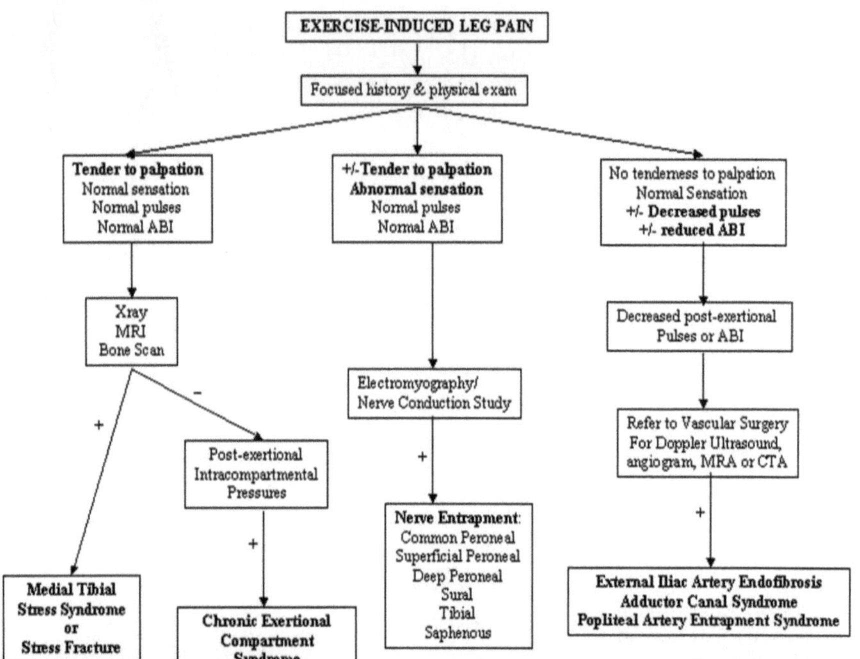

Fig. 13.11 Diagnostic algorithm for an athlete presenting with exercise-induced lower extremity pain

mere practice of considering vascular disease on the differential diagnosis of an athlete with lower limb pain, paresthesias, fatigue, or swelling can prevent the severe consequences of early retirement from sport, loss of limb function, or loss of the limb itself.

References

1. Darling RC, Buckley CJ, Abbott WM, et al. Intermittent claudication in young athletes: popliteal artery entrapment syndrome. J Trauma 1974;14:543–52.
2. Rich NM, Mattox KL, Hirshberg A. Vascular Trauma. 2nd ed. Philadelphia: Elsevier Saunders; 2004.
3. Sriussadaporn S. Arterial injuries of the lower extremity from blunt trauma. J Med Assoc Thai 1997;80:121–9.
4. Vasdekis SN, Kakisis JD, Lazaris AM, et al. Common femoral artery injury secondary to tennis ball strike. J Vasc Surg 2006;44:1350–2.
5. Muck PE, Nunez TC, Hruska L, et al. Blunt injury to the external iliac artery: a case report. Am Surg 2002;68(1):11–4.
6. Sarfati MR, Galt SW, Treiman GS, et al. Common femoral artery injury secondary to bicycle handlebar trauma. J Vasc Surg 2002;35:589–91.
7. McDonald EJ, Goodman PC, Winestock DP. The clinical indications for arteriography in trauma to the extremity: a review of 114 cases. Radiology 1975;116:45–7.
8. Rutherford RB. Diagnostic evaluation of extremity vascular injuries. Surg Clin North Am 1998;68:683–91.
9. Martin LC, McKenny MG, Sosa JL, et al. Management of lower extremity arterial trauma. J Trauma 1994;37:591–8.
10. Frykberg ER. Popliteal vascular injuries. Surg Clin North Am 2002;82:67–89.
11. Kennedy, TC. Complete dislocation of the knee joint. J Bone Joint Surg Am 1963;45:889.
12. Varnell RM, Coldwell DM, Sangeorzan BJ, et al. Arterial injury complicating knee disruption. Am Surg 1989;55(12):699–704.
13. Miller HH, Wech CS. Quantitative studies on the factor in arterial injuries. Am Surg 1949;130:538.
14. Jones S, Journeaux SF. Pure hyperextension of the knee causing popliteal artery injury. Injury 1996;27(5):355–6.
15. Kendall RW, Taylor DC, Salvian AJ, et al. The role of arteriography in assessing vascular injuries associated with dislocation of the knee. J Trauma 1993;35:875.
16. Skudder PA, Gelfand ML, Blumenberg RM, et al. Tibial artery false aneurysm: uncommon result of blunt injury occurring during athletics. Ann Vasc Surg 1999;13:589–91.
17. Lee AT, Fanton GS, McAdams TR. Acute compartment syndrome of the thigh in a football athlete: a case report and the role of the vacuum-assisted wound closure dressing. J Orthop Trauma 2005;19:748–50.
18. Machold W, Muellner T, Kwasny O. Is the return to high-level athletics possible after fasciotomy for a compartment syndrome of the thigh? A case report. Am J Sports Med 2000;28:407–10.
19. Burns BJ, Sproule J, Smyth H. Acute compartment syndrome of the anterior thigh following quadriceps strain in a footballer. Br J Sports Med 2004;38:218–20.
20. Mithofer K, Lhowe DW, Vrahas MS, et al. Clincal spectrum of acute compartment syndrome of the thigh and its relation to associated injuries. Clin Orthop 2004;425:223–9.
21. Zweifach SS, Hargens AR, Evans KL, et al. Skeletal muscle necrosis in pressurized compartments associated with hemorrhagic hypotension. J Trauma 1980;20:941–7.
22. Hilberg T, Jeschke D, Gabriel HHW. Hereditary thrombophilia in elite athletes. Med Sci Sports Med 2002;34:218–21.
23. Roberts WO, Christie DM. Return to training and competition after deep venous calf thrombosis. Med Sci Sports Exerc 1992;24:2–5.
24. Laroche GP. Steroid anabolic drugs and arterial complications in an athlete: a case history. Angiology 1990;41:964–9.
25. Echlin PS, Upshur REG, McKeag DB, et al. Traumatic deep vein thrombosis in a soccer player: a case study. Thromb J 2004;2:8.
26. Goodacre S, Sutton A, Sampson F. Meta-analysis: the value of clinical assessment in the diagnosis of deep venous thrombosis. Ann Intern Med 2005;143(2):129–39.
27. Anand SS, Wells PS, Hunt D, et al. Does this patient have deep vein thrombosis? JAMA 1998;279:1094–9.
28. Hyers TM. Management of venous thrombembolism: past, present, and future. Arch Intern Med 2003;163:759–68.
29. Bates SM, Ginsberg JS. Treatment of deep-vein thrombosis. N Engl J Med 2004;351:268–77.
30. Kahn SR, Ginsberg JS. The post-thrombotic syndrome: current knowledge, controversies, and directions for future research. Blood Rev 2002;16:155–65.
31. Thompson TL, Robinson AK, Gilbert C. Deep vein thrombosis of the lower extremity in a football player: a case report. Clin J Sport Med 2006;16:372–4.
32. Karahan M, Isbir S, Baltacyoglu F, et al. False Aneurysm of the common femoral vein in a footballer. Br J Sports Med 2005;39:8.
33. Abraham P, Saumet JL, Chevalier JM. External iliac endofibrosis in athletes. Sports Med 1997;24:221–6.
34. Schep G, Bender MHM, Kaandorp D, et al. Flow limitations in the iliac arteries in endurance athletes—current knowledge and directions for the future. Int J Sports Med 1999;20:421–8.
35. Chevalier JM, Enon B, Walder J, et al. Endofibrosis of the external iliac artery in bicycle racers: an unrecognized pathological state. Ann Vasc Surg 1986;1:297–303.
36. Kral CA, Han DC, Edwards WD, et al. Obstructive external iliac arteriopathy in avid bicyclists: new and variable histopathologic features in four women. J Vasc Surg 2002;36:565–70.
37. Giannoukas AD, Berczi V, Unnikrishnan A, et al. Endofibrosis of iliac arteries in high-performance athletes: diagnostic approach and minimally invasive

endovascular treatment. Cardiovasc Intervent Radiol 2006;29:866–9.
38. Bender MHM, Schep G, de Vries WR, et al. Sports-related flow limitations in the iliac arteries in endurance athletes: aetiology, diagnosis, treatment and future developments. Sports Med 2004;34(7):427–42.
39. Abraham P, Saumet JL, Chevalier JM. External iliac endofibrosis in athletes. Sports Med 1997;24:221–6.
40. Schep G, Schmikli SL, Bender MHM, et al. Recognising vascular causes of leg complaints in endurance athletes. Part I: Validation of a decision algorithm. Int J Sports Med 2002;23:313–21.
41. Taylor AJ, George KP. Exercise induced leg pain in young athletes misdiagnosed as pain of musculoskeletal origin. Manual Ther 2001;6(1):48–52.
42. Ford SJ, Rehman A, Bradbur AW. External iliac endofibrosis in endurance athletes: a novel case in an endurance runner and a review of the literature. Eur J Vasc Endovasc Surg 2003;26:629–34.
43. Taylor AJ, George KP. Ankle to brachial pressure index in normal subjects and trained cyclists with exercise-induced leg pain. Med Sci Sports Exerc 2001;33:1862–7.
44. Abraham P, Leftheriotis G, Bourre Y, et al. Echography of external iliac artery endofibrosis in cyclists. Am J Sports Med 1993;21(6):861–3.
45. Lomis NNT, Miller FJ, Whiting JH, et al. Exercise-induced external iliac artery intimal fibrosis: confirmation with intravascular ultrasound. J Vasc Interv Radiol 2000;11:51–3.
46. Ehsan O. Non-traumatic lower limb vascular complications in endurance athletes: review of literature. Eur J Vasc Endovasc Surg 2004;28:1–8.
47. Mosely JG. Arterial problems in athletes. Br J Surg 2003;90:1461–9.
48. Goh BKP, Tay KH, Tan SG. Diagnosis and surgical management of popliteal artery entrapment syndrome. ANZ J Surg 2005;75:869–73.
49. Hoffman U. Popliteal artery compression and force of active plantar flexion in young healthy volunteers. J Vasc Surg 1997;26:281–7.
50. Stager A, Clement D. Popliteal artery entrapment syndrome. Sports Med 1999;28(1):61–70.
51. Olson SK, Parker DG, Reul GJ. Popliteal artery entrapment: a diagnosis that may be overlooked. Tex Heart Inst J 1983;10:305–10.
52. Erdoes LS, Devine JJ, Bernhard VM, et al. Popliteal vascular compression in a normal population. J Vasc Surg 1994;20:978–86.
53. Ohara N, Miyata T, Oshiro H, et al. Surgical treatment for popliteal artery entrapment syndrome. Cardiovasc Surg 2001;9:141–4.
54. Do DD, Braunschwei M, Baumgartner I, et al. Adventitial cystic disease of the popliteal artery: percutaneous US-guided aspiration. Radiology 1997;203:743–6.
55. Tsolakis IA, Walvatne CS, Caldwell MD. Cystic adventitial disease of the popliteal artery: diagnosis and treatment. Eur J Vasc Endovasc Surg 1998;15(3):188–94.
56. Mhuircheartaigh MN, Kavanagh E, O'Donohoe M, et al. Pseudo compartment syndrome of the calf in an athlete secondary to cystic adventitial disease of the popliteal artery. Br J Sports Med 2005;39:e36.
57. Wilder RP, Sethi S. Overuse injuries: tendinopathies, stress fractures, compartment syndrome and shin splints. Clin Sports Med 2004;23:55–81.
58. Mars M, Hadley GP. Raised intracompartmental pressure and compartment syndromes. Injury 1998;29:403–11.
59. Verleisdonk EJ. At what tissue pressure, measured immediately after exercise, should the diagnosis of chronic exertional compartment syndrome of the lower leg be made: the exertional compartment syndrome [PhD thesis]. Utrecht, the Netherlands: University Medical Center; 2000:111–27.
60. Lauder TD, Stuart MJ, Amrami KK, et al. Exertional compartment syndrome and the role of magnetic resonance imaging. Am J Phys Med Rehabil 2002;81:315–9.
61. Van den Brand JG, Nelson T, Verleisdonk EJ, et al. The diagnostic value of intracompartmental pressure measurement, magnetic resonance imagine and near-infrared spectroscopy in chronic exertional compartment syndrome. Am J Sports Med 2005;33:699–704.
62. Schmitt HE, Mihatsch MJ. Thrombosis of the popliteal vein. Cardiovasc Intervent Radiol 1992;15(4):234–9.
63. Hilberg T, Jeschke D, Gabriel HH. Hereditary thrombophilia in elite athletes. Med Sci Sports Exerc 2002;34(2):218–21.

Index

MIX
Papier aus verantwortungsvollen Quellen
Paper from responsible sources
FSC® C105338

If you have any concerns about our products,
you can contact us on
ProductSafety@springernature.com

In case Publisher is established outside the EU,
the EU authorized representative is:
Springer Nature Customer Service Center GmbH
Europaplatz 3, 69115 Heidelberg, Germany

Printed by Libri Plureos GmbH
in Hamburg, Germany